T0259412

Practical Guidelines in Antiviral Therapy

Edited by

CHARLES A.B. BOUCHER

GEORGE A. GALASSO

Contributing Editors

DAVID A. KATZENSTEIN

DAVID A. COOPER

2002

ELSEVIER

AMSTERDAM – LONDON – NEW YORK – OXFORD – PARIS – SHANNON – TOKYO

ELSEVIER SCIENCE B.V.
Sara Burgerhartstraat 25
P.O. Box 211, 1000 AE Amsterdam, The Netherlands

1st edition 2002

Library of Congress Cataloging in Publication Data
A catalog record from the Library of Congress has been applied for.

Printed and bound by CPI Antony Rowe, Eastbourne

ISBN: 0-444-508848

TABLE OF CONTENTS

PREFACE

This text was developed with the practicing physician in mind, but we believe it will be of considerable interest to the virologist, pharmacologist, chemist and all scientists interested in antiviral agents. It is proposed that, approximately a year after its publication, this volume will be available in an online version through the publisher Elsevier and will be kept updated by the authors. This is to make it readily available in an updated version for the practicing physician to review what the current status of antiviral research is, so that he/she can utilize this information in making their decisions. It is not intended as a recommended treatment syllabus but as a source of current information. It is also intended for the involved scientist to keep abreast of developments in subspecialties other than his/her own.

Progress in the field of antiviral development, in the past has been slow, but we are pleased to see that it is now moving rapidly and we hope that there will be successful treatment modalities for most viral diseases. The future is indeed bright. However, with progress, we have also learned of the pitfalls we need be aware of, such as resistance and toxicity, to which we must remain alert. Research continues at a rapid rate to find improved drugs and safe treatment regimens. An additional challenge will be to make treatment for viral disease available for those individuals who live in countries that cannot afford some of the current antiretroviral drugs.

We are most grateful to the internationally renowned experts who have agreed to participate in this volume, sharing their information on the latest developments. We have tried to select experts on both sides of the ocean for each chapter so as to capture the worldwide practices. We would also like to thank The Macrae Group for helping with the initial development of this book.

Charles A.B. Boucher
George J. Galasso, Editors

CHAPTER 1

CLASSES OF ANTIVIRAL DRUGS

MIREILLE VAN WESTREENEN and CHARLES A. B. BOUCHER

Table of Contents

Introduction

Being obligate intracellular parasites, viruses are dependent on the metabolic pathways of the host cell for their replication. So, virus and host cell are intimately connected and an effective antiviral agent must be able to distinguish virus related enzymes from host cell material itself. The search for antitumour agents generated a great deal of interest in DNA synthesis inhibitors. The first drugs capable of inhibiting viral DNA *in vitro* were described in the 50s, but real progress was not made until the 70s. In the last decades we have come to know more about the biochemistry of viral replication and this has led to a more rational approach to the search for antiviral agents. When reviewing the possibilities for antiviral chemotherapy, the best guideline is the viral replicative cycle, which can be divided in ten steps (Figure 1). First a virus binds to the cell surface of the host cell and penetrates the cell membrane and shed its protein coat (1-3 *binding and entry*). The genetic material of the virus uses the biochemical mechanisms of the host cell to replicate the genetic material of the virus (4-8 *replication*). This replication step differs in RNA and DNA viruses, but mRNA is produced in all. Then the genetic material is capsulated and the newly formed particles are released out of the host cell (9-10 *release*). Although all viruses follow this replicative cycle, different virus families may differ considerably from one another at one or more steps of the cycle. Useful inhibitors are generally specific for one family of virus and, in some cases, to individual members of that family (e.g. particular members of the herpesviruses).

1

Practical Guidelines in Antiviral Therapy Ed. by Charles A.B. Boucher and George J. Galasso. 1 — 12
© 2002 *Elsevier Science. Printed in the Netherlands.*

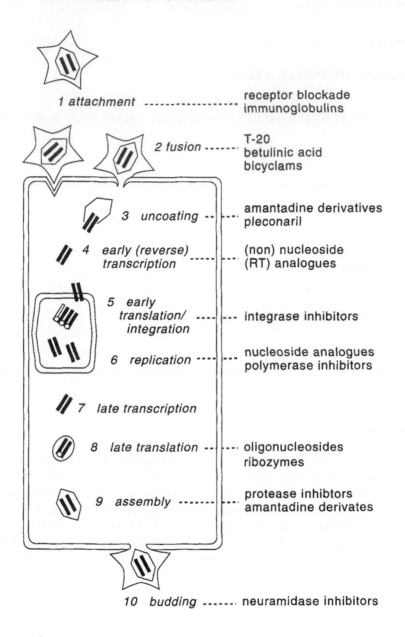

Figure 1.   Sites of potential action for most classes of virus inhibitors.

The target of these antiviral agents can be (I) specific viral proteins, (II) host cellular enzymes or (III) modulation of host immune responses. This chapter will summarize the various optional compounds, which interact with the viral replicative cycle.

I.   Inhibition of Viral Proteins

Binding and Entry

1.   *Attachment of The Virus Particle*

The first event in viral infection of the host cell is binding of the virus to the cell surface. This binding of the virus particle to the cell-surface molecule, the receptor, involves numerous interactions between the virion surface and the receptor. A wide variety of cell-surface molecules that normally serve the host cells as receptors for other molecules such as protein molecules, carbohydrates, or glycolipids are used by viruses for entry. Some receptor molecules are widely distributed. To block initial aspecific binding of virus to cells, polyanionic compounds (i.e. polysulfates, polysulfonates, polycarboxylates, polyoxometalates) were suggested. Although polyanionic compounds may interfere with processes other than virus adsorption (particularly virus–cell fusion and the reverse transcription process), their mechanism of action can be attributed primarily to inhibition of virus-cell binding. Dextran sulfate, as prototype of the sulfated polysaccharides, was found to inhibit the *in vitro* replication of HIV and other enveloped viruses [1]. A series of sulfated polymers were potent and selective inhibitors of respiratory syncytial virus and influenza A virus in mice [2]. The fact that the polysaccharides and polymers are inhibitory to some myxoviruses and retroviruses but not to others seems to depend on the composition of the amino acid sequences of the viral envelope glycoproteins that are involved in virus-cell binding and fusion.

Another form of receptor blocking can be achieved by specific molecules such as the CD4 protein molecule, which serves as the receptor for HIV on T-lymphocytes. Various forms of recombinant CD4 were assayed against *in vitro* and *in vivo* HIV infection [3]. To block the attachment of rhinovirus to the cellular protein, intracellular adhesion molecule-1 (ICAM-1) was tested. Because 90% of all rhinoviruses use ICAM-1 as a mechanism to gain entry to the host cell, antagonism of the virus-receptor interaction would appear to be an effective way to inhibit a broad spectrum of rhinoviruses [4].

Another way of preventing binding of the virus to the host cell is by using antibodies against the infecting agent. These antibodies are specific immunoglobulins against an infecting agent and can be obtained by passive or active immunization (vaccination). Passive immunization with for instance CMV-, hepatitis B-, tetanus-, or RSV immunoglobulin can only protect the host during a short time. Vaccins against measles, rubella, mumps, hepatitis A, hepatitis B, influenza and poliomyelitis protects the host from infection during a time span ranging from a couple of years to lifetime [5].

2.   *Virus-cell Fusion*

After binding to its surface receptor, a virus must enter the cell. Two general pathways have been defined for virus entry: 1) surface fusion between the viral lipid envelope and the cell plasma membrane and 2) as an alternative strategy for nonenveloped viruses; receptor-mediated endocytosis. Some compounds are assumed to interact with the postbinding virus-cell fusion process by affecting syncytium formation. Syncytia results from the fusion of the infected cell with neighboring cells, which is a feature of infection by lentiviruses, paramyxoviruses, some herpesviruses, and other viruses. This may represent an important mechanism of spread which avoids exposure of virions to antibodies. Several compounds effectively block syncytium formation by interfering with the junction of the viral envelope glycoprotein (gp120) and the (CD4) cell-receptor. Examples of such virus-cell fusion inhibitors are T-20, betulinic acid, bicyclams and negatively charged albumins [6-9]. The most promising compound in preclinical development is T-20, a synthetic peptide, which blocks HIV-1 entry into the host cell by binding to the viral glycoprotein gp41.

3.   *Uncoating of The Viral Capsid*

The process of disassembly or uncoating requires that the virion is stable to survive the conditions that exist in the new intracellular environment. However, the virion should not be as stable as to withstand the receptor and pH-induced conformational changes that must occur to allow efficient DNA or RNA release. The uncoating-blocking agents retain the virus in the encapsulated state by increasing the stability of the virion, and in this way the infection cycle is effectively blocked. Uncoating inhibitors such as the amantadine derivatives (**amantadine** and **rimantadine**) specifically prevent release of influenza A virus in the cells. Amantadine and rimantadine operate through physical blockade of the proton channels formed by the protein M2, which is a minor component of the influenza viral envelope that is thought to play a key role in stabilizing the viral hemagglutinin. This blockade affects the proton flow through the M2 protein channels, which leads to inhibition of virus uncoating [10].

Other uncoating inhibitors have been shown to prevent the uncoating of picornaviruses [4]. These compounds can prevent uncoating of the virion by binding within a hydrophobic pocket of the virus. In this way these agents increase the stability of the viral capsid to receptor and pH induced conformational changes which normally occur during the process of cellular entry. These events prevent the disassembly and release of viral ribonucleic acid. **Pleconaril** is one such antipicornaviral agent with potential therapeutic applications in the treatment of viral meningitis, upper respiratory disease, and other enteroviral infections [11, 12]. Conformational changes in the presence of calcium ions are also suggested by data indicating that calcium mediates a tighter interaction of hepatitis A receptors with hepatitis A particles. Calcium ions were found to destabilize hepatitis A virus particles [13]. Hepatitis A virus replication in cultured cells was studied in the presence of other potential uncoating inhibitors. Strong inhibition was observed in the presence of chlorpromazine and chloroquine.

Replication

Different events occur in the replication cycle of DNA or RNA viruses. The genetic material of DNA viruses is translated into mRNA by RNA polymerase. The genetic material of RNA viruses is transcribed into mRNA by a virus-coded RNA polymerase or the RNA is modulated by a viral reverse transcriptase into viral DNA, which is integrated into the host cell DNA. After activation of the cell, viral mRNA can be produced. Antiviral drugs that inhibit the replication steps can be therefore divided into reverse transcriptase inhibitors (4), integrase inhibitors (5), nucleoside analogues, DNA polymerase inhibitors or RNA polymerase inhibitors (6) and viral protein synthesis (mRNA) antagonists (7, 8).

4.   *Reverse Transcriptase*

The emergence of HIV and of human cancer caused by retroviruses quickened interest in the search for inhibitors of the crucial retroviral enzym, reverse transcriptase (RT). Two classes of drugs act on the reverse transcriptase; the nucleoside reverse transcriptase inhibitors (NRTIs) and the non-nucleoside reverse transcriptase inhibitors (NNRTIs). The first acts at the substrate (dNTP) binding site and is active against retroviruses. NRTIs either directly inhibit the enzyme or serve as alternative substrates for catalysis. The earliest compounds to display sufficient antiviral activity *in vivo* were nucleoside analogues; the first to be licensed for human use was **zidovudine** (AZT). **Abacavir, didanosine** (ddI), **lamivudine** (3TC), **stavudine** (d4T), and **zalcitabine** (ddC) are all dideoxynucleoside analogues. Nucleoside analogues can either act by inhibiting viral reverse transcription (HIV), inhibiting viral DNA or RNA polymerases synthesis. For example, lamivudine is also used as monotherapy in the treatment of hepatitis B virus infection [14]. The acyclic nucleoside phosphonate (ANP) analogues such as **cidofovir** (HPMPC), **adefovir** (PMEA) and PMPA (tenofovir) act also with the dNTP binding site of HIV-1 reverse transcriptase and inhibit the replication of other retroviruses and hepadnaviruses (e.g. hepatitis B). The ANP analogues, if incorporated into the growing DNA chain, terminate the chain growth and thus act as DNA chain terminator [15].

The second class of drugs inhibits reverse transcriptase by binding to sites other than which normally interact with the nucleosides. These compounds act at the aspecific binding site and are active against HIV-1 but not other retroviruses. The NNRTIs bind to HIV reverse transcriptase and disrupt the catalytic site to block viral replication. They do not inhibit human polymerases, which makes them less toxic than the NRTIs. The NNRTIs have shown to be potent partners for antiretroviral combined therapies, resistance may develop early when given alone. A benzodiazepine-like drug with the shortened name **TIBO** was the first of the NNRTIs to be identified. Subsequently several other NNRTIs were found to behave like TIBO: **HEPT, nevirapine, delaviridine** and many others [16].

5.   *Early Translation/Integration*

During integration, viral DNA is inserted into the host genome in a process catalyzed by the virus-encoded integrase. Thus, integration is leading to the formation of progeny viral particles. Integration is also essential for maintenance of persistent infection by keeping the provirus in the host cell genome, ready for production of new infectious particles [17]. HIV integrase is being intensively explored as a potential target for anti-HIV agents [18]. As no cellular homologue of HIV integrase has been described, potential inhibitors could be relatively nontoxic. Development of HIV-1 integrase inhibitors could have favorable implication for combination therapy, as well as prevention of the chronic carrier state and the emergence of resistant mutants. Although several classes of putative integrase inhibitors has been described, still no clinically useful anti-integration drugs are available. It is the structural and functional complexity of the integration process together with the limitations of the available *in vitro* assays that has made it problematic to develop inhibitors of the HIV integrase [19].

6.   Replication

The DNA polymerase responsible for the replication of the genome of herpesviruses (HSV-1, HSV-2, VZV, CMV, EBV, and human herpesvirus-6) is a target for several compounds that could collectively be referred to as the antiherpetic compounds [20]. Structurally the antiherpetic compounds fall into one of the following categories: pyramidine nucleoside analogues (**brivudin, sorivudine**); acyclic nucleoside analogues (**acyclovir, ganciclovir, penciclovir**); carbocyclic nucleoside analogues (**lobucavir**); and acyclic nucleoside phoshonates (**cidofovir, adefovir**) [21]. In addition to the nucleoside analogues, the pyrophosphate analogue **foscarnet** also has been pursued for the treatment of CMV infections. Whereas foscarnet is able to interact directly with its target (the viral DNA polymerase), the nucleoside analogues must first be phosphorylated to their triphosphate form before they can interact with the viral DNA polymerase. Idoxuridine (IDU) and trifluorothymidine (TFT) were the first pyrimidine nucleoside analogues ever shown to be effective against herpesviruses in particular, HSV-1. They were the first to be approved for clinical use, and are still used as eyedrops in the topical treatment of HSV-1 keratitis. Neither IDU nor TFT can be used systemically because they are too toxic, especially for the bone marrow. The antiviral activity spectrum of brivudin and sorivudine is essentially limited to HSV-1, VZV, and EBV; that of acyclovir and penciclovir encompasses HSV-1, HSV-2, and VZV, whereas for ganciclovir it extends to CMV (because the specific phosphorylation by phosphotransferase). The activity spectrum of cidifovir, however, includes most herpesviruses and extends to other DNA viruses (i.e. papillomaviruses, poxviruses and adenoviruses). Furthermore, cidifovir induces a much longer lasting antiviral response than the other nucleoside analogues, and this may be ascribed to the unusually long intracellular half-life of its metabolites [22]. Herpesviruses can develop resistance to the antiherpetic compounds by mutations either in the thymidine kinase (HSV and VZV) or phosphotransferase (CMV) gene. These mutations can affect the phosphorylation of the compounds, or in the viral DNA polymerase gene, affect the interaction with their target site.

A rather different nucleoside analogue is ribavirin. The fact that ribavirin inhibits the cellular enzym IMP hydrogenase and in this way inhibits mRNA synthesis, suggest that it may be acting on cellular pathways and will be discussed later.

7.   Late Transcription

On the reasonable assumption that many or most viruses will carry regulatory genes, the approach to block these regulatory genes by antiviral chemotherapy is considerable appealing. Products of these regulatory genes; like the *tat* and *rev* proteins play an important role in the expression of the HIV genome. Both proteins engage in a highly specific binding to regulatory elements in the viral mRNA. An agent capable of binding to the *tat* protein would be expected to be an effective inhibitor of HIV replication. In particular, the late transcription process (DNA→mRNA) is considered to be the target for transactivation (Tat) antagonists [23].

8.   *Viral mRNA Translation*

Antisense oligonucleotides (ODNs) are short pieces of DNA that are complementary to a target mRNA and can block the expression of specific genes involved in the development of human disease. The viral mRNA could be targeted by antisense therapy by blocking the translation of viral mRNA to viral protein. In principle, any sequence of any viral mRNA could serve as target, and complementary oligos to each of them could be synthesized. However, for a successful outcome, the oligos must meet several criteria: easily synthesized, stable *in vivo*, able to enter the target cell, able to interact with their cellular target, and no interaction with other macromolecules [24]. Modifications of ODNs lead to altered lipophilicity and binding stability to its RNA target and resistance against serum nucleases. Their uptake occurs via receptor-mediated endocytosis and after release from the endosomes, ODNs may exert their effects by interaction with cytosolic or nuclear structures [25]. Side effects can occur when interaction affects intra- or extracellular targets essential for biological cell function. Several trials with ODNs targeted against HIV-1 and hepatitis viruses are performed [26]. The new drug **vitravene** (fomivirsen), based on a phosphorothiote oligonucleotide designed to inhibit CMV, promises that some substantial successes can be achieved with the antisense technique.

Ribozymes, or catalytic RNAs, could be considered as a special class of antisense ODNs and are involved in the processing of RNA precursors [27]. They recognize their target RNA in a highly sequence-specific manner and therefore can be used to inhibit gene expression by cleavage of the target mRNA. Antisense ODNs in general, and ribozymes in particular, also can be taken up in gene therapy strategies, whereby they are introduced in the cells through retroviral vectors. This then allows constitutive expression of the ribozyme, leading to inhibition of HIV gene expression in the cell that have already been infected by HIV and conferring "intracellular immunity" of noninfected cells against subsequent HIV infection.

Release

9.   *Assembly*

Maturation of the viral proteins in infected cells involves mostly host-cell metabolic pathways, including proteolytic cleavage. Cleavage of viral proteins by proteases is required at several stages in the viral replication cycle: activation of some viral enzymes, posttranslational cleavage, activation of envelope fusion glycoproteins, and maturation of the viron. This latter process has proved to be a highly specific intervention point for HIV protease inhibitors [28]. The HIV protease enzyme is responsible for the post translational processing of *gag* and *gag-pol* polyprotein precursors into their functional products. Inhibition of this enzyme results in the production of non infectious virus. Examples of these agents are **indinavir, ritonavir, saquinavir, amprenavir**, and **nelfinavir**. Currently, a number of viral encoded proteases have emerged as new targets for antiviral intervention in the treatment of herpes-, retro-, hepatitis C and human rhinovirus infections [29]. Optimal use involves combination with reverse transcriptase inhibitors.

Alteration in the cellular enzyme activity is necessary for efficient assembly of infectious virus particles. As mentioned above, **rimantadine** inhibit the proton flow through the M2 pore, which depending on whether this occurs early or late in the infectivity cycle, leads also to inhibition of virus maturation and release [10].

10.   Budding

Besides haemagglutinin, neuramidase is also a surface influenza virus glycoprotein, that interact with cell-receptors. Specific inhibitors of neuramidase have been developed, and two (**zanamivir** and **oseltamivir**) are used in humans. Unlike the amantadine derivates, these drugs inhibit replication of both influenza A and B viruses. In the presence of the NA inhibitors virions stay attached to the membrane of infected cells and thus virus spread is inhibited [30]. The neuramidase inhibitors are effective for both prevention and treatment of acute influenza.

II.   Inhibition of Virus Replication By Cellular Enzymes

1.   IMP Dehydrogenase Inhibitors

IMP (inosinate 5´-monophosphate) dehydrogenase is involved in *de novo* synthesis of GTP, the direct substrate for RNA synthesis. In the presence of IMP dehydrogenase inhibitors, the RNA synthesis is suppressed and this affect virus-infected and rapidly growing cells, where the need for RNA synthesis is greatest [31]. However, this is not thought to be the single inhibitory mechanism. There may be also one or more important cellular effects that are not virus-specific. IMP dehydrogenase inhibitors such as **ribavirin** and its derivatives have shown broad-spectrum antiviral activity against many RNA and DNA viruses, particularly, ortho- and paramyxoviruses [32]. Clinically, aerosolized ribavirin has been reported to be efficacious for treating respiratory syncytial virus infection of infants. Oral ribavirin in combination with interferon also reduces mortality from infections with hepatitis C virus [33].

2.   SAH Hydrolase Inhibitors

SAH (S-adenosyl-homocysteine) hydrolase is a key enzym in methylation reactions, required for the maturation of viral mRNAs. SAH hydrolase is a target for a variety of adenosine analogues, which eventually lead to inhibition of the methylation of viral mRNA [34]. SAH hydrolyse inhibitors (neplanocin A derivatives) are particularly effective against poxvirus, paramyxovirus, rhabdovirus, and reovirus. This activity spectrum also extends to human CMV [35].

3.   OMP Decarboxylase and CTP Synthetase Inhibitors

OMP (orotidine 5´-monophosphate) decarboxylase and CTP (cytidine 5`-triphosphate) synthetase are involved in the biosynthetic pathway of the pyrimidine mononucleotides [36]. OMP and CTP are the substrates for cellular and viral RNA synthesis. OMP decarboxylase inhibitors (**pyrazofurin**), and CTP synthetase inhibitors (carbodine, and its more potent counterpart cyclopentylcytosine) are active against a broad range of DNA and RNA virus. Carbodine was first described as an anti-influenza virus agent.

4.   *Hydroxyurea*

Hydroxyurea is a compound extensively used in medical practice, mainly for treating chronic myelogenous leukemia, sickle cell anemia, and other diseases. This agent has been shown to inhibit retroviral reverse transcription by targeting a cellular enzym responsible for the synthesis of dNTP. The intracellular concentration of dNTP decreases, and the incorporation of other drugs such as NRTIs (chiefly of didanosine but also of stavudine and lamivudine) increases [37]. Hydroxyurea have synergistic effects that prove promising, though larger clinical studies are needed to define the role in the treatment of HIV.

III.   Immunomodulators

Immunomodulators are substances that modify the response of immune competent cells through signaling mechanisms. They are administered to augment or restore host immune responses to infectious agents or malignancies [38]. Cytokines play an important role in the defense against viral infections, both indirectly, through determination of the host response, and directly, through inhibition of viral replication. One class of cytokines are the interferons (IFNs). In response to IFN, cells develop an antiviral state in which the replication of viruses is inhibited [39]. The binding of IFN to specific receptors leads to the activation of signal transduction pathways that stimulate genes, whose products are eventually responsible for the antiviral effects. The steps of the viral replication cycle that are affected by interferon have been identified for several families of viruses. It has been reported that IFNs restrict virus growth at the levels of penetration, uncoating, synthesis of mRNA, protein synthesis and assembly [40]. Viruses differ in their sensitivity to IFN, which initially were discovered on the basis of their antiviral activity against influenza virus. There are four major classes of human interferons, including IFN-∀, IFN-∃, IFN-α and IFN-T. Only **IFN-∀** has been approved for use in the treatment of certain viral infections. IFN-∀, as a recombinant protein produced in bacteria, has proved to be effective in the treatment of diseases caused by papillomaviruses [41], hepatitis B and C virus [42, 43]. **Imiquimod**, a member of the class of imidazoquinolinamines, is a novel immune response modifier, inducing interferons and a number of other endogenous cytokines. Topical use of imiquimod has been shown to be efficacious in both molluscum contangiosum and genital warts [44].

Colony-stimulating factors (CSFs) are natural occurring cytokines that stimulate the reproduction and differentiation of granulocytes (G-CSF) or granulocytes, monocytes, and macrophages (**GM-CSF**). Studies have shown both CSFs to be very effective in correcting the neutropenias seen with for example AZT therapy alone or combined with interferon. In monocytes, GM-CSF stimulates virus replication *in vitro*, an effect consistent with the cell stimulatory properties of cytokines. Only the two immunomodulators, IFN-∀ and GM-CSF, are commercially available in the treatment of HIV infection. Many others are in the early phases of investigation. Isoprinisone, diethyldithiocarbamate, and IMREG-1, have been administered to patients in controlled trials and have shown some possible short-term effects in decreasing progression of the disease [38]. Other agents such as thymic hormones, enkephalins, interleukin-2, and activated natural killer cells are in earlier stages of investigations. Reconsideration of existing immunomodulating drugs like cyclosporin and thalidomide in the treatment of HIV infection is currently under investigation [45]. Cyclosporin blocks the activation of T-cells and also prevents proper HIV virion maturation. However, clinical studies have produced conflicting results with regard to immunological and disease effects and toxicity. Thalidomide may have antiretroviral effects as result of its inhibitory effects on the production of tumour necrosis factor-∀ (TNF-∀). TNF-∀ and also interleukin-6 have been shown *in vitro* to induce expression of HIV from chronically infected cells.

Conclusion

In the last decade there has been rapid progress in both our understanding of antiviral therapy and the number of antiviral agents on the market. Increasingly, combinations of agents are being used to achieve synergistic inhibition of viruses, to delay resistance, and to decrease dosages of toxic drugs. Future directions include the use of molecular biologic techniques to identify enzymes unique in viral replication and computer-aided drug design to interfere with these enzymes or receptors.

References

1. Hosoya M, Balzarini J, Shigeta S, De Clercq E. Differential inhibitory effects of sulfated polysaccharides and polymers on the replication of various myxoviruses and retroviruses, depending on the composition of the target amino acid sequences of the viral envelope glycoproteins. *Antimicrob Agents Chemother* 1991; 35(12): 2515-20.
2. Ikeda S, Neyts J, Verma S, Wickramasinghe A, Mohan P, De Clercq E. *In vitro* and *in vivo* inhibition of ortho- and paramyxovirus infections by a new class of sulfonic acid polymers interacting with virus-cell binding and/or fusion. *Antimicrob Agents Chemother* 1994; 38(2): 256-9.
3. Damonte EB. [Antiviral agents that act in the early phases of the viral cycle] Agentes antivirales que actuan en las etapas tempranas del ciclo viral. *Rev Argent Microbiol* 1996; 28(4): 204-16.
4. McKinlay MA, Pevear DC, Rossmann MG. Treatment of the picornavirus common cold by inhibitors of viral uncoating and attachment. *Annu Rev Microbiol* 1992; 46: 635-54.
5. van der Sijs H, Wiltink EH. Antiviral drugs: present status and future prospects. *Int J Biochem* 1994; 26(5): 621-30.
6. Schols D, Este JA, Henson G, De Clercq E. Bicyclams, a class of potent anti-HIV agents, are targeted at the HIV coreceptor fusin/CXCR-4. *Antiviral Res* 1997; 35(3): 147-56.
7. Soler F, Poujade C, Evers M, et al. Betulinic acid derivatives: a new class of specific inhibitors of human immunodeficiency virus type 1 entry. *J Med Chem* 1996; 39(5): 1069-83.
8. Kuipers ME, Huisman JG, Swart PJ, et al. Mechanism of anti-HIV activity of negatively charged albumins: biomolecular interaction with the HIV-1 envelope protein gp120. *J Acquir Immune Defic Syndr Hum Retrovirol* 1996; 11(5): 419-29.
9. De Clerq. Novel compounds in preclinical/early clinical development for the treatment of HIV infections. *Rev Med Virol* 2000; 10(4): 255-77.
10. Lin TI, Heider H, Schroeder C. Different modes of inhibition by adamantane amine derivatives and

natural polyamines of the functionally reconstituted influenza virus M2 proton channel protein. *J Gen Virol* 1997; 78(Pt 4): 767-74.

11. Pevear DC, Tull TM, Seipel ME, Groarke JM. Activity of pleconaril against enteroviruses. *Antimicrob Agents Chemother* 1999; 43(9): 2109-15.

12. Schiff GM, Sherwood JR. Clinical activity of pleconaril in an experimentally induced coxsackievirus A21 respiratory infection. *J Infect Dis* 2000; 181(1): 20-6.

13. Bishop NE. Examination of potential inhibitors of hepatitis A virus uncoating. *Intervirology* 1998; 41(6): 261-71.

14. Jarvis B, Faulds D. Lamivudine. A review of its therapeutic potential in chronic hepatitis B. *Drugs* 1999; 58(1): 101-41.

15. De Clercq E. Acyclic nucleoside phosphonates in the chemotherapy of DNA virus and retrovirus infections. *Intervirology* 1997; 40(5-6): 295-303.

16. Katlama C. Review of NNRTIs: 'today and tomorrow'. *Int J Clin Pract Suppl* 1999; 103: 16-20.

17. Pommier Y, Neamati N. Inhibitors of human immunodeficiency virus integrase. *Adv Virus Res* 1999; 52: 427-58.

18. Thomas M, Brady L. HIV integrase: a target for AIDS therapeutics. *Trends Biotechnol* 1997; 15(5): 167-72.

19. Pani A, Marongiu ME. Anti-HIV-1 integrase drugs: how far from the shelf? *Curr Pharm Des* 2000; 6(5): 569-84.

20. Matthews JT, Terry BJ, Field AK. The structure and function of the HSV DNA replication proteins: defining novel antiviral targets. *Antiviral Res* 1993; 20(2): 89-114.

21. De Clercq E. Trends in the development of new antiviral agents for the chemotherapy of infections caused by herpesviruses and retroviruses. *Rev Med Vir* 2000; 5: 149-64.

22. Aduma P, Connelly MC, Srinivas RV, Fridland A. Metabolic diversity and antiviral activities of acyclic nucleoside phosphonates. *Mol Pharmacol* 1995; 47(4): 816-22.

23. Hsu MC, Schutt AD, Holly M, et al. Inhibition of HIV replication in acute and chronic infections *in vitro* by a Tat antagonist. *Science* 1991; 254(5039): 1799-802.

24. Stein CA, Cheng YC. Antisense oligonucleotides as therapeutic agents--is the bullet really magical? *Science* 1993; 261(5124): 1004-12.

25. Caselmann WH, Eisenhardt S, Alt M. Synthetic antisense oligodeoxynucleotides as potential drugs against hepatitis C. *Intervirology* 1997; 40(5-6): 394-9.

26. Galderisi U, Cascino A, Giordano A. Antisense oligonucleotides as therapeutic agents. *J Cell Physiol* 1999; 181(2): 251-7.

27. Tanner NK. Ribozymes: the characteristics and properties of catalytic RNAs. *FEMS Microbiol Rev* 1999; 23(3): 257-75.

28. Deeks SG, Smith M, Holodniy M, Kahn JO. HIV-1 protease inhibitors. A review for clinicians. *JAMA* 1997; 277(2): 145-53.

29. Patick AK, Potts KE. Protease inhibitors as antiviral agents. *Clin Microbiol Rev* 1998; 11(4): 614-27.

30. Gubareva LV, Kaiser L, Hayden FG. Influenza virus neuraminidase inhibitors. *Lancet* 2000; 355(9206): 827-35.

31. Andrei G, De Clercq E. Molecular approaches for the treatment of hemorrhagic fever virus infections. *Antiviral Res* 1993; 22(1): 45-75.

32. Gilbert BE, Knight V. Biochemistry and clinical applications of ribavirin. *Antimicrob Agents Chemother* 1986; 30(2): 201-5.

33. Heathcote J. Antiviral therapy of patients with chronic hepatitis C. *Sem Liver Disease* 2000; 20(2):

185-99.

34. Wolfe MS, Borchardt RT. S-adenosyl-L-homocysteine hydrolase as a target for antiviral chemotherapy. *J Med Chem* 1991; 34(5): 1521-30.

35. Snoeck R, Andrei G, Neyts J, et al. Inhibitory activity of S-adenosylhomocysteine hydrolase inhibitors against human cytomegalovirus replication. *Antiviral Res* 1993; 21(3): 197-216.

36. De Clercq E. Antiviral agents: characteristic activity spectrum depending on the molecular target with which they interact. *Adv Virus Res* 1993; 42: 1-55.

37. Zala C, Rouleau D, Montaner JS. Role of hydroxyurea in treatment of disease due to human immunodeficiency virus infection. *Clin Infect Dis* 2000; 30(S2): S143-50.

38. Bean B. Antiviral therapy: current concepts and practices. *Clin Microbiol Rev* 1992; 5(2): 146-82.

39. Dorr RT. Interferon-alpha in malignant and viral diseases. A review. *Drugs* 1993; 45(2): 177-211.

40. Landolfo S, Gribaudo G, Angeretti A, Gariglio M. Mechanisms of viral inhibition by interferons. *Pharmacol Ther* 1995; 65(3): 415-42.

41. Friedman Kien AE, Eron LJ, Conant M, et al. Natural interferon alfa for treatment of condylomata acuminata. *JAMA* 1988; 259(4): 533-8.

42. Davis GL, Balart LA, Schiff ER, et al. Treatment of chronic hepatitis C with recombinant interferon alfa. A multicenter randomized, controlled trial. Hepatitis Interventional Therapy Group. *N Engl J Med* 1989; 321(22): 1501-6.

43. Perrillo RP, Schiff ER, Davis GL, et al. A randomized, controlled trial of interferon alfa-2b alone and after prednisone withdrawal for the treatment of chronic hepatitis B. The Hepatitis Interventional Therapy Group [see comments]. *N Engl J Med* 1990; 323(5): 295-301.

44. Zerr DM, Frenkel LM. Advances in antiviral therapy. *Curr Opin Pediatr* 1999; 11(1): 21-7.

45. Ravot E, Lisziewicz J, Lori F. New uses for old drugs in HIV infection: the role of hydroxyurea, cyclosporin and thalidomide. *Drugs* 1999; 58(6): 953-63.

CHAPTER 2

PHARMACOLOGY

SAYE KHOO, DAVID BACK and CONCEPTA MERRY

Table of Contents

Introduction

Why do clinicians need to understand pharmacology when treating infections? It could reasonably be argued that for the standard bacterial infection, prescribing of an appropriate antibiotic with little more than a rudimentary knowledge of pharmacology usually results in successful eradication. The same is alas not true of antiviral drugs. Unlike most bacteria, viruses utilise host cell mechanisms for their own replication and are as a general rule harder to treat. Drugs not only have to penetrate inside the cell and target these processes, but must also achieve this with minimum detriment to host cell metabolism. Toxicity is consequently increased. Many viruses (e.g. herpesviruses) have the capacity to undergo latency and are difficult to eradicate. Others such as hepatitis C produce chronic infection and require prolonged treatment. Therapeutic alternatives are more limited than for bacterial infection and pharmacological manipulation may be required to minimise toxicity or maximise efficacy. HIV infection in particular has transported pharmacology from the dusty bookshelf to the clinic and the bedside. No physician treating HIV-infected patients can afford to be ignorant of the potential for

Practical Guidelines in Antiviral Therapy Ed. by Charles A.B. Boucher and George J. Galasso. 13 — 35
© 2002 *Elsevier Science. Printed in the Netherlands.*

drug interaction (particularly with protease inhibitors), the importance of maintaining adequate drug levels at all times to prevent virus breakthrough, and the concept of 'pharmacological resistance' i.e. reservoirs and sanctuary sites not adequately targeted by drugs. This chapter will provide an overview of pharmacological principles relevant to the treatment of viral infections, citing examples from the treatment of HIV and other viral infections.

Mechanism of Drug Action

Viruses are obligate intracellular parasites, lacking the means to replicate without the mechanisms for protein synthesis provided by the host cell. A generalised representation of the cycle of infection is shown in Figure 1. The infecting virion first attaches to the cell membrane and is then internalised through processes that differ between viruses. There follows a process of uncoating and release of viral nucleic acid. DNA viruses (e.g. herpesviruses, adenovirus and hepatitis B) have their nuclear material transcribed to mRNA. Early proteins have a regulatory function that serve to enhance viral replication and the production of later (structural) proteins through the use of host enzymes and the Golgi apparatus. Virally-encoded enzymes also play an important part in these processes. For RNA viruses, mRNA is synthesised by viral enzymes or else derives directly from viral nucleic acid. RNA retroviruses (such as HIV) encode reverse transcriptase, generating DNA which is then transcribed and translated to produce structural proteins. Many viruses such as herpesviruses and HIV lay down 'archival' DNA material incorporated within the host cell nucleus. No therapeutic intervention has yet been utilised to target this process, which if successful would result in eradication of infection. One possible strategy may be the use of 'intracellular immunisation' using genes whose products may prevent transactivation of viral replication.

Antiviral drugs target different stages of this process (Figure 1). Immunoglobulin, hyperimmune serum or specific monoclonal antibodies form complexes with free virus which are then inactivated. Pleconaril, a promising compound which exhibits broad enterovirus and rhinovirus activity, binds within a hydrophobic pocket leading to inhibition of viral capsid protein function, thus interrupting viral attachment and uncoating of viral RNA. The fusion inhibitor T-20 disrupts the interaction between the HIV glycoprotein gp120 and its co-receptor on the cell surface, inhibiting an essential process in the attachment and fusion of HIV. Amantadine blocks the ionic channel formed by influenza A M2 protein, inhibiting both viral uncoating and maintenance of pH neutral haemagglutinin in the trans-Golgi network. Many antiviral drugs (e.g. foscarnet, non-nucleoside reverse transcriptase inhibitors and competitive analogues of endogenous nucleosides such as aciclovir, zidovudine and lamivudine) inhibit the production of viral mRNA, by inhibiting either viral DNA or RNA polymerases or in the case of HIV, reverse transcriptase. Unlike DNA polymerase, HIV reverse transcriptase is virally encoded and reverse transcriptase inhibitors act directly upon a viral product before replication of nucleic acid. Interferon has a multiplicity of antiviral effects, one important one being inhibition of mRNA translation. Other drugs (e.g. HIV protease inhibitors and neuraminidase inhibitors such as zanamivir and oseltamivir) interfere

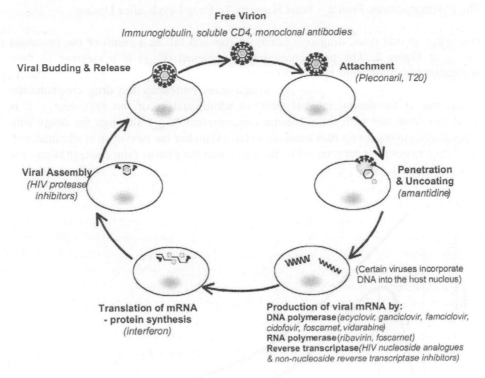

Figure 1. The viral life cycle with targets for drug intervention.

later on in the process with viral assembly, budding or release. From Figure 1, it is clear that apart from those compounds acting upon free virions or cell membrane attachment and penetration, it is necessary to achieve sufficient concentrations of antiviral agents *inside* virally-infected cells to successfully interfere with viral replication.

Determinants of Drug Activity

For most antiviral drugs, activity is directly related not just to the ability to penetrate to target organs but also to the ability to achieve sufficient concentrations of active drug at the site of action (usually intracellular). Many factors may influence this, such as the bioavailability and lipid-solubility of the compound, plasma protein binding, whether the drug requires metabolic activation, pharmacokinetics of all active metabolites, the mode of action of the drug and interactions with other compounds [1]. Also of importance are the mechanisms of active fluxing of drug into- and out of cells (cellular 'influx' and 'efflux' transporters). These are discussed in further detail below.

The Pharmacokinetic Profile – What Happens To Drug Levels after Dosing

Following an oral dose, drug concentrations rise and fall as a result of the processes shown in Figure 2. The peak concentration achieved (C_{max}) is a measure of drug absorption and subsequent tail-off in concentrations is influenced by tissue distribution, drug metabolism and excretion. The trough level represents the drug concentration at the end of the dosing interval, prior to administration of the next dose – it is usual to equate this with the minimum concentration (C_{min}) although for drugs with delayed absorption, levels may continue to fall even after the next dose is administered. Total drug exposure is represented by the area under the plasma drug concentration-time curve (AUC) [2].

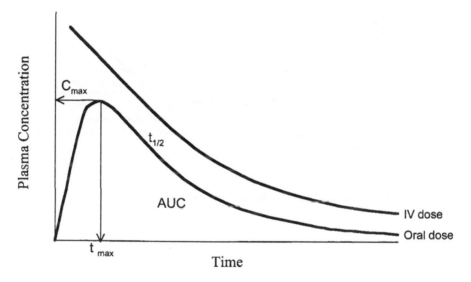

Figure 2.   Pharmacokinetic profile following oral and i.v. administration of a drug.

Absorption

This is dependent upon several factors [3]. Orally administered drugs are clearly dependent upon the absorptive capacity of the gut. Any process that affects intestinal surface area, blood flow or transit time will impair absorption. The 'bioavailability' of a drug (which gives a measure of how much drug gets into the systemic circulation) is calculated from the difference between the AUC of unaltered drug after identical i.v. and oral dosing. The lipid solubility of a compound will influence its bioavailability. This is determined by its size and molecular structure as well as the degree of ionisation at intestinal or gastric pH (the fraction of unionised drug is more lipid-soluble and will be better absorbed). Gastric acidity also plays a role in drug absorption. For example, the HIV nucleoside analogue didanosine is acid-labile and is not absorbed without the co-administration of an antacid buffer. This has resulted in an increase in the bulk of the tablets and some side effects e.g. bloating and diarrhoea. The presence of food may also affect bioavailability, by affecting gastric emptying, or binding of drug to food particles. Food may increase the absorption of certain drugs (lipid solubility is increased by fatty meals), for example the protease inhibitor saquinavir achieves significantly higher blood levels when taken with meals.

Food may alter drug absorption [4] e.g. calcium binds to tetracycline. Enzymes present in intestinal secretions or the gut wall may inactivate the compound [5] ('first pass metabolism' – see Figure 3) but may themselves be inactivated by dietary components. One interesting example is grapefruit juice which inhibits intestinal cytochrome p450 enzymes (CYP3A4 isoform). CYP3A4 together with other molecules such as the efflux transporter P-glycoprotein (see below) constitutes a barrier to intestinal absorption, and the co-administration of grapefruit juice was found to increase plasma levels of felodipine and nifedipine. Prior to the availability of a new soft-gel formulation, grapefruit juice when given to patients receiving the HIV protease inhibitor saquinavir led to an average doubling in the plasma AUC of saquinavir.

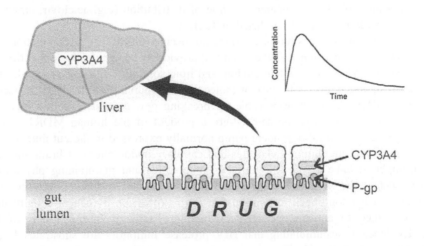

Figure 3.   First pass loss of drug following oral administration. Principle components of the first pass effect are *a*) metabolism in the gut wall and liver and *b*) efflux transport by P-glycoprotein (P-gp).

Distribution

Plasma protein binding is a key consideration [6], [7]. The amount of drug present in plasma is made up of free drug and drug complexed to plasma proteins such as albumin (acidic compounds) or the acute phase protein α_1-acid glycoprotein (basic compounds). Conditions that either decrease (e.g. nephrotic syndrome, liver disease) or increase (e.g. acute infection with α_1-acid glycoprotein) the levels of these proteins will affect the fraction of unbound drug (i.e. the amount of free drug able to produce a pharmacological effect) although often without an appreciable change in free drug concentrations. However, this becomes important when considering the role of therapeutic drug monitoring (e.g. for HIV protease inhibitors, which may be >98% bound to α_1-acid glycoprotein), since higher total concentration of drug in plasma will be necessary to maintain the same steady state free concentration. Extensively protein-bound drugs may be displaced by other drugs which are highly bound to the same protein, again altering the fraction of the unbound drug although the overall effect of this is usually minor.

Distribution into tissue compartments also depends upon lipid solubility of the drug – hydrophilic drugs highly ionised at physiological pH penetrate poorly across cell membranes compared to lipophilic compounds. The apparent volume of distribution (V_D) of a drug is defined as the volume of fluid required to contain the total amount of drug in the body at the same concentration as that present in plasma. This gives an indirect measure of the tissue distribution of a drug. Drugs which remain largely in the circulation (e.g. foscarnet) have an apparent volume of distribution close to the plasma volume (~3.5 litres in an average adult) whereas drugs which concentrate in tissues will have a considerably larger apparent volume of distribution (e.g. aciclovir, amantadine and ribavirin). Further details are listed in Table 1.

Considerable interest has recently centred on mechanisms of drug accumulation within cells and tissue compartments. Whereas it had previously been considered that the major determinants were plasma protein binding and lipid solubility, the role of cellular transporters mediating influx and efflux of molecules has increasingly been recognised [8]. Here again, HIV has been responsible for breaking new ground. The best recognised efflux transporter is P-glycoprotein (P-gp, a product of the human MDR1 gene see Table 2). P-gp is an ATP-dependent pump normally expressed in the gut mucosa, liver, kidney, placenta, circulating leukocytes and capillary endothelium of brain and testes. It is thought to have a role for excreting xenobiotics and maintaining physiological barriers such as the blood-brain barrier, the blood-testes barrier and between the mother and foetus. It has long been recognised that P-gp expression by cancer cells results in class resistance to anti-tumour agents, which are actively 'pumped out' of these cells. Evidence is accumulating that HIV protease inhibitors are substrates for, and inhibitors of P-gp [9-12]. This may explain in part the poor absorption of some protease inhibitors (e.g. saquinavir) from the gut. Protease inhibitors in general have poor penetration into the central nervous system but in *mdr1a* knockout mice (lacking P-gp), plasma concentrations of orally administered indinavir, saquinavir, and nelfinavir were increased 2-5 fold, and brain concentrations 7-36 fold. Moreover, the addition of ritonavir markedly increases plasma concentration of saquinavir (~10-fold) and indinavir (~5-fold). A related family of efflux transporters, MRP (MDR-related protein) has been characterised, for which HIV protease inhibitors (MRP-1) and nucleoside analogues (MRP4) appear to be substrates *in-vitro*. The clinical relevance of all these transporters in HIV therapy has not yet been ascertained, nor has it been established whether influx transporters may also play a role.

Metabolism

Some antiviral agents are excreted largely unchanged (e.g. aciclovir) while others undergo extensive biotransformation prior to removal from the body. Although metabolites generally lack pharmacological activity, there are important exceptions with antiviral agents.

Metabolic activation.   Firstly, the bioavailability of drugs such as aciclovir and ganciclovir is relatively poor [13]. This becomes a problem when the virus is less sensitive (e.g. varicella zoster virus is less sensitive to aciclovir than herpes simplex) and when prolonged courses of therapy are required (e.g. maintenance therapy for CMV disease in AIDS patients). Modification of aciclovir to its L-valine ester, valaciclovir (which is then hydrolysed almost completely to aciclovir) increases absorption from 20% to 54%. The resulting AUC after dosing with valaciclovir 3g/day is comparable with i.v. aciclovir. Similarly, valganciclovir (which is converted to ganciclovir) has improved bioavailability of compared to ganciclovir, and has been successfully used in treatment and maintenance of CMV retinitis in AIDS patients. Famciclovir is converted to penciclovir and has a bioavailability of >70%.

Secondly many antiviral agents (e.g. aciclovir, ganciclovir, famciclovir, ribavirin and all the HIV nucleoside analogues) are analogues of the endogenous cellular nucleosides such as thymidine, cytidine, guanosine and adenosine [14]. These agents require conversion by intracellular phosphorylation to their active triphosphate compounds which compete directly with endogenous nucleoside triphosphate for incorporation by viral enzymes such as DNA or RNA polymerase and reverse transcriptase. The intracellular activation pathway for the HIV nucleoside analogues is shown in Figure 4.

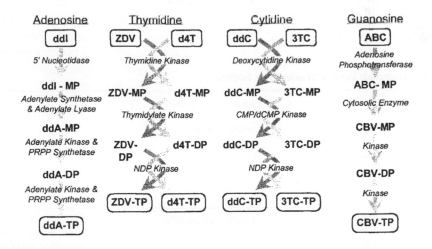

Figure 4.   Nucleoside analogue phosphorylation.

20   S. Khoo, D. Back and C. Merry

Table 1.   Pharmacokinetic characteristics of antiviral drugs

Drug	Indication	Site of Action	Active Metabolite ?
Aciclovir	HSV, VZV	Intracellular. Inhibits viral DNA polymerase	Intracellular phosphates
Amantadine	Influenza A	Extra and intracellular. Inhibits viral uncoating and proton transport channel of influenza A	No
Cidofovir	CMV	Intracellular	
Famciclovir	HSV, VZV, (HBV)	Intracellular. Inhibits viral DNA polymerase	Pro-drug of penciclovir
Foscarnet	CMV	Intracellular. Inhibits viral DNA and RNA polymerase	No
Ganciclovir	CMV, resistant HSV	Intracellular. Inhibits viral DNA polymerase	Intracellular phosphates
Ribavirin	wide range of DNA and RNA viruses including HCV and RSV	Intracellular. Inhibits viral DNA and RNA polymerase	Intracellular phosphates
Valaciclovir	(As aciclovir)	(As aciclovir)	Pro-drug of aciclovir
Valganciclovir	(As ganciclovir)	(As ganciclovir)	Pro-drug of ganciclovir
Zanamivir	Influenza A and B	Administered topically, inhibits neuraminidase impairing release and propagation of new virions	No

HIV Nucleoside Analogues

Abacavir	HIV	Intracellular. Inhibits HIV reverse transcriptase	Intracellular phosphates
Didanosine	HIV		
Lamivudine	HIV (also HBV)		
Stavudine	HIV		
Zalcitabine	HIV		
Zidovudine	HIV		

HIV Non-nucleoside Reverse Transcriptase Inhibitors

Delavirdine	HIV	Intracellular. Inhibits HIV	No
Efavirenz	HIV	reverse transcriptase	
Nevirapine	HIV		

HIV Protease Inhibitors

Amprenavir	HIV	Probably intracellular	No, apart from nelfinavir which has an active (M8) metabolite
Indinavir	HIV		
Nelfinavir	HIV		
Ritonavir	HIV		
Saquinavir	HIV		

Bioavailability	Protein Binding	Plasma half-life	V_D (L/kg)	Clearance	Notes/Interactions
10-20%	9-33%	2.5-3.3 h		Renal (unchanged)	Initial phosphorylation by viral enzymes, concentrates 40-100× in infected cells.
>90%	67%	15 h	5-10	Renal (unchanged)	
	<11%	2.2 h	0.4	Renal (unchanged)	
77%	<20%	2-3 h	1.08	Renal (unchanged)	
20%	15%	18 h		Renal (unchanged)	Oral/i.v. hydration reduces risk of renal toxicity.
5%	1-2%	3.5-4.8 h	0.74	Renal (unchanged)	
45-65%	does not bind	79 h	64	Renal	Also reduces endogenous dGTP pool (against which ribavirin triphosphate competes) thus potentiating its own effect.
~55%	13-18%	2.5-3.3 h		Renal (as aciclovir)	
	<10%	2.5-5.1 h		Renal (unchanged)	Administered by diskhaler. 4-17% of inhaled dose is systemically absorbed.
83%	~49%	1.5 h	0.8	Renal (80%)	
~42%		1.5 h	1.08	Renal (50%)	
80-85%	<36%	5-7 h	1.3	Renal (70%)	
~86%		1.3-1.4 h	0.66	Renal (40%)	
>80%	<4%	2.0 h	0.53	Renal (75%)	
60-70%	34-38%	1.1 h	1.6	Hepatic	Metabolite renally excreted.
not determined	~98%	6 h			Delavirdine is an inhibitor of CYP3A4.
not determined	>99%	45 h			Efavirenz both induces and inhibits CYP3A4.
~93%	~60%	25-30 h	1.21	Hepatic	Nevirapine is an inducer of CYP3A4.
not determined	90%	7-10 h	6.1	All PIs mainly	
~65%	60%	2		cleared hepatically,	
not determined	>98%	3-5	2-7	only indinavir	
not determined	98-99%	3-5	~0.3-0.6	undergoes significant	
12%	97%	12	10	renal clearance	

Table 2.   Key features of the efflux transporters P-glycoprotein (P-gp) and multi-drug resistance protein
(MRP)

P-gp	MRP
• ATP-dependent pump	• ATP-dependent pump
• ABC superfamily of transporters	• ABC superfamily of transporters
• Encoded by MDR-1	• Six sub-types (MRP1-6)
• Protease inhibitors are substrates and inhibitors	• Protease inhibitors are substrates
• Physiological role is protection of cells from toxic substances	• MRP1, 2, 3 & 5 transport glutathione conjugates
• Important in limiting bioavailability and blood brain barrier	• MRP2 is at apical membrane and MRP1, 3 & 5 are at basolateral membraneblood brain barrier
• Basolateral transporters important in testes and choroid plexus	

Incorporation of drug triphosphate results in chain termination; Figure 5 shows
lamivudine as an example (the completeness of chain termination varies between
compounds, e.g. with aciclovir it is nearly 100%, but with famciclovir, ~3 penciclovir
nucleotides are incorporated before chain termination).

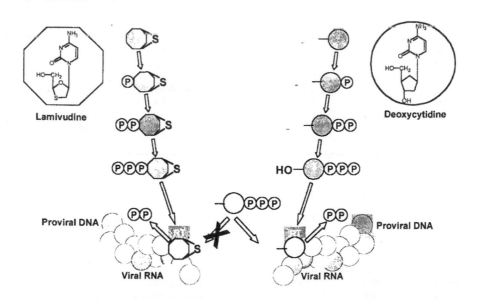

Figure 5.   Mechanism of action of 3TC (lamivudine). Phosphorylation occurs stepwise and the 3TC-TP
competes with endogenous dTTP for incorporation into the growing proviral DNA. This is the basic
mechanism of action for all nucleoside analogues.

Clearly, the potency of a drug will be influenced by the amount of its triphosphate metabolite relative to the competing endogenous nucleosides. For example, the *ratios* of zidovudine triphosphate: dTTP or lamivudine triphosphate:dCTP or aciclovir triphosphate:dGTP will most clearly reflect their activity [15]. This ratio may be influenced by drugs which alter the amount of endogenous nucleoside or else affect drug phosphorylation. Hydroxyurea lowers dATP levels by inhibiting ribonucleotide reductase thereby potentiating the action of didanosine, and ribavirin reduces dGTP levels thereby potentiating its own action, however, dTTP levels are increased [16]. This is potentially an important mechanism for enhancing drug activity and much interest centres on adding hydroxyurea to didanosine, or mycophenolic acid [17] (which like ribavirin inhibits inosine monophosphate dehydrogenase thereby lowering dGTP levels) to abacavir (Figure 6). On the other hand, drugs which share the same activation pathway may competitively reduce the formation of their respective triphosphate metabolites.

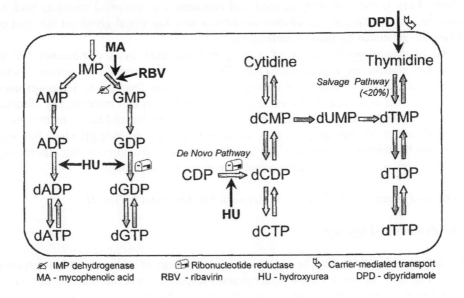

Figure 6.   Metabolic pathways of endogenous cellular nucleosides and potential sites of drug manipulation.

Biotransformation and clearance. The metabolic biotransformation of a drug generally involves the conversion of molecules into more polar, water-soluble compounds that may be eliminated in urine or bile. Most of these processes take place in the liver, and are broadly classified into phase I and phase II reactions. Phase I reactions include oxidation, reduction and hydrolysis and mainly involve the cytochrome P450 family of enzymes. There are many different isoforms of cytochromes P-450 with substrate

specificity determined by the individual isoforms. The nomenclature for cytochromes
P-450 has been developed to help understand their interrelationships.

- The capital letters 'CYP' abbreviate the cytochrome P450 and indicate a human
  isoform.
- CYP is followed by an Arabic number to indicate the isoform's family (i.e. CYP3)
- Subfamilies are then designated by a capitalised letter of the alphabet (i.e. CYP3A).
- Finally there is another Arabic number to designate an individual gene product in
  the subfamily (i.e. CYP3A4).

The families of cytochrome P450 so far identified as important contributors to drug
metabolism are shown in Table 3. The CYP3A subfamily is the major form of P450 in
human liver and is also expressed in the intestine. CYP2D6 is a polymorphic enzyme
with approximately 5-10% of Caucasians having deficient phenotypic expression.

Phase 2 reactions are also referred to as conjugation and occur in a wide variety of
tissues. They involve the enzyme-mediated attachment of activated moieties such as
glucuronic acid, sulphate, glutathione and acetate to a functional group on the drug or
metabolite generated by Phase 1 metabolism.

The pharmacological activity of a drug is terminated by a combination of its
metabolic inactivation and EXCRETION. Drugs can be excreted by several routes
including the kidneys (urine), the intestinal tract (bile and faeces), the lungs (exhaled
air), breast milk and sweat. Renal excretion is the most important route for any elimination and is determined by glomerular filtration, active secretion and active reabsorption.
Renal clearance of some drugs is very sensitive to change in urine pH since this will
determine the fraction of drug that will be in the ionised and unionised state. Increasing
the urine flow will also increase the urinary clearance of some drugs.

Pharmacodynamics – The Interaction Between The Drug and its Target

Drug Potency and Efficacy

The activity of a drug may be represented in the form of a concentration-response
curve. Figure 7 shows a typical concentration-response curve for three drugs (a-c).
Drug a is more potent than b or c, since it achieves the maximum response at lower
concentrations. However, the maximum efficacy of drugs a and b is identical, and
greater than that of drug c. It is important not to confuse 'efficacy' with 'effectiveness'
which describes the clinical usefulness of a drug, based upon clinical studies (phase III
and IV) in relevant patient groups.

Table 3. Substrates, inhibitors and inducers of known CYP450s (list not exhaustive)

Substrates

1A2	2C9	2C19	2D6	2E1	3A4
clozapine	diclofenac	diazepam	codeine	acetaminophen	alprazolam
fluvoxamine	ibuprofen	lansoprazole	metoprolol	dapsone	astemizole
haloperidol	naproxen	nelfinavir	oxycodone	ethanol	cyclosporine
propranolol	tolbutamide	omeprazole	thioridazine	halothane	HIV protease inhibitors
tacrine	warfarin		venlafaxine		lovastatin
theophylline					midazolam
					many steroids

Inhibitors

1A2	2C9	2C19	2D6	2E1	3A4
cimetidine	fluconazole	cimetidine	fluoxetine	disulfiram	HIV protease inhibitors
erythromycin	metronidazole	lansoprazole	quinidine		ketoconazole
ciprofloxacin	paroxetin	omeprazole	ritonavir		macrolides
			sertraline		

Inducers

1A2	2C9	2C19	2D6	2E1	3A4
rifampicin	phenobarbital	carbamazepine		chronic ethanol	rifabutin
tobacco	rifampicin	rifampicin			rifampicin
					ritonavir
					St John's Wort

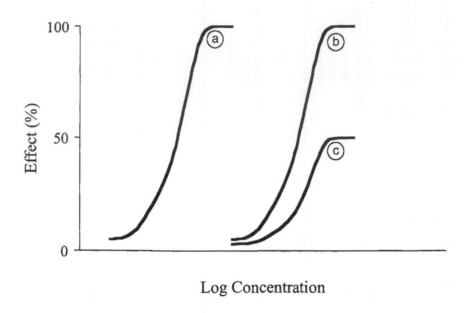

Figure 7.   Typical log dose response curves for 3 drugs (a-c).

Drug failure – The role of 'pharmacological resistance' [18]

Treatment failure is frequently associated with the acquisition of virological resistance. This has been well-characterised for many viruses e.g. mutation or deletion of viral thymidine kinase in aciclovir-resistant herpes simplex. However, viral resistance is not always the cause of treatment failure and other factors such as inadequate potency, poor penetration of drug into the target site, impaired drug activation, suboptimal pharmacokinetics and poor adherence by the patient to the allocated regimen may lead to failure. This introduces the concept of 'pharmacological resistance' – patients may remain refractory to treatment despite infection with drug-sensitive strains of virus [19]. Indeed, pharmacological resistance may precede virological resistance more often than we care to consider.

    This is yet another area of interest that HIV has opened up. One of the major goals of combination anti-retroviral therapy is to achieve suppression of plasma viral load to below the level of quantification. Even when this is achieved, the virus is detected elsewhere e.g. lymph node or central nervous system. Replication-competent HIV has been identified in small circulating subsets of circulating lymphocytes in peripheral blood, in the absence of detectable viraemia [20]. Detailed studies in lymphoid tissue from HIV-positive patients with 'successful' virological suppression demonstrate that the virus continues to evolve and replicate in these reservoirs or 'sanctuary sites'.

Surprisingly, genetic mutations associated with resistance to nucleoside analogues or protease inhibitors were not detected suggesting that the viral evolution takes place without any appreciable drug selection pressure. It is not known why this is the case but processes may exist within individual cells or at privileged anatomical sites that prevent the drug from reaching its target. The major challenge in the coming years is to identify and characterise these mechanisms, so that strategies may be found to overcome them.

Individualising Therapy

Individual Variability

Individuals differ in their response to drugs (inter-individual variability) and there may also be differences within an individual (intra-individual variability). The reasons are manifold and include, genetics, disease, age, concomitant administration of other drugs and a variety of environmental factors. In addition, it is important to consider non-compliance as an important factor contributing to variability in drug response. Non-compliance includes the taking of drug at the wrong time, the omission of a prescribed dose, and the stopping of therapy either because the patient begins to feel better or because of side effects considered unacceptable. Whatever the reasons, patient counselling and education are essential.

Age [21]

The foetus is able to metabolise drugs early in its development, but the expression of drug metabolising enzymes differs from that of the adult and is usually less efficient. Premature infants also have a deficiency of drug metabolising enzymes and renal function is also not fully developed. Drug therapy in such infants is difficult. A few months after birth, oxidative drug metabolising pathways increase dramatically and by 2 years of age children can metabolise some drugs more rapidly than adults. However, the ability to glucuronidate develops more slowly. There are other problems to be considered at the other extreme of age i.e.. when prescribing for the elderly. These include changes in circulating albumin (increasing the free fraction of drug in the plasma), decrease in lean body mass, decrease in expression of some enzymes with changes in hepatic clearance.

Genetics [22], [23]

Genetic factors may account for a large part of inter-individual variability. Examples of inherited variability in pharmacokinetics have been almost exclusively restricted to drug metabolism. Renal excretion of drugs does not appear to show genetic polymorphisms. Several genetic polymorphisms of drug metabolism have been identified involving oxidation (CYP isozymes) and acetylation (Table 3). CYP2D6 is associated with the oxidative metabolism of many CVS and CNS active drugs. The polymorphism of

CYP2D6 has been thoroughly characterised on the molecular level. The CYP2D6 gene locus has proven to be highly polymorphic e.g. both the extensive metaboliser (EM) and poor metaboliser (PM) phenotype are encoded by numerous allelic variants which range from complete deletion of the entire CYP2D6 gene to gene amplification leading to up to 12 copies of the CYP2D6 gene in one individual. The latter phenomenon has been identified as the molecular base for the ultrarapid metaboliser phenotype. Approximately 5-10% of Caucasians have deficient phenotypic expression of the CYP2D6 enzyme. There are also racial differences in expression of CYP2D6 [24]. The pharmacokinetic implications of an individual being a 'poor metaboliser' is that plasma levels of parent drug will remain elevated throughout the dosing interval and this may well have implications for adverse effects.

Disease

Hepatic [25] [26, 27]

Because the liver is the major site for drug metabolism, care should be taken when administering drugs to patients with disease states modifying hepatic function. However, hepatic disorders are not a single entity and different diseases affect various levels of hepatic organisation to a different extent. Generally, hepatic clearance of drugs is decreased in cirrhosis. In contrast, in acute viral hepatitis, there are those drugs for which clearance is decreased or half-life prolonged and those for which no change is detected. Drug elimination will also be reduced in obstructive jaundice, particularly for drugs removed by biliary excretion.

Another consideration is that the oral bioavailability of drugs highly cleared by the liver will be increased in cirrhosis. There are two reasons for this. One is a diminished first pass hepatic loss due to reduced enzyme activity and the other is the development of portal bypass (portocaval shunts).

Renal [28]

In patients with compromised renal function, urinary excretion of drugs is diminished. The degree of reduction in renal elimination depends on the reduction in renal function. The extent of drug accumulation in plasma depends on the frequency of administration and the half-life of the drug. With a longer half life the time to reach steady state is prolonged compared to a patient with normal renal function. Obviously to avoid excessive accumulation dosage of drug must be reduced in the patient with renal dysfunction. The clinician needs information on which drugs accumulate excessively in renal dysfunction and also how to adjust drug administration to achieve an optimal therapeutic response.

Renal abnormalities are common in HIV-infected patients. These disorders range from asymptomatic proteinuria of unknown clinical significance to HIV-associated nephropathy. Dose reduction recommendations are usually based on estimated creatinine clearance with estimations derived from standard equations. With HIV-related muscle wasting, creatinine clearance may be overestimated (due to low serum creatinine values) and timed urine collections will give a more accurate determination. Dose adjustment of nucleoside analogue reverse transcriptase inhibitors is dependent on whether renal failure is mild (CrCl 50-80 ml/min), moderate (CrCl 10-50 ml/min) or severe (CrCl < 10 ml/min). There is currently limited data on elimination by peritoneal dialysis or hemodialysis. In contrast to nucleoside analogues, protease inhibitors are predominantly metabolised in the liver with only a small percentage undergoing renal elimination, hence dosage adjustments are not considered necessary. However, there is some concern among clinicians on how to use the drugs optimally in patients with severe renal failure.

Drug Interactions

Drug interactions may be either pharmacokinetic with alteration of plasma drug concentrations, or pharmacodynamic with no alteration of drug concentration but an effect on either drug activity or drug toxicity. The most important pharmacokinetic drug interactions involve:

• Induction of metabolism
• Inhibition of metabolism
• Altered drug absorption
• Inhibition of renal excretion

Each of the above will be considered in turn. An example of a pharmacodynamic interaction is the enhanced bone marrow suppression in patients given concurrent zidovudine and ganciclovir.

Enzyme Induction [29-32]

This is particularly important for CYP450 enzymes but also takes place with glucuronyl transferase. A P450 inducer increases the amount of enzyme in the cell (hepatocyte, enterocyte) by binding directly to promoter elements in the DNA region that regulates expression of the gene. There is an increase in transcription of the gene with a subsequent increase in the amount of protein. With more enzyme present it means a drug that is a substrate for the enzyme will be more rapidly cleared. Maximal induction will normally take about 10 days to reach as new enzyme is synthesised. Importantly when an enzyme inducer is withdrawn from therapy it will take at least another 10 days to return to the original steady state (this being dependent on the half-life of breakdown of the enzyme). Inducers can switch on several genes at the same time. So, for example, rifampicin (a potent inducer) induces CYP1A2, CYP2C9, and CYP3A4. Other potent inducers are phenobarbital and rifabutin. Ritonavir, nelfinavir, efavirenz and nevirapine are moderate P450 inducers. The crucial thing to realise when considering co-administering an enzyme inducer with another drug is that therapeutic efficacy can readily be compromised. In some cases an increase in dose will be necessary but in other cases there is definite contraindication. So, because of the magnitude of the enzyme-inducing effects, rifampicin should not be given to patients who require treatment with protease inhibitors. Concurrent administration of rifabutin with ritonavir or saquinavir is not recommended.

Enzyme Inhibition [33-35]

An enzyme inhibitor is any drug that inhibits the metabolism of another drug by the same enzyme. This process is nearly always competitive and reversible which means that inhibition only occurs when the drug is actually present in the cell. As soon as the inhibitor is cleared metabolism returns to normal. Examples of CYP450 inhibitors include:

- All protease inhibitors (ritonavir > indinavir = nelfinavir = amprenavir > saquinavir).
- Some non-nucleoside reverse transcriptase inhibitors e.g., delavirdine.
- Macrolide antibiotics (e.g., clarithromycin, erythromycin)
- Azole antifungal drugs (e.g., ketoconazole, itraconazole, and to a lesser extent fluconazole).

The main concern with inhibition interactions is elevated plasma drug concentrations as a consequence of reduced hepatic clearance and prolonged half life. Many drugs are actually contraindicated in patients who are receiving antiviral therapy (for key information in this area the reader is encouraged to look at the following: http://www.medscape.com and http://www.hiv-druginteractions.org). Note however, that it is also possible to reverse the deleterious effect of an induction interaction. For example adding ritonavir to efavirenz plus amprenavir reverses the decrease in area under the curve produced by efavirenz.

Not all inhibition drug interactions are regarded as being a problem. In fact there is considerable interest in HIV therapy in the use of ritonavir as a pharmacoenhancing drug [36-38]. In this case a low dose of ritonavir is used to boost the plasma concentration of another PI and prevent its concentrations from falling sufficiently low so that viral replication may take place. In the case of saquinavir the boosting effect of ritonavir is on bioavailability so that C_{max} is markedly increased. For indinavir, the effect is to reduce hepatic clearance thereby increasing the half-life and minimum concentrations at the end of the dosing interval.

Lopinavir (ABT378r) will be the first licensed protease inhibitor containing a low dose of ritonavir (100 mg) in the formulation [39].

Ritonavir may also be useful in some situations to salvage a failing regimen without the need to switch the patient. This is because the elevated concentrations will be above the IC_{90} of even resistant viruses. There is also the possibility of once daily dosing of boosted protease inhibitors although further clinical trials are essential.

Given the complexity of induction and inhibition interactions it is essential that clinicians keep up-to-date on this area in relation to antiviral drugs so that treatment is optimised in individual patients [35], [40].

Absorption Interactions

As previously indicated, drug absorption may be altered by changes in the pH of the gastrointestinal tract, the presence (or absence) of food and the influence of, for example calcium and magnesium ions in buffers. Some drugs require an acidic environment to be absorbed so that if the pH of the stomach is increased – by antacids, buffers found in the formulation of some drugs, H_2 antagonists or proton pump inhibitors – absorption will be reduced. Food-drug interactions are difficult to predict because food can inhibit the absorption of some drugs and increase it in others.

Elimination

Elimination interactions involve drugs which are excreted via the kidney and occur either by inhibition of active tubular secretion of drug or by decreased elimination as a consequence of a decline in renal function. Since a number of potentially nephrotoxic drugs are used in the treatment of patients with viral diseases, monitoring of renal function is important.

Therapeutic Drug Monitoring [41], [42]

Despite the fact that therapeutic drug monitoring (TDM) is a relatively new scientific discipline, it is now established as the standard of care in the management of certain diseases as it has been demonstrated to impact positively on a variety of surrogate end-points [43]. TDM is based on the principle that drugs exhibit a positive concentration-effect relationship and aims specifically to maximise clinical efficacy while minimising drug related toxicity. The approach to the TDM of anti-infective agents differs to that of other therapeutic agents as it must embrace the complex triangular relationship between the host, drug and pathogen and not just the host-drug relationship in order to prevent the emergence of drug resistant isolates [44]. Such an approach is a synthesis of pharmacokinetics and pharmacodynamics and a number of PK-PD surrogate markers of clinical outcome have been defined for infectious disease therapeutics [45]. The TDM of antiviral agents is further complicated by the fact that meaningful PK data for some drugs (e.g. nucleoside analogues) would necessitate bedside cell separation for the determination of intracellular drug levels (note there is a poor correlation between the plasma concentration of parent drug and the intracellular concentration of the active triphosphate anabolite). This technique is costly, time consuming and demands considerable expertise which effectively precludes routine TDM of many antiviral agents. A notable exception to this is the protease inhibitor class of drugs that, as substrates for CYP3A4 and P-gp exhibit wide inter and intra-patient variability in plasma drug levels. There is increasing interest in the potential of TDM in the management of HIV disease as a number of recent studies have demonstrated that low PI plasma levels may be a contributing factor to virological failure in this patient population [46],[47]. Emerging concerns about the long-term toxicities of these drugs in addition to preliminary data that suggests a relationship between drug exposure and adverse effects supports the fact that TDM may be beneficial in this clinical setting [48]. Our current understanding of the PK-PD of PI therapy is incomplete. In the absence of such data, it is difficult at this time to determine the optimum timing of blood sampling for TDM or the appropriate interpretation of the resultant plasma levels. However, it is possible that in the near future, monitoring of PI levels in conjunction with viral phenotyping may allow us to individualise antiretroviral therapy in order to optimise the response to therapy in HIV infected patients.

Adverse Drug Reactions

An adverse drug reaction (ADR) may be defined as any undesirable effect of a drug beyond its anticipated therapeutic effects occurring during clinical use [49]. ADRs are common and account for a significant number of hospital admissions. A recent meta-analysis has suggested that ADRs are the fourth commonest cause of death in the USA [50]. There are 2 main types of ADRs, type A and type B. Type A reactions represent an augmentation of the pharmacological actions of the drug, are dose-dependent and will be reversible on drug withdrawal or dose reduction. In contrast, type B reactions (also known as idiosyncratic adverse reactions), are bizarre, and cannot be predicted from the pharmacology of the drug. Type A reactions are most frequently seen and account for over 80% of all ADRs.

There are many factors which predispose to ADRs but in the context of pharmacokinetics it is important to recognise the role of enzyme inhibition and enzyme induction in this regard. Both type A and B reactions may arise as a result of modulation of enzyme activity (particularly of P450 enzymes). For example co-administration of a drug with a narrow therapeutic index (e.g. astemizole or terfenadine) together with an enzyme inhibitor (such as ritonavir) can lead to adverse drug reactions which could be severe and sometime fatal.

In other situations it is possible that inhibition of detoxication enzymes could decrease the bioinactivation of a toxic metabolite and thereby increase the likelihood of an idiosyncratic reaction. With several of the antiretroviral drugs (e.g. abacavir and nevirapine) there are hypersensitivity reactions (rash) with mechanisms currently under investigation.

Enzyme induction increases the clearance of a drug and therefore should protect against dose-dependent toxicity. However, if the toxicity is due to an active metabolite, then enzyme induction will increase the risk of toxicity. Through knowledge of metabolic pathways and the properties of co-administered drugs it may be possible to anticipate and avoid type A ADRs. For type B ADRs this is clearly more difficult and indicates the importance of constant vigilance when prescribing.

Conclusion

Pharmacology may not be the most highly regarded subject in medical school but a sound grounding in the principles of pharmacokinetics and pharmacodynamics is absolutely vital if we are to understand the key issues relating to the efficacy and adverse effects of antiviral drugs.

Acknowledgements

The authors are grateful to Dr PE Klapper for helpful suggestions to this chapter.

References

1. Barry M, et al. Pharmacokinetics and potential interactions amongst antiretroviral agents used to treat patients with HIV infection. [Review] [101 refs]. Clinical Pharmacokinetics 1999; 36(4): 289-304.

2. Rowland M, Tozer T, eds. Clinical Pharmacokinetics: Concepts & Applications. 3rd ed. 1995, Williams & Wilkins: Philadelphia.

3. Fleisher D, et al. Drug, meal and formulation interactions influencing drug absorption after oral administration. Clinical implications. Clin Pharmacokinet 1999; 36(3): 233-54.

4. Welling PG. Effects of food on drug absorption. Annu Rev Nutr 1996; 16: 383-415.

5. Hall SD, et al. Molecular and physical mechanisms of first-pass extraction. Drug Metab Dispos 1999; 27(2): 161-6.

6. Sansom LN, Evans AM. What is the true clinical significance of plasma protein binding displacement interactions? Drug Saf 1995; 12(4): 227-33.

7. Bilello JA, Drusano GL. Relevance of plasma protein binding to antiviral activity and clinical efficacy of inhibitors of human immunodeficiency virus Protease. Journal of Infectious Diseases 1996; 173: 1524-1525.

8. Tanigawara Y. Role of P-glycoprotein in drug disposition [In Process Citation]. Ther Drug Monit 2000; 22(1): 137-40.

9. Huisman MT. Smit JW, Schinkel AH. Significance of P-glycoprotein for the pharmacology and clinical use of HIV protease inhibitors [editorial] [see comments]. Aids 2000; 14(3): 237-42.

10. Profit L, Eagling VA, Back DJ. Modulation of P-glycoprotein function in human lymphocytes and Caco-2 cell monolayers by HIV-1 protease inhibitors. Aids 1999; 13(13): 1623-7.

11. Washington CB, et al. Interaction of anti-HIV protease inhibitors with the multidrug transporter P-glycoprotein (P-gp) in human cultured cells. J Acquir Immune Defic Syndr Hum Retrovirol 1998; 19(3): 203-9.

12. Choo EF, et al. Pharmacological inhibition of P-glycoprotein transport enhances the distribution of HIV-1 protease inhibitors into brain and testes [In Process Citation]. Drug Metab Dispos 2000; 28(6): 655-60.

13. Snoeck R, Andrei G, De Clercq E. Current pharmacological approaches to the therapy of varicella zoster virus infections: a guide to treatment. Drugs 1999; 57(2): 187-206.

14. Sommadossi J-P. Nucleoside analogs: similarities and differences. Clinical Infectious Diseases 1993; 16 (suppl 1): S7-S15.

15. Moore KH, et al. The pharmacokinetics of lamivudine phosphorylation in peripheral blood mononuclear cells from patients infected with HIV-1. Aids 1999; 13(16): 2239-50.

16. Lori F, Lisziewicz J. Mechanisms of human immunodeficiency virus type 1 inhibition by hydroxyurea. J Biol Regul Homeost Agents 1999; 13(3): 176-80.

17. Heredia A, et al. Abacavir in combination with the inosine monophosphate dehydrogenase (IMPDH)-inhibitor mycophenolic acid is active against multidrug-resistant HIV-1 [letter] [published erratum appears in J Acquir Immune Defic Syndr 2000 Jan 1;23(1):105]. Journal of Acquired Immune Deficiency Syndromes 1999; 22(4): 406-7.

18. Back, D.J., Pharmacological issues relating to viral resistance. Infection 1999; 27(Suppl. 2): S42-S44.
19. Markowitz M. Resistance, fitness, adherence, and potency: mapping the paths to virologic failure [editorial; comment]. Jama 2000; 283(2): 250-1.
20. Zhang L, et al. Quantifying residual HIV-1 replication in patients receiving combination antiretroviral therapy [see comments]. N Engl J Med 1999; 340(21): 1605-13.
21. Kinirons MT. Variability in human drug reponses: Age as a source of variability, in Variability in Human Drug Response, GT Tucker, Editor. 1999; Excerpta Medica: Amsterdam. 109-120.
22. Tucker GT. Clinical aspects of polymorphic drug metabolism, in Variability in Human Drug Response, G.T. Tucker, Editor. 1999; Excerpta Medica: Amsterdam. 11-28.
23. Benitez J. Role of phenotyping and genotyping in the measurement of variability in human drug response, in Variability in Human Drug Response, G.T. Tucker, Editor. 1999; Excerpta Medica: Amsterdam. 231-238.
24. Wood AJJ. Ethinic differences in drug response: A model for understanding interindividual variability, in Variability in Human Drug Response, GT Tucker, Editor. 1999; Excerpta Medica: Amsterdam. 133-140.
25. Reidenberg M. Drugs and the liver. Symposium proceedings. 21-24 April 1998. Br J Clin Pharmacol 1998; 46(4): 351-9.
26. Glue P, et al. The single dose pharmacokinetics of ribavirin in subjects with chronic liver disease. Br J Clin Pharmacol 2000; 49(5): 417-21.
27. Rodighiero V. Effects of liver disease on pharmacokinetics. An update. Clin Pharmacokinet 1999; 37(5): 399-431.
28. Jayasekara D, et al. Antiviral therapy for HIV patients with renal insufficiency. J Acquir Immune Defic Syndr 1999; 21(5): 384-95.
29. von Bahr C, et al. Time course of enzyme induction in humans: effect of pentobarbital on nortriptyline metabolism. Clin Pharmacol Ther 1998; 64(1). 18-26.
30. Lin JH, Lu AY. Inhibition and induction of cytochrome P450 and the clinical implications. Clin Pharmacokinet 1998; 35(5): 361-90.
31. Burman WJ, Gallicano K, Peloquin C. Therapeutic implications of drug interactions in the treatment of human immunodeficiency virus-related tuberculosis. Clin Infect Dis 1999; 28(3): 419-29; quiz 430.
32. Flexner C. Drug Interactions: Better Living Through Pharmacology? 2000, Medscape.
33. Bertz RJ, Granneman GR. Use of in vitro and in vivo data to estimate the likelihood of metabolic pharmacokinetic interactions. Clin Pharmacokinet 1997; 32(3): 210-58.
34. Dresser GK, Spence JD, Bailey DG. Pharmacokinetic-pharmacodynamic consequences and clinical relevance of cytochrome P450 3A4 inhibition. Clin Pharmacokinet 2000; 38(1): 41-57.
35. Flexner C. Drug Interactions 1999, Medscape.
36. Hsu A, et al. Pharmacokinetic interaction between ritonavir and indinavir in healthy volunteers. Antimicrob Agents Chemother 1998; 42(11): 2784-91.
37. van Heeswijk RPG, et al. Once-daily dosing of saquinavir and low-dose ritonavir in HIV-1-infected individuals: a pharmacokinetic pilot study. Aids 2000; 14(9): F105-F110.
38. Merry C, et al. Saquinavir pharmacokinetics alone and in combination with ritonavir in HIV-infected patients. AIDS 1997; 11: F29-F33.
39. Kumar GN, et al. Potent inhibition of the cytochrome P-450 3A-mediated human liver microsomal metabolism of a novel HIV protease inhibitor by ritonavir: A positive drug-drug interaction. Drug Metab Dispos 1999; 27(8): 902-8.
40. Piscitelli SC, et al. Indinavir concentrations and St John's wort [letter]. Lancet 2000; 355(9203): 547-8.

41. Back DJ, et al. Therapeutic drug monitoring of antiretrovirals in human immunodeficiency virus infection [In Process Citation]. Ther Drug Monit 2000; 22(1): 122-6.

42. Back DJ, et al. Therapeutic Drug Monitoring of Antiretrovirals: Ready for the Clinic? Journal of the International Association of Physicians in AIDS Care 2000; 6(2): 34-37.

43. Ensom MH, et al. Clinical pharmacokinetics in the 21st century. Does the evidence support definitive outcomes? Clin Pharmacokinet 1998; 34(4): 265-79.

44. Li RC, Zhu M, Schentag JJ. Achieving an optimal outcome in the treatment of infections. The role of clinical pharmacokinetics and pharmacodynamics of antimicrobials. Clin Pharmacokinet 1999; 37(1): 1-16.

45. Hyatt JM, et al. The importance of pharmacokinetic/pharmacodynamic surrogate markers to outcome. Focus on antibacterial agents. Clin Pharmacokinet 1995; 28(2): 143-60.

46. Descamps D, et al., Mechanisms of virologic failure in previously untreated HIV-infected patients from a trial of induction-maintenance therapy. Trilege (Agence Nationale de Recherches sur le SIDA 072) Study Team) [see comments]. Jama 2000; 283(2): 205-11.

47. Havlir DV, et al. Drug susceptibility in HIV infection after viral rebound in patients receiving indinavir-containing regimens [see comments]. Jama 2000; 283(2): 229-34.

48. Gatti G, et al. The relationship between ritonavir plasma levels and side-effects: implications for therapeutic drug monitoring. Aids 1999; 13(15): 2083-9.

49. Pirmohamed M, et al. Adverse drug reactions. Bmj 1998; 316(7140): 1295-8.

50. Lazarou J, Pomeranz BH, Corey PN. Incidence of adverse drug reactions in hospitalized patients: a meta-analysis of prospective studies [see comments]. Jama 1998; 279(15): 1200-5.

CHAPTER 3

MOLECULAR DIAGNOSTICS

STEVEN THIJSEN and ROB SCHUURMAN

Table of Contents

Practical Guidelines in Antiviral Therapy Ed. by Charles A.B. Boucher and George J. Galasso. 37 — 63
© 2002 *Elsevier Science. Printed in the Netherlands.*

General Introduction

Molecular diagnostics assays are based on the detection of specific nucleic acid sequences in biological material. These type of assays are of increasing importance in the diagnosis, monitoring and characterization of infectious agents. This chapter aims to shortly review the processes involved in molecular diagnostics and summarizes most of the technical options available (Figure 1). Since these methods are generally based on the use of amplification technologies and their intrinsic high sensitivity, it is inevitable that laboratories should be well educated and trained in performing these types of laboratory measures. Moreover, special attention should be taken to the physical setup and organization of the laboratories, with regards to prevention of sample contamination. This should include the use of at least three different separated areas for sample preparation (I), amplification (II) and post-amplification analysis (III). Personnel should plan their activities such that they work from area I to III and do not go back to one of the previous areas on the same day. This asks for extreme laboratory discipline, but is an essential prerequisite for the successful implementation and routine use of molecular diagnostics.

Molecular assays are relatively new in the diagnostic microbiological laboratory. The assays have a rapid turnover and new improvements are being developed continuously. The assays in general involve a high number of laboratory manipulations, which, at present, are mainly manual. This may result in a relatively high chance of significant inter and intra-laboratory variation, also given the fact that assay standardization in many cases has not yet been achieved. Therefore, adequate, regular and extensive quality assurance and control are essential.

This chapter will now review the different aspects and options and applications of molecular diagnostics, with special attention to its practical application.

Qualitative and Quantitative Molecular Diagnostics

Qualitative Molecular Diagnostics

Molecular diagnostic assays can be applied for either the (qualitative) detection of pathogens or for determination of the amount of pathogen present (quantitative). Qualitative assays are generally developed with the aim to achieve ultimate sensitivity. However, given their diagnostic application, there should also be strong emphasis on specificity. Therefore most diagnostic approaches consist of an amplification reaction using target specific oligonucleotides, followed by a specificity control step. This specificity control may either consist of a hybridization step, using a target specific nucleic acid probe, or consist of a second round of amplification using a second (nested) set of amplification primers, as described later in this chapter.

In general, these specificity control steps are primarily aimed to confirm specific detection of the target nucleic acid, but may also help to further improve the sensitivity of the applied assay. With the introduction of real-time PCR (described in one of the next paragraphs), specificity control subsequent to a first round of amplification

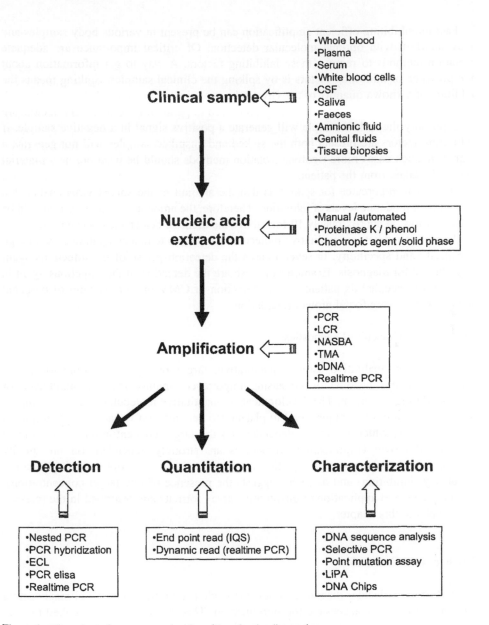

Figure 1. Flow chart of processes and options for molecular diagnostics.

is no longer necessary. Amplification and detection are performed and determined in real-time, i.e. during the amplification reaction, omitting the need for any post-PCR sample manipulations. This approach is an important new development that helps to improve the quality of the results generated in a diagnostic laboratory.

Factors inhibiting efficient amplification can be present in various body samples and may interfere with optimal molecular detection. Of critical importance are adequate isolation methods to remove these inhibiting factors. A way to get information about the presence of inhibiting factors is by spiking the clinical samples. Spiking means the addition of a known quantity of the virus to be investigated to a part of the sample. Both spiked and unspiked samples should be processed in parallel. If no inhibiting factors are present, only the spiked sample will generate a positive signal in a negative sample. If inhibiting factors are present both the spiked and unspiked samples will not generate a signal. In such cases more rigorous isolation methods should be used ore new material should be taken from the patient.

Of critical importance for spiking is that the amount of the spiked virus enables the detection of moderate levels of inhibition. Therefore, the amount of spiked virus should be relatively low, at approximately 10-fold above the minimal detectable concentration.

As mentioned before, qualitative molecular assays aim to detect a pathogen with high sensitivity and specificity. In several cases the detection per se of the infectious agent is sufficient for diagnosis. Examples of these are the detection of the infectious agent in the CSF of encephalitis patients or the detection of CMV in amnion fluid of pregnant women with severe foetal growth retardation.

Quantitative Molecular Diagnostics

In addition to qualitative assays, quantitative, target or signal amplification based molecular assays become of increasing importance, mainly for the monitoring of patients during treatment. The development of quantitative molecular assays is complex since amplification techniques tend to plateau (to become non-linear) at high amplicon concentrations, which in turn is dependent on the target concentration in the clinical sample. Moreover amplification efficiencies are strongly dependent on the quality of the sample. Poor sample quality may result in a less optimal amplification efficiency (inhibition) and as such, suggests the presence of low target concentrations. Development and application of quantitative assay formats are described in the relevant paragraphs of this chapter.

Nucleic Acid Extraction

To perform a molecular diagnostic assay, the nucleic acid present in the clinical sample should first be made accessible for amplification. This is achieved by so called nucleic acid extraction methods. In general these methods results in lysis of membrane structures (cell membranes, virus envelopes and core structures, nucleus membranes, etc) present in biological materials (cells, viruses or bacteria) and subsequent purification of the nucleic acid material. In this extraction and purification process, any components that may prevent or inhibit efficient amplification of the nucleic acid present should be efficiently removed. Such components include nucleases (RNAse and DNAse) that may degrade the RNA and or DNA present, biological components that inhibit the amplification reaction (e.g. haem) or inhibitory anti-coagulants such as heparin.

Several commercial and non-commercial methods for nucleic acid extraction are now available. Originally these methods were based on the use of proteinase-K to destruct the proteins present in the sample, followed by phenol-chloroform extraction to separate the proteins from the nucleic acid. Most of the currently used assays are based on sample lysis using a high molar chaotropic agent, e.g. guanidinium-thiocyanate, and subsequent binding of the nucleic acid to a solid phase [1]. Upon extensive washing of the captured nucleic acid, to remove proteins and cell debris, the nucleic acid can be eluted from the solid phase using a low salt buffer or water, after which the nucleic acids are ready to be amplified. At present most of these methods are manual and laborious and as such contribute a significant amount of hands-on time to the diagnostic assay. Currently, several attempts are made to try and automate the extraction process, in particular for nucleic acid isolation from the most commonly used biological materials, like plasma, White Blood Cells (WBCs) and CSF. The major complicating factors for automation of nucleic acid extraction has long been the absence of generic methods for nucleic acid isolation from different biological materials, as well as the risk for sample cross-contamination.

Although automated extraction devices currently consist of first generation equipment, they start being implemented in routine practice of molecular diagnostic laboratories, as is the case in blood banking laboratories performing nucleic acid testing on blood donations. Evaluation studies have demonstrated that the equipment may speed up and improve the quality of molecular diagnostic results [2, 3].

Assay Approaches

PCR

The polymerase chain reaction (PCR) was the first *in vitro* amplification system making the detection of nucleic acids feasible for clinical practice [4]. The principle of PCR is based on repeated cycles of DNA synthesis (*in vitro* replication) for both complementary strands of a specific nucleic acid sequence (target sequence, Figure 2). The amount of synthesized DNA is doubled with every cycle and, as such, results in an exponential amplification of the target sequence. The first step of the process is the annealing of oligonucleotide primers to each of both target DNA strands. These oligonucleotides are chemically synthesised, 20-30 nucleotides long and complementary to the DNA template strand. After annealing to the DNA template, the primer is elongated using a DNA dependent DNA polymerase, generating double stranded DNA, Finally, the double stranded DNA molecule is heat-denatured thereby generating 2 single stranded DNA molecules, each of which can be used as target in the next round of amplification. Typically primer annealing is performed between 40°C and 65°C; template denaturation at 94°C and strand elongation (DNA synthesis) at 72°C. This whole cyclic process can be performed in a closed reaction vessel, using dedicated amplification devices and a thermostable DNA-polymerase (e.g. Taq-polymerase, derived from *Thermus aquaticus*). The identification of these thermostable enzymes and equipment has been essential for the further development of PCR as a diagnostic tool.

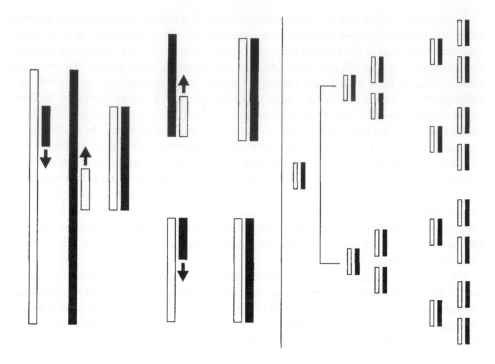

Figure 2.   Polymerase chain reaction. The left side of the figure represents the first part of the PCR. Starting from a (denatured) single-strand target DNA molecule, sequence-specific oligonucleotides (primers) anneal to the target DNA strands and initiate second strand DNA synthesis by the Taq-polymerase. After denaturation of the newly synthesized double-stranded DNA molecules, additional primers, directed towards another, anneal to both strands and upon elongation result in the production of double stranded target DNA molecules, harboring both primer sequences, one at each end of the molecule. The right side of the figure demonstrates the doubling of these target DNA molecules with each cycle of the PCR, resulting in logarithmic amplification.

Theoretically, under ideal circumstances, the template DNA is amplified by a factor two during each cycle. This leads to a 2^{25} fold (33, 554, 432) amplification in a standard PCR of 25 cycles and an almost billion-fold amplification after 35 cycles (2^{35}). Initial specificity is provided by the requirement for two specific hybridization reactions, for the forward and reverse primers, to generate a PCR product. The sensitivity and specificity can be further enhanced by performing an additional PCR on an aliquot of the amplified material obtained in the first round PCR. In this second round of amplification primers are used which are located nested within the first round primers. As such, the amplification product of this so-called nested-PCR is the result of 4 specific oligonucleotide hybridizations.

Successful amplification reactions are strongly dependent on the use of perfectly matching primers. Any nucleotide variation between a primer and the target sequence will reduce or even prevent efficient amplification of the target. Therefore, in the development of a (diagnostic) PCR reaction careful selection of the amplification primers is extremely important. In particular for some viruses, natural variation in the target sequences for amplification may be extensive and can cause a major hurdle in the development of new PCR assays.

Using PCR one can detect single target copies in a given sample. This high sensitivity also is a drawback of PCR technology, since the risk of contamination of the PCR mixture with previously amplified DNA and a subsequent false positive result is paramount. In order to prevent such events, strict measurements should be taken, such as working in different rooms for DNA preparation and PCR [5].

In addition to the logistical measures, the risk of sample cross-contamination can further be reduced by daily laboratory and equipment cleaning using bleach and by using Uracil-N-glycosylase (UNG) in combination with incorporation of dUTP in the amplification reaction. As such, dUTP, not being a natural component of DNA, will only be present in the amplified DNA and not in the original target DNA. Upon incubation with UNG, any Uracil containing (amplified) DNA will be destroyed and as such can not be amplified in subsequent amplification reactions. Thymidine containing DNA in the clinical samples will not be affected by UNG.

In addition to amplification of a DNA target sequence, RNA can be used for amplification, but only after an initial reverse-transcription step, generating a single stranded copy-DNA (cDNA) of the RNA target.

Qualitative and quantitative assay formats have been developed for an infinite number of target sequences. Quantitative PCR is widely used for the monitoring of plasma viral load in HIV-1, HCV or HBV infected individuals.

The development of quantitative molecular assays is complex since amplification techniques tend to plateau (to become non-lineair) at high amplicon concentrations, which in turn are dependent on the target concentration present in the clinical sample. Moreover amplification efficiencies are strongly dependent on the quality of the sample. Poor sample quality may result in a less optimal amplification efficiency (inhibition) and as such, suggests the presence of low target concentrations. These limitations can be overcome by inclusion of an internal quantitation standard (IQS) in the amplification reaction. The IQS is subsequentely co-amplified with the target nucleic acid. The concentration of the IQS, which is added at a low copy number, is exactly known and its amplification efficiency should be identical to that for the nucleic acid target in the clinical sample [17]. In general these IQS molecules harbor the same primer-binding sites as used for the target organism, but the sequence in between these sites are generally re-shuffled. Subsequent to amplification, the relative amounts of amplified IQS and that of the target organism can be measured separately by using specific probes for both sequences. Given that the IQS copy number added to the amplification reaction was known, one could now, based on the IQS/sample amplification ratio, calculate the absolute concentration of target DNA in the sample. In general the linear range of such assays are limited to approximately 3 to 5 orders of magnitude and have a detection limit at around 50-400 genome copies/ml plasma.

Recent developments in real-time PCR have demonstrated that the linear range of such assays is much broader and may cover 6-8 orders of magnitude [18]. In these assays, quantitation is based on the direct relation between the amount of amplification product and the amount of probe hybridization. In general, assays are run without an IQS. Quantitation is achieved using an external calibration curve. However, as a consequence of the absence of an IQS, there is no (internal) control for amplification inhibition, which may be a major drawback when using these techniques for clinical purposes. External spiking of the samples with a low amount of target DNA may only be helpful in case of significant inhibition of amplification in a sample; moderate levels of inhibition will hardly be detected but may affect the level of sensitivity achieved in a sample.

LCR

Ligase chain reaction (LCR) is an amplification technique that has no need for polymerase enzymes. It is based on the annealing of two oligonucleotide probes immediately adjacent to each other on a target DNA molecule [6]. Subsequently, a DNA ligase enzyme covalently joins the two probes and thus synthesizes a second strand. The last step in this cyclic process is the denaturation of the double strand DNA molecule. The newly synthesized strand consisting of two ligated oligonucleotide probes is now itself a target for annealing of two complementary immediately adjoining oligonucleotide probes and again the ligase ensures the covalent linkage between these two molecules (Figure 3). Doubling of the target molecule is achieved with each round of amplification. Like PCR, the use of thermostable ligase enzymes enables to add these enzymes once, at the start of the LCR reaction. LCR amplification can be performed on DNA, as well as on RNA after reverse-transcription.

As with PCR, contamination is a great problem in daily practice of LCR, making strict protective measures to avoid LCR products carryover an essential part of the entire assay set-up.

A diagnostic assay for the detection of Chlamydia trachomatis currently is the most widely applied LCR assay.

NASBA

Nucleic Acid Sequence Based Amplification (NASBA) and Transcrpition Mediated Amplification (TMA) are additional examples of template amplification procedures, but, in contrast to PCR and LCR, do not require thermal cycling and generally start from an RNA template [7]. The technology makes use of an ingeniously isothermal amplification biochemistry (Figure 4), performed at 41°C, with 3 different enzymes and a set of 2 oligonucleotide primers. In the first step of the reaction a reverse transcriptase converts the single stranded RNA molecules into cDNA. The RNAse H enzyme subsequently digests the RNA from the RNA-DNA hybrid and thereafter the reverse transcriptase also synthesizes the second strand DNA. Since one of the oligonucleotide primers used is extended with the promoter sequence of T7 RNA polymerase, this enzyme, also present in the mixture of the NASBA reaction, now starts generating multiple RNA copies, using the double stranded DNA molecule as a template. All these newly synthesized RNA molecules can now be processed in a continuous cyclic amplification starting with the synthesis of cDNA by the reverse transcriptase.

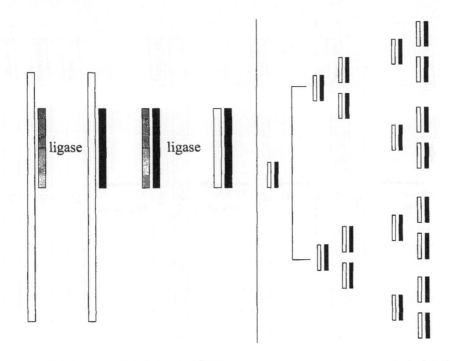

Figure 3. Ligase chain reaction. The left side of the figure represents the first part of the LCR. Two synthetic target specific oligonucleotides anneal adjacent to one another on the target DNA. Ligase present in the reaction mixture will covalently link both probes, thereby generating a double stranded DNA molecule. After denaturation both strands are target for annealing of two adjacent complementary oligonucleotide probes. After ligation, two double stranded DNA molecules are formed. The right side of the figure demonstrates the doubling of target DNA with each cycle of the LCR, resulting in logarithmic amplification.

Since amplification is not dependant on thermal cycling, costly thermocyclers are not needed. The sensitivity of NASBA or TMA is comparable to PCR, but cannot be performed on double stranded DNA templates. Amplification products mainly consist of RNA. Given the sensitivity of RNA for RNAse degradation, the use of the amplification products in further characterizations asks for specific measures preventing RNA degradation.

Qualitative and quantitative formats of these assays have been described and applied in the detection and monitoring of infectious agents such as HIV-1, HCV and CMV.

Branched DNA

Branched DNA technology (bDNA) is based on signal amplification, whereas PCR, LCR and NASBA all are template amplification technologies [8] (Figure 5). Signal amplification is achieved by a complex hybridization scheme. First, the target sequences are captured onto a solid phase, by using an array of specific probes complementary

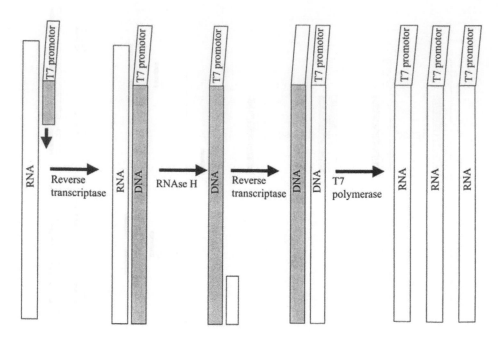

Figure 4. Nucleic acid sequence based amplification (NASBA, essentially similar for TMA). Upon annealing of a target-specific oligonucleotide extended with a T7-promotor sequence, the first enzymatic step in the NASBA reaction consists of reverse transcription of the template RNA by reverse transcriptase. The resulting RNA-DNA hybrid molecule subsequently is a target for RNAse H, which digests the RNA part of the hybrid. After annealing of a reverse oligonucleotide, the DNA polymerase activity of the reverse transcriptase will generate double stranded DNA molecule containing a T7-promotor sequence. Finally, T7-RNA-polymerase will transcribe multiple RNA copies from the target nucleic acid. All these RNA transcripts can subsequently be a target in the next round of amplification by the combined action of reverse transcriptase, RNAse H and T7 polymerase, thereby providing unprecedented sensitivity.

to several parts of the (viral) sequences to be detected. Subsequently, a set of target specific DNA probes, each containing a number of branches with all identical sequences is hybridized to the captured target. Thereafter, alkaline phosphatase labelled probes complementary to the sequences of the DNA branches are hybridized and the amount of hybridization is subsequently quantitatively detected enzymatically.

A big advantage of this technique is that target DNA is not amplified so that contamination risk is reduced, compared to PCR. Additionally, due to the usage of multiple capture and extender probes, this technology is less sensitive to sequence variation in the target genes.

The method has been developed and applied for several infectious agents like HIV-1, HCV and HBV and can be used quantitatively to determine patient plasma viral load, in some instances down to 50 genome copies/ml

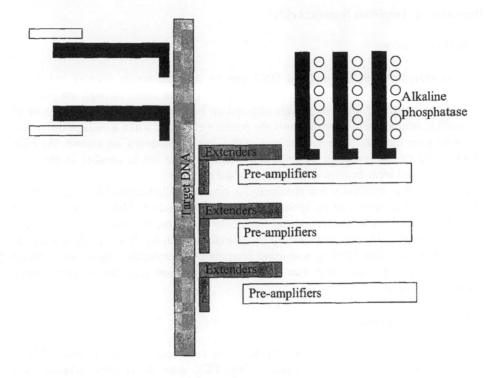

Figure 5. Branched DNA. Target DNA is captured by synthetic capture oligonucleotide probes which are bound to sequences bound to a solid carrier. Multiple probe extenders sandwich the target DNA. Extender probes harbor extender sequences, which can bind pre-amplifier probes, which can bind multiple copies of branched DNA molecules. Branched DNA molecules are labeled with alkaline phosphatase. This enzyme can process substrates into a reaction product that can be easily detected.

Non-amplification Based Methods

With the availability of nucleic acid amplification technologies, the use of non-amplification based systems for the detection and quantitation of viral targets has greatly reduced. These systems are/were based on the use of nucleic acid hybridizations techniques and subsequent detection. The absence of an amplification step results in a significant reduction in sensitivity as compared to amplification based assays. In general hybridization assays have a lower limit of detection around 10.000 to 100.000 genome equivalents and as such can only be applied for viral infection expressing high viral loads, e.g. HBV or HCV, and in some cases for CMV. A detection limit like this makes these assays less applicable for sensitive monitoring of viral infections during highly suppressive antiviral therapy.

Detection of Amplified Nucleic Acids

PCR Hybridization

For the analysis of PCR, amplified DNA can be detected on an agarose gel. DNA can be separated on size, since small DNA products move faster through the pores of the agarose matrix. DNA is negatively charged on basis of the phosphate backbone of the nucleic acid and will move towards the positive electrode when a voltage difference is placed over the gel. Since in most cases DNA target sequences are known, the PCR product size can be predicted. A molecular weight marker run in parallel on the same gel allows rapid identification of the PCR product on size.

For additional sensitivity and specificity, a labeleled oligonucleotide probe specific for the amplified target can be hybridized to the PCR product. Therefore the DNA in the gel first needs to be transferred and fixed onto a membrane (Southern blotting) [9]. The transferred DNA can subsequently be hybridized with the labeled oligonucleotide probe. In general this labeling nowadays consists of a molecule (digoxigenin, biotin or alkaline phosphatase) that can be detected enzymatically, for instance using chemiluminescence.

Enhanced Chemiluminescence

Enhanced chemiluminescence is a very sensitive technique, which has been able to replace radioactive detection techniques [10]. ECL uses digoxigenin labeled PCR products, which can be detected using anti-digoxigenin coupled to peroxidase enzyme.

In the presence of peroxide, the peroxidase oxidises the substrate luminol, thereby creating a temporary excitation of this molecule. In the presence of enhancers the emitted light from luminol can be detected using a luminescence detector or an X-ray film. ECL detection can be applied in combination with hybridization reactions performed in solution, thereby omitting the need for laborious techniques such as southern blotting and hybridization.

PCR Elisa

In general, agarose gel electrophoresis of PCR products and subsequent hybridization is laborious and harbour the risk of spreading amplicons (contamination). Instead of immobilizing the amplicons on a membrane it is also possible to immobilize the hybridization probe to a solid carrier. This approach has led to the development of Microchip-arrays where oligonucleotide probes are bound onto a silicon carrier [11]. At present a more general approach is the use of coated microwell plates that capture the, for instance biotin-labeled PCR product by using microtiter wells coated with avidin [12] and performing a so called PCR-Elisa. The captured DNA can subsequently be detected using enzyme labeled oligonucleotide probes. Many variations on this theme have been developed using for example Digoxigenin labelled probes or by coating the bottom of microtiter wells with capture oligonucleotide probes.

New Developments for Diagnosis and Monitoring

Real Time PCR

All of the aforementioned detection methods are based on the detection of the amplification products subsequent to amplification reaction (end-point detection). The recent development of new methods enable the detection of amplification products during the amplification reaction (real-time amplification). These developments have further revolutionarized the application of amplification technology. Several techniques have now been developed to monitor amplicon production during the proceeding of the PCR, thereby omitting the need for post-PCR amplicon manipulations (eg gel electrophore). A further important advantage is that the process of amplification can be monitored dynamically, with a direct relationship between the amount of amplification signal and the amount of input nucleic acid in the sample. As such, quantification of the PCR can be achieved without the need for laborious competitor DNA techniques (Figure 6).

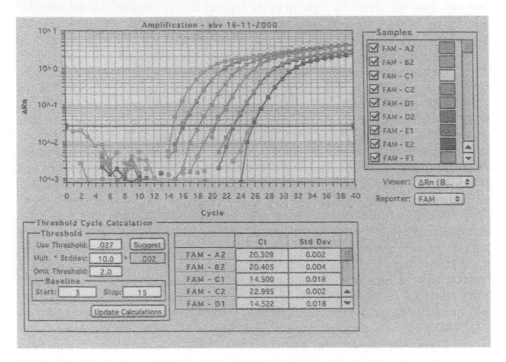

Figure 6. Results of real-time PCR assay. Graphical read-out of real-time PCR results, using a dilution series of input DNA. Horizontal axis: number of PCR cycles performed, vertical axis: relative fluorescence intensity (dR). Ct: cycle at which the dR reaches the threshold for amplification. Ct values decline with increased amounts of input DNA.

Available real-time techniques make use of the detection of fluorochromes present in the reaction mixture. These fluorochromes can be target specific or target non specific.

An example of a target non-specific dye is SYBR-green [13]. This fluorochrome will only emit light after it is bound to double stranded DNA, comparable with the use of Ethidium bromide as an intercalating dye in agarose gel electrophoreses. The amount of fluorescence for SYBR-green is directly related to the amount of double stranded DNA present. During the PCR, fluorescence activity is measured in real-time at each cycle. The drawback of this system is that there is no specificity control in the reaction; any double stranded DNA molecule will bind SYBR-green and emit fluorescnce. Thus, aspecific amplification and/or primer dimer formation cannot be distinguished from the formation of specific products. Thus, spatially control will be necessary in some cases.

Several approaches have been developed to monitor real time PCR using sequence specific probes. The so called Taqman system uses an oligonucleotide probe located in between the amplification primers and is labeled with two different fluorochromes; a quencher and a reporter dye (Figure 7) [14]. When present on the same oligonucleotide, these fluorescent dyes are in close proximity of one another, leading to energy exchange between these two dyes: the light from the reporter dye is absorbed by the quencher dye and no fluorescence is emitted. During PCR, the labeled probe will hybridise to the target DNA. The Taq polymerase, engaged in elongating the amplification primer and synthesizing the second strand DNA, will encounter the hybridised probe. Due to the 5'→ 3'-nuclease activity of the Taq polymerase the hybridized probe will be degraded into separate nucleotides thereby separating the quencher dye from the reporter due, and enabling the reporter dye to emit a fluorescent signal. For each synthesized DNA strand the emission of one reporter dye molecule can be detected using a fluorimeter. As such, the amount of amplified DNA is directly related to the amount of fluorescence.

The assays are performed in a 96 well format with optical caps enabling transmission of UV excitation light and the transmission of the emitted light of the reporter dye. Fluorescence is automatically measured and collected for every well during each cycle. One assay run takes approximately 2 hours.

A different approach has been adopted in the LightCycler, another type equipment for real-time PCR. In this format two internal oligonucleotide probes hybridize onto the target DNA [15]. Probes are labeled with the fluorochromes FITC or Red-640 and after hybridization these dyes are in close proximity of one another. Upon excitation by UV light the FITC dye emits light, which can excite the Red-640 dye, which subsequently emits light of a certain wavelength and can be measured using a fluorometer. During polymerisation the probes are displaced from the DNA by the polymerase. Again, the fluorescence intensity is a direct measure of the amount of target DNA formed.

The LightCycler format uses glass capillaries, with a maximum of 32 capillaries per run. Samples inside the capillaries are heated using air, enabling very rapid cycling. A PCR of 30-40 cycles takes less than 30 minutes to be completed. The glass capillaries allow for UV excitation of the fluorochromes and the detection of the emission wavelengths.

Yet another approach for detection of amplification products during real-time PCR is using molecular beacons [16]. These are oligonucleotide probes which can fold back and form a hairpin structure due to complementary sequences at the ends of the probes. These ends are labeled with fluorochrome dyes, which quench one another.

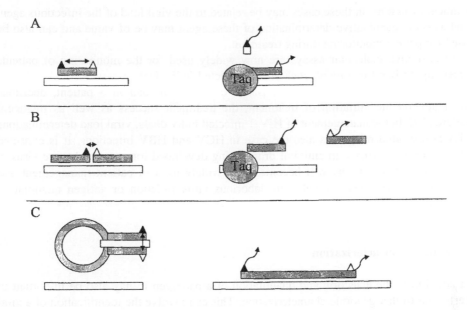

Figure 7. Real-time PCR. Three formats of realtime detection of amplification are depicted. Part A depicts the Taqman system. The nuclease activity of the Taq polymerase digests the probe and fluorescence activity is no longer quenched. Part B depicts the Lightcycler format. The two hybridized probes labeled with fluorescent dyes are quenched. Only after displacement by the Taq enzyme fluorescence can be detected. Part C depicts the format using molecular beacons. Upon hybridization quenching of the fluorochromes is abolished and fluorescence activity can be detected. ▲: quencher dye; Δ: reporter dye

After hybridization to the target, the quencher and reporter dyes become relatively distant and are to wide apart for quenching to be effective. As such, the fluorescence intensity can be measured as a direct measure for the amount of DNA present.

Clinical Applications of Molecular Diagnostic Assays

Qualitative molecular assays are used in the detection and diagnosis of (primary) infections, like those causing the CSF and causing neurological symptoms, e.g. HSV, CMV, JC- virus, enteroviruses or Toxoplasma gondii. The detection of these pathogens per se is sufficient proof to identify the causative agent with high probability. Similar approaches can be followed in the identification of the infectious agents causing respiratory infections. In general, also in these infections qualitative detection of the infectious agent is sufficient for diagnosis. A more complex situation exists in the diagnosis and monitoring of infections upon solid organ of bone marrow transplantation. In particular for CMV (and EBV), the detection of these agents per se may not be sufficient, since antiviral treatment options for the infection are available but rather toxic.

Clinical symptoms in these cases may be related to the viral load of the infectious agent and as such, quantitative determination of these agent may be of value and can also be used for patient monitoring during treatment.

Quantitative molecular assays are now widely used for the monitoring of patients receiving antiviral treatment, such HIV-1 infected individuals receiving Highly Active Anti-Retroviral Therapy (HAART). Based on the viral load in a patient, decisions are made on the initiation of treatment, the treatment success as well as treatment failure [19]. In the management of HIV-1 infected individuals, viral load determinations play an essential role, as is also the case in HCV and HBV infections. It is expected that, given the increase in antiviral drugs being developed for more and more viruses, viral load determinations will become more widely used in patient management and will replace less sensitive and more laborious virus isolation or antigen quantitation techniques.

Molecular Characterization

In addition to the detection and quantitation of a pathogen it may also be important to perform a further genomic characterization. This can involve the identification of a viral subtype, as for example in case of HCV infections. Different HCV subtypes circulate in different part of the world and clinical studies suggest antiviral treatment for some of these subtypes to be less successful than for other subtypes. Also for HIV different subtypes have been identified based on variation in several parts of the genome. Based on this, a subtype classification has been generated. In addition to HIV-1 sub-typing, genetic characterization of this virus plays an essential role upon in HIV-1 treatment. The presence or absence of so called drug-resistance mutations plays a critical role in clinical decisions with respect to subsequent treatment regimes. In addition to these examples genetic characterization of pathogens becomes of increasing importance for individual patient management but also for epidemiological purposes.

Several methods have been developed for genetic characterization of pathogens, some more generic than others. We will now review some of most frequently used approaches. Which methodology to choose is strongly dependent on the question to be answered.

DNA Sequencing

DNA sequencing, in most cases using automated sequencing devices, is widely applied for the genetic characterization of genes and organisms. A number of hardware technologies based on fluorescent detection of chain-terminated sequencing products upon electrophoresis, is currently available (e.g. Applied Biosystems Visible genetics, Pharmacia Upjohn and others). Instrument specific chemistry is applied for the labeling of the nucleic acid sequences to be analyzed. Labeling of the sequencing products can either be performed using fluororescently labeled sequencing primers or by incorporating labeled (di)deoxynucleotides into the growing DNA strand during the actual sequencing reaction.

One innovative technology, developed by Affymetrix Inc., that is currently under evaluation involves the differential hybridization of nucleic acid sequences with short oligonucleotide probes present on micro-chips [20, 21]. Each microchip has the capacity to contain several thousands of different oligonucleotide probes (arrays) and as such these arrays can be used to scan the target sequence for variation at the level of single nucleotides. A first generation of this technology has been developed and evaluated for the detection of HIV-1 drug resistance mutations, however this technology can, in principal, be applied to any nucleic acid target.

Sequencing is especially appropriate for the simultaneous identification of new resistance mutations and their interactions with other mutations. Population sequencing approaches enable the genotypic analysis of the entire viral population (quasispecies) circulating in a patient, whereas analysis of (individual) cloned genes generates detailed insight in the interaction of mutations present on the same genome.

The high mutation rate of some viruses, like HIV, results in dynamic changes in the composition of the viral population (quasi-species). Therefore, heterogeneities (sequence mixtures) are common among the viral genome of HIV. In general the sensitivity of sequencing in the detection of minority virus populations is highly variable [30]. It is generally assumed that the lower limit for detection of minority populations in a mixture is about 25% and dependent on the applied technology. Confirmation of the heterogeneity by analysis of both strands is still inevitable. Dye labeled sequencing primers used to give better estimates than dye-terminator chemistry due to more equal fluorescence signals for each of the nucleotides. Recent developments on sequencing enzymes (e.g. the development of Amplitaq-FS) and alternative fluorescent labels (e.g. Big-Dye terminators) have demonstrated to improve reproducibility in the detection of sequence heterogeneities using dye terminator chemistry.

DNA sequencing used to be performed by research laboratories, but now is increasingly being applied in diagnostic laboratories, since in some cases DNA typing may have clinical benefit [22, 23, 24]. Diagnostic application asks for simple and highly standardized technologies with a well-controlled sensitivity and specificity. Attempts have been made by Visible Genetics and Applied Biosystems, to develop complete sequencing kits, at present dedicated for the detection of drug-resistance mutations in HIV-1. In addition to the sequencing kit, containing amplification and sequencing primers, assay reagents and reaction controls, specific software has been developed to assist in data analysis (Figure 8). These improvements are essential for the diagnostic implementation of these complex technologies.

Alternative Genotyping Strategies

Instead of full sequence analysis, alternative genotyping strategies can be applied for the identification of specific, 'known', mutations. Alternative genotypic analysis offers an advantage over sequence analysis because, despite an accurate detailed characterization of the viral genome, sequence analysis also provides a significant quantity of possibly irrelevant information, especially when trying to apply the method diagnostically. Several alternatives to full sequence analysis are currently available and will be reviewed in the next paragraphs. Most of these methods have been developed in the

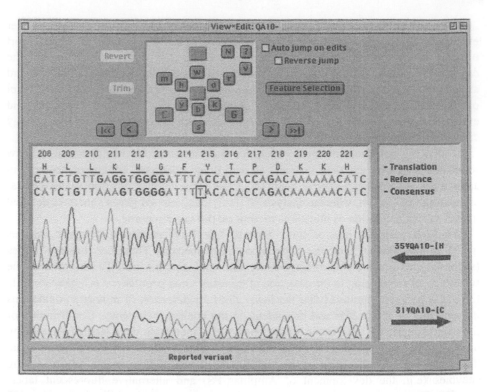

Figure 8. DNA Sequence analysis. Example of automated DNA sequence analysis for the identification of mutations. Upper and lower electropherograms demonstrate the nucleotide sequence pattern for the upper and lower DNA strands of the clinical sample. These electropherograms result in a consensus nucleotide sequence for the clinical sample (as indicate on the right hand site in the middle of the figure), which is subsequently compared to a reference sequence to identify mutations. Amino acid codes and numbers are indicated above the reference sequences.

area of HIV-1 drug-resistance, but can be applied for any given target with known specific sequence heterogeneities.

Selective PCR Assay

One of the earliest alternative approaches for the detection of drug resistance mutations is the so-called selective PCR assay [25]. This assay, which is still applied [26, 27, 28, 29] is based on a nested PCR approach in which the second (nested) amplification is performed using a pair of oligonucleotide which specifically amplifies either the wild type or the mutant allele. Specificity is achieved by the extreme 3'-nucleotide of the selective primer, being complementary to either the wild type or the drug resistant genotype. The result is qualitative and indicates the presence of wild type genotype, mutant genotype or a mixture of both, though at undefined relative quantity. The method is highly sensitive for the detection of minority populations, in some instances being capable to detect minority species present at a frequency of less than 1 in a 1000 to 10000. This makes the method useful for screening of (drug-naive) patients for the presence of minority quantities of pre-existing drug resistant viral quasispecies [31]. However, extensive optimization of the reaction conditions is frequently needed in adapting the assay to a new resistance mutation. Moreover, the analysis is restricted to one nucleotide position per test.

Point Mutation Assay

Another alternative method for the determination of individual drug resistance mutations, is the so called point mutation assay (PMA) [32]. The assay is based on single nucleotide primer extension, performed with DNA bound to a solid phase. In primer extension reactions either 35S- labeled or a fluorescently labeled (di-)deoxynucleotide is incorporated upon elongation of a template bound oligonucleotide primer with its 3' end one nucleotide in front of the resistance mutation of interest. Semi-quantitative information (i.e. the proportion of wild type and mutant phenotype) is obtained by measuring the amount of incorporated label (either a radioactive or fluorescent) in the primer extension reactions for the wild type and mutant genotypes. Using this technology, the dynamics of viral turnover have been extensively studied (Figure 9) [33, 34, 35] and it enables studying the dynamics of viral turnover, by coupling the relative amount of mutant genotype to the viral load in the sample present. The method is rather generic and needs no optimization for the analysis of new mutations, though only generates information for a single nucleotide position.

Median absolute RNA copy numbers

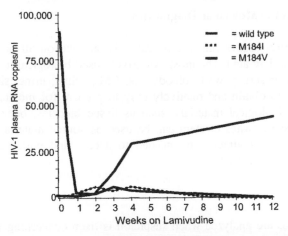

Figure 9. Turnover of HIV-1 in plasma. Median wildtype and resistant HIV-1 RNA concentrations in patients on Lamivudine monotherapy. HIV-1 RNA concentrations were determined using the HIV-1 Amplicor Monitor assay (Roche Diagnostics), The presence of Lamivudine resistance mutations (M184I an M184V) was determined using the point mutation assay. Figure demonstrates the rapid turnover of wildtype virus, being replaced in a few weeks by a lamivudine resistant virus population (M184V).[33]

HIV-1 RT Line Probe Assay

Another approach for the simultaneous analysis of multiple codons associated with drug-resistance to HIV-1 RT inhibitors was introduced some years ago [36, 37, 38, 39]. The assay, based on reverse (selective) hybridization of a biotinylated amplified part of the RT gene with specific probes present as lines on a nitrocellulose filter (line-probes), has been applied earlier for the typing of HCV strains and HLA genotypes. Currently, the HIV-1 RT LiPA is capable of detecting an array of mutations associated with resistance mutations to nucleoside and non-nucleoside inhibitors, as well as for protease inhibitors. In small studies comparing the HIV-1 RT LiPA with sequencing, it was demonstrated that the LiPA assay was highly specific and that general concordance existed between both technologies [36, 37, 40, 26], although the technology is extremely sensitive to sequence variation in the probe regions and as such is dependent on the careful selection of the probe sequences. Concordant results were obtained upon comparing the LiPA HCV sub-typing assay to sequence analysis.

The LiPA assay, in contrast to all earlier described "alternative approaches", is capable of detecting a spectrum of mutations within one run. This makes it a good candidate for diagnostic laboratories as a first line screen for the presence of resistance mutations in clinical samples, either before patients start antiretroval treatment, or during treatment when treatment failure is observed. With the continuous development of antiviral drugs and new combination therapies, new resistance mutations will continuously be identified. Therefore, the LiPA assay, as well as the other alternative approaches, need to be updated regularly, in order to keep of relevance to the clinician treating the patient. LiPA assays for HCV genotype determination are widely applied diagnostically.

Clinical Materials for Molecular Diagnostics

Molecular diagnostics assays can, theoretically, be applied on all biological material containing intact nucleic acid. The most extensively used biological materials are body fluids like plasma or serum, white blood cells, CSF, saliva, urine, since all of these materials are easy to obtain and relatively easy to prepare for molecular approaches. In addition, other biological materials, such as tissue biopsies, bone marrow, feces, sputum, nasal washes, swabs etcetera can be used as source material. In some cases specific sample (pre-) treatments are needed to access and purify the nucleic acid present in these tissues or fluids.

CSF

Cerebrospinal fluids are analyzed when suspicion is risen concerning viral meningitis. Worldwide common agents of viral meningitis are Mumps and enteroviruses [41]. When suspicion is raised concerning viral encephalitis, analysis of CSF can also be of value, although sensitivity/specificity might be lower as compared to the analysis of brain biopsies [42]. In case of HSV encephalitis, PCR on CSF has been shown to be equally sensitive to the analysis of brain biopsies [43].

Important agents include members of the Flaviviridae (such as the West Nile virus [44]), Herpes simplex virus and Varizella zoster virus. The list of possible pathogens is even longer when immunocompromised patients are involved, such as bone marrow transplantation patients. In these cases pathogens such as Cytomegalovirus, Ebstein-Barr virus, Herpes 6 virus, myeloma viruses (JC) should be included in the diagnostic procedure [45].

Except in cases of buoyant bacterial meningitis, CSF fluid is of low protein content, therefore it can be processed simply by heating to free nucleic acids for molecular detection. Otherwise simple isolation procedures are sufficient since in most cases no substances are present which suppress molecular detection.

Serum and Plasma

Only those viruses that produce a viremia are of concern when analyzing serum or plasma samples. In general, substances interfering with coagulation are not added to the bloodsample. Plasma samples are treated with EDTA, heparin, or Citrate to avoid coagulation. Advantage of this approach is that apart from the plasma, also the white blood cells can be isolated to analyze cell bound viruses. However, the addition of heparin, which is most suitable for preserving white blood cells, can interfere with PCR because heparin itself can inhibit Taq polymerase [46]. Not all isolation methods are capable of removing heparin from plasma samples and thus isolation methods should be chosen with care. Isolation methods such as described by Boom offer an excellent tool to isolate high grade nucleic acids from serum and plasma [1]. Plasma viremia can be evaluated for example for HIV, HCV, HBV, enteroviruses and EBV. Quantitative plasma viral load determinations are common practice now for the monitoring of HIV, HCV or HBV infected individuals on treatment.

In addition, analysis of serum/plasma in some cases has the advantage that the presence of the virus correlates with active viral replication. For instance in case of EBV, this has lead to the regular monitoring of EBV plasma loads in patients after a bone-marrow transplantation, in order to determine EBV reactivation [47].

White Blood Cells

Analysis of white blood cells is warranted in some special cases. Examples are the suspicion of vertical transmission of HIV or the suspicion of a patient with a recently acquired HIV infection prior to antibody development (window phase). Analysis of HIV proviral DNA in leukocytes is critical in new-born children since antibody based tests are inadequate, due to the presence of maternal antibodies, and analysis of viremia is not always adequate due to the lag phase for the production of cell free viremia. Proviral DNA can also be of value for the diagnosis of an HTLV-1 infection. HTLV infections can become manifest years after infection, by the development of T-cell leukemia. In cases where HTLV-1 serology is inconclusive, the detection of proviral DNA can be diagnostic. Other examples for the analysis of white blood cells include CMV status when serology is not reliable.

Faeces

Analysis of feces for the presence of nucleic acids from pathogens of interest, has long been hampered by the presence of inhibiting factors in feces [48]. Probably these inhibitors belong to the same group of molecules as the heparin inhibitors and are derived from plant polysaccharides. However the emergence of more robust isolation methods enable molecular analysis of this material. Since than, methods have been published to detect "difficult to culture" organisms such as Norwalk-like viruses. Until recently Norwalk-like virus infections could only be diagnosed by electron-microcopy. Application of molecular tests will greatly enhance insight in the epidemiology of these infections. Finally, molecular analyses on feces are also applied for the detection of adenoviruses and CMV.

Urine

Analysis of urine is of importance for those pathogens that are excreted reliably in the urinary tract, such as is the case with CMV and BK virus. Although inhibiting factors in urine are present and should be eliminated during the extraction process. Indications for urine analysis are suspicion of vertical CMV transmission In those cases CMV excretion in urine of the newborn child is indicative for vertical transmission.

BKV excretion should be investigated when immune-compromised patients develop hemorrhagic cystitis. Culture of BKV is tedious molecular detection can improve on a timely diagnosis.

Tissue Specimens/Biopsies

Several approaches can be used to make solid tissue specimens applicable for molecular diagnostic analysis. Tissue can be grinded using a mortar, leading to high recovery of nucleic acid, but intrinsically this method also has a high risk of contamination. Alternatively, tissues can be enzymatically treated, for instance using Proteinase-K, to degrade the cell structures. When this is performed in the presence of a high concentration of guanidinium-thio-cyanate, degradation of the nucleic acid itself, in particular of RNA, can be prevented. However, robust and reproducible recovery of nucleic acid from tissue remains complex and needs extensive experience and control.

Conclusion

Molecular methods in the diagnosis of viral infections, although relatively recently introduced, nowadays play an important role in the diagnostic virology laboratory. At present, most of these assays are still complex, involve numerous manual steps and, given the contamination risks, require well-disciplined and dedicated laboratory personnel. It is expected that, with the development of automated equipment for sample preparation and real-time approaches for amplification and detection, molecular diagnostics become easier to apply in the diagnostic laboratory. Given the need for diagnosis using molecular assays in various body fluids and body tissues, it is a prerequisite that nucleic acids can be easily and reliably obtained from these compartments. Further improvements in nucleic acid extraction procedures are needed and expected.

Various amplification technologies are available, PCR being by far the most widely applied technique. In addition to qualitative molecular assays for diagnosis, quantitative assays become of increasing importance. This is mainly because of the development of antiviral agents against an increasing number of viruses and the associated need for monitoring of treatment efficiency. Additionally, natural history studies investigating the relationship between the amount of virus during the course of the infection and its clinical symptoms also ask for quantitative information. Technological improvements such as real-time PCR have facilitated the development of quantitative assays formats.

Finally, in addition to the qualitative and quantitative determination of viral infections, detailed genomic characterization is applied using various technologies. The reasons for these analyses may be either epidemiological or may be used in individual patient treatment management.

Some important steps forward, towards the integration of molecular diagnostic approaches for qualitative, quantitative determination as well as genetic characterization can be expected in the next decade. The use of so-called micro-arrays using sequence specific probes on a solid phase, may enable such an integrated approach and may even have the potential to identify, quantitate and characterize the infectious agent.

Given their high potential and important role in viral diagnostics, there is no doubt molecular diagnostic essays are here to stay.

References

1. Boom R, Sol CJ, Salimans MM, Jansen CL, Wertheim-van Dillen PM, van der Noordaa J. Rapid and simple method for purification of nucleic acids. J Clin Microbiol 1990; 28(3): 495-503.
2. Jongerius JM, Bovenhorst M, van der Poel CL, van Hilten JA, Kroes AC, van der Does JA, van Leeuwen EF, Schuurman R. Evaluation of automated nucleic acid extraction devices for application in HCV. Transfusion 2000 Jul; 40(7): 871-4.
3. Beld M, Habibuw MR, Rebers SP, Boom R, Reesink HW. Evaluation of automated RNA-extraction technology and a qualitative HCV assay for sensitivity and detection of HCV RNA in pool-screening systems. Transfusion 2000 May; 40(5): 575-9.
4. Saiki RK, Scharf S, Faloona F, Mullis KB, Horn GT, Erlich HA, Arnheim N. Enzymatic amplification of beta-globin genomic sequences and restriction site analysis for diagnosis of sickle cell anemia. Science 1985 20; 230(4732): 1350-4.
5. Kwok S, Higuchi R. Avoiding false positives with PCR. Nature 1989. 339: 237-238.
6. Wu DY, Wallace RB The ligation amplification reaction (LAR)--amplification of specific DNA sequences using sequential rounds of template-dependent ligation. Genomics 1989 May; 4(4): 560-9.
7. Kievits T, van Gemen B, van Strijp D, Schukkink R, Dircks M, Adriaanse H, Malek L, Sooknanan R, Lens P. NASBA isothermal enzymatic *in vitro* nucleic acid amplification optimized for the diagnosis of HIV-1 infection. J Virol Methods 1991 Dec; 35(3): 273-86
8. Collins ML, Irvine B, Tyner D, Fine E, Zayati C, Chang C, Horn T, Ahle D, Detmer J, Shen LP, Kolberg J,

Bushnell S, Urdea MS, Ho DD. A branched DNA signal amplification assay for quantification of nucleic acid targets below 100 molecules/ml. Nucleic Acids Res 1997 1; 25(15): 2979-84.

9. Southern EM, Detection of specific sequences among DNA fragments separated by gel electrophoresis. J Mol Biol 1975; 98: 503-517.

10. Mansfield ES, Worley JM, McKenzie SE, Surrey S, Rappaport E, Fortina P. Nucleic acid detection using non-radioactive labelling methods. Mol Cell Probes 1995; 9(3): 145-56

11. Schena M, Shalon D, Davis RW, Brown PO. Quantitative monitoring of gene expression patterns with a complementary DNA microarray. Science 1995; 270: 467-70

12. Landgraf A, Reckmann B, Pingoud A. Direct analysis of polymerase chain reaction products using enzyme-linked immunosorbent assay techniques. Anal Biochem 1991; 198(1): 86-91

13. Schmittgen TD, Zakrajsek BA, Mills AG, Gorn V, Singer MJ, Reed MW. Quantitative reverse transcription-polymerase chain reaction to study mRNA decay: comparison of endpoint and real-time methods. Anal Biochem 2000 Oct 15; 285(2): 194-204

14. Heid CA, Stevens J, Livak KJ, Williams PM Real time quantitative PCR. Genome Res 1996; 6(10): 986-94

15. Loeffler J, Henke N, Hebart H, Schmidt D, Hagmeyer L, Schumacher U, Einsele H. Quantification of fungal DNA by using fluorescence resonance energy transfer and the light cycler system. J Clin Microbiol 2000; 8(2): 586-90

16. Leone G, van Schijndel H, van Gemen B, Kramer FR, Schoen CD. Molecular beacon probes combined with amplification by NASBA enable homogeneous, real-time detection of RNA. Nucleic Acids Res 1998; 26(9): 2150-5

17. M Mulder J, McKinney N, Christopherson C, Sninsky J, Greenfield L, Kwok S. Rapid and simple PCR assay for quantitation of human immunodeficiency virus type 1 RNA in plasma: application to acute retroviral infection. J Clin Microbiol 1994 Feb; 32(2): 292-300.

18. Pas SD, Fries E, De Man RA, Osterhaus AD, Niesters HG. Development of a quantitative real-time detection assay for hepatitis B virus DNA and comparison with two commercial assays. J Clin Microbiol 2000 Aug; 38(8): 2897-901.

19. Carpenter CC, Cooper DA, Fischl MA, Gatell JM, Gazzard BG, Hammer SM, Hirsch MS, Jacobsen DM, Katzenstein DA, Montaner JS, Richman DD, Saag MS, Schechter M, Schooley RT, Thompson MA, Vella S, Yeni PG, Volberding PA. Antiretroviral therapy in adults: updated recommendations of the International AIDS Society-USA Panel. JAMA 2000 Jan 19; 283(3): 381-90. Review.

20. Lipshutz RJ, Fodor SP, Gingeras TR, Lockhart DJ. High density synthetic oligonucleotide arrays. Nat Genet 1999 Jan; 21(1 Suppl): 20-4. Review.

21. Kozal MJ, Shah N, Shen N, Yang R, Fucini R, Merigan TC, Richman DD, Morris D, Hubbell E, Chee M, Gingeras TR. Extensive polymorphisms observed in HIV-1 clade B protease gene using high-density oligonucleotide arrays. Nat Med 1996 Jul; 2(7): 753-9.

22. DeGruttola V, Dix L, D'Aquila R, Holder D, Phillips A, Ait-Khaled M, Baxter J, Clevenbergh P, Hammer S, Harrigan R, Katzenstein D, Lanier R, Miller M, Para M, Yerly S, Zolopa A, Murray J, Patick A, Miller V, Castillo S, Pedneault L, Mellors J. The relation between baseline HIV drug resistance and response to antiretroviral therapy: re-analysis of retrospective and prospective studies using a standardized data analysis plan. Antivir Ther 2000 Mar; 5(1): 41-8.

23. Durant J, Clevenbergh P, Halfon P, Delgiudice P, Porsin S, Simonet P, Montagne N, Boucher CA, Schapiro JM. Dellamonica P. Drug-resistance genotyping in HIV-1 therapy: the VIRADAPT randomised controlled trial. Lancet 1999 Jun 26; 353(9171): 2195-9.

24. Hirsch MS, Brun-Vezinet F, D'Aquila RT, Hammer SM, Johnson VA, Kuritzkes DR, Loveday C,

Mellors JW, Clotet B, Conway B, Demeter LM, Vella S, Jacobsen DM, Richman DD. Antiretroviral drug resistance testing in adult HIV-1 infection: recommendations of an International AIDS Society-USA Panel. JAMA 2000 May 10; 283(18): 2417-26.

25. Boucher CA, O'Sullivan E, Mulder JW, Ramautarsing C, Kellam P, Darby G, Lange JM, Goudsmit J, Larder BA. Ordered appearance of zidovudine resistance mutations during treatment of 18 human immunodeficiency virus-positive subjects. J Infect Dis 1992 Jan; 165(1): 105-10

26. Schmit JC, Ruiz L, Stuyver L, Van Laethem K, Vanderlinden I, Puig T, Rossau R, Desmyter J, De Clercq E, Clotet B, Vandamme AM. Comparison of the LiPA HIV-1 RT test, selective PCR and direct solid phase sequencing for the detection of HIV-1 drug resistance mutations. J Virol Methods 1998 Jul; 73(1): 77-82.

27. de Jong MD, Loewenthal M, Boucher CA, van der Ende I, Hall D, Schipper P, Imrie A, Weigel HM, Kauffmann RH, Koster R, et al. Alternating nevirapine and zidovudine treatment of human immunodeficiency virus type 1-infected persons does not prolong nevirapine activity. J Infect Dis 1994 Jun; 169(6): 1346-50.

28. Van Vaerenbergh K, Van Laethem K, Albert J, Boucher CA, Clotet B, Floridia M, Gerstoft J, Hejdeman B, Nielsen C, Pannecouque C, Perrin L, Pirillo MF, Ruiz L, Schmit JC, Schneider F, Schoolmeester A, Schuurman R, Stellbrink HJ, Stuyver L, Van Lunzen J, Van Remoortel B, Van Wijngaerden E, Vella S, Witvrouw M, Yerly S, De Clercq E, Destmyer J, Vandamme AM. Prevalence and characteristics of multinucleoside-resistant human immunodeficiency virus type 1 among European patients receiving combinations of nucleoside analogues. Antimicrob Agents Chemother 2000 Aug; 44(8): 2109-17.

29. Van Laethem K, Van Vaerenbergh K, Schmit JC, Sprecher S, Hermans P, De Vroey V, Schuurman R, Harrer T, Witvrouw M, Van Wijngaerden E, Stuyver L, Van Ranst M, Desmyter J, De Clercq E, Vandamme AM. Phenotypic assays and sequencing are less sensitive than point mutation assays for detection of resistance in mixed HIV-1 genotypic populations. J Acquir Immune Defic Syndr 1999 Oct 1; 22(2): 107-18.

30. Schuurman R, Demeter L, Reichelderfer P, Tijnagel J, de Groot T, Boucher C. Worldwide evaluation of DNA sequencing approaches for identification of drug resistance mutations in the human immunodeficiency virus type 1 reverse transcriptase. J Clin Microbiol 1999 Jul; 37(7): 2291-6.

31. Fontaine E, Lambert C, Servais J, Ninove D, Plesseria JM, Staub T, Arendt V, Kirpach P, Robert I, Schneider F, Hemmer R, Schmit JC. Fast genotypic detection of drug resistance mutations in the HIV-1 reverse transcriptase gene of treatment-naive patients. J Hum Virol 1998 Nov-Dec; 1(7): 451-6.

32. Kaye S, Loveday C, Tedder RS. A microtitre format point mutation assay: application to the detection of drug resistance in human immunodeficiency virus type-1 infected patients treated with zidovudine. J Med Virol 1992 Aug; 37(4): 241-6.

33. Schuurman R, Nijhuis M, van Leeuwen R, Schipper P, de Jong D, Collis P, Danner SA, Mulder J, Loveday C, Christopherson C, et al. Rapid changes in human mmunodeficiency virus type 1 RNA load and appearance of drug-resistant virus populations in persons treated with lamivudine (3TC). J Infect Dis 1995 Jun; 171(6): 1411-9.

34. Brun-Vezinet F, Boucher C, Loveday C, Descamps D, Fauveau V, Izopet J, Jeffries D, Kaye S, Krzyanowski C, Nunn A, Schuurman R, Seigneurin JM, Tamalet C, Tedder R, Weber J, Weverling GJ. HIV-1 viral load, phenotype, and resistance in a subset of drug-naive participants from the Delta trial. The National Virology Groups. Delta Virology Working Group and Coordinating Committee. Lancet 1997 Oct 4; 350(9083): 983-90.

35. de Jong MD, Veenstra J, Stilianakis NI, Schuurman R, Lange JM, de Boer RJ, Boucher CA. Host-parasite dynamics and outgrowth of virus containing a single K70R amino acid change in reverse transcriptase are

responsible for the loss of human immunodeficiency virus type 1 RNA load suppression by zidovudine. Proc Natl Acad Sci USA 1996 May 28; 93(11): 5501-6.

36. Clarke JR, Kaye S, Babiker AG, Hooker MH, Tedder R, Weber JN. Comparison of a point mutation assay with a line probe assay for the detection of the major mutations in the HIV-1 reverse transcriptase gene associated with reduced susceptibility to nucleoside analogues. J Virol Methods 2000 Aug; 88(2): 117-24.

37. Descamps D, Calvez V, Collin G, Cecille A, Apetrei C, Damond F, Katlama C, Matheron S, Huraux JM, Brun-Vezinet F. Line probe assay for detection of human immunodeficiency virus type 1 mutations conferring resistance to nucleoside inhibitors of reverse transcriptase: comparison with sequence analysis. J Clin Microbiol 1998 Jul; 36(7): 2143-5.

38. Stuyver L, Wyseur A, Rombout A, Louwagie J, Scarcez T, Verhofstede C, Rimland D, Schinazi RF, Rossau R. Line probe assay for rapid detection of drug-selected mutations in the human immunodeficiency virus type 1 reverse transcriptase gene. Antimicrob Agents Chemother 1997 Feb; 41(2): 284-91.

39. Rusconi S, La Seta Catamancio S, Sheridan F, Parker D. A genotypic analysis of patients receiving Zidovudine with either Lamivudine, Didanosine or Zalcitabine dual therapy using the LiPA point mutation assay to detect genotypic variation at codons 41, 69, 70, 74, 184 and 215. J Clin Virol 2000 Oct 1; 19(3): 135-142.

40. Wilson JW, Bean P, Robins T, Graziano F, Persing DH. Comparative evaluation of three human immunodeficiency virus genotyping systems: the HIV-GenotypR method, the HIV PRT GeneChip assay, and the HIV-1 RT line probe assay. J Clin Microbiol 2000 Aug; 38(8): 3022-8. Chernesky MA, Jang D, Sellors J, Luinstra K, Chong S, Castriciano S, Mahony JB Urinary inhibitors of polymerase chain reaction and ligase chain reaction and testing of multiple specimens may contribute to lower assay sensitivities for diagnosing Chlamydia trachomatis infected women. Mol Cell Probes 1997 Aug; 11(4): 243-9

41. Poggio GP, Rodriguez C, Cisterna D, Freire MC, Cello J Nested PCR for rapid detection of mumps virus in cerebrospinal fluid from patients with neurological diseases. J Clin Microbiol 2000 Jan; 38(1): 274-8

42. Dorries K, Arendt G, Eggers C, Roggendorf W, Dorries RNucleic acid detection as a diagnostic tool in polyomavirus JC induced progressive multifocal leukoencephalopathy. J Med Virol 1998; 54(3): 196-203.

43. Lakeman FD, Whitley RJ. Diagnosis of herpes simplex encephalitis: application of polymerase chain reaction to cerebrospinal fluid from brain-biopsied patients and correlation with disease. National Institute of Allergy and Infectious Diseases Collaborative Antiviral Study Group. J Infect Dis 1995; 171(4): 857-63

44. Lanciotti RS, Kerst AJ, Nasci RS, Godsey MS, Mitchell CJ, Savage HM, Komar N, Panella NA, Allen BC, Volpe KE, Davis BS, Roehrig JT. Rapid Detection of West Nile Virus from Human Clinical Specimens, Field-Collected Mosquitoes, and Avian Samples by a TaqMan Reverse Transcriptase-PCR Assay.J Clin Microbiol.

45. Casas I, Pozo F, Trallero G, Echevarria JM, Tenorio A Viral diagnosis of neurological infection by RT multiplex PCR: a search for entero- and herpesviruses in a prospective study. J Med Virol 1999; 7(2): 145-51

46. Yokota M, Tatsumi N, Nathalang O, Yamada T, Tsuda I. Effects of heparin on polymerase chain reaction for blood white cells. J Clin Lab Anal 1999; 13(3): 133-40

47. Niesters HG, van Esser J, Fries E, Wolthers KC, Cornelissen J, Osterhaus AD. Development of a real-time quantitative assay for detection of Epstein-Barr virus. J Clin Microbiol 2000 Feb; 38(2):

712-5.

48. Boom R, Sol C, Weel J, Lettinga K, Gerrits Y, van Breda A, Wertheim-Van Dillen P. Detection and quantitation of human cytomegalovirus DNA in faeces. J Virol Methods 2000 Jan; 84(1): 1-14.

CHAPTER 4

HOST DEFENSES AGAINST VIRAL INFECTION

BRIGITTE AUTRAN, LUCILLE MOLET
and MICHAEL M. LEDERMAN

Table of Contents

Practical Guidelines in Antiviral Therapy Ed. by Charles A.B. Boucher and George J. Galasso. 65 — 94
© 2002 *Elsevier Science. Printed in the Netherlands.*

Introduction

Host Defenses and Viral Pathogenesis Are Intimately Linked

The relationship between humans and viruses is intimate and complex. Incapable of extracellular growth, viruses must parasitize host cells for replication to take place. Thus viruses have evolved numerous creative mechanisms for cellular entry and for utilization of cellular factors for successful replication. Many viruses utilize cell surface receptors that are key molecules in host immune defense mechanisms for cellular entry. As examples, Epstein Barr virus (EBV) utilizes complement receptors, the human immunodeficiency virus (HIV) utilizes the CD4 molecule and chemokine receptors and rhinovirus utilizes adhesion molecules for cellular entry. All viruses must utilize host substrates for synthesis of macromolecules and host cellular machinery for protein synthesis and many utilize host cellular factors to activate and regulate replication. Thus it is not surprising that host immunity and viral pathogenesis are intimately linked.

Host defenses against viruses include both simple innate non-immune defense mechanisms and complex adaptive defense mechanisms that define the principles of immunity.

Adaptive Immune Responses – Key to the Survival of Complex Organisms

The survival of complex and simple organisms is a constant struggle. Those organisms that can best adapt to environmental stresses or competition are most likely to survive and propagate. If we assume that long term adaptation to stresses is mediated primarily through random germ line mutations, then the ability of complex organisms such as humans to survive when competing with microbes that are fully capable of fatal infections is remarkable. As key examples, compare the generation times, the number of offspring per generation and the fidelities of DNA polymerases among bacteria, viruses and humans. In each instance the arithmetic clearly favors the microbes. Humans must develop at least 10 years or more before becoming capable of reproduction and then may generate one to a dozen or fewer offspring over the next twenty to thirty years. In contrast bacteria are fully capable of logarithmic expansion with a generation time measured in minutes to hours and viruses express thousands of progeny with each replication cycle that can be completed within several hours to days. Human DNA polymerases generally have an error rate of approximately one base pair per 10^{12} per cellular division; bacterial DNA polymerases of approximately one base pair per 10^6 and the reverse transcriptase of HIV-1 for example has an estimated error rate of approximately one base pair per $10^3 - 10^4$ per replication. Now, we (humans) love our offspring more than viruses and bacteria do and for us, the survival of each of our offspring is critically important. In contrast, bacteria and viruses are fully prepared to generate many defective offspring with null mutations just to assure that rare mutations confer some degree of survival advantage. Clearly, there must be a mechanism in place to assure that humans and other complex species with slow and infrequent germ line evolution can compete with and respond to the challenges posed by rapidly replicating and evolving organisms such as viruses. Indeed it is the enormously adaptable immune defense system that permits a rapid response to infectious agents without the need for reproduction and germ line mutation. The intrinsic non-adaptive host defenses discussed below also play roles in protection from microbial infection. These non-immune defenses however are limited in scope and not capable of rapid adaptation to microbial evolution. Thus development of the ability to "evolve" an immune response that is directed specifically to a pathogen without the need for germ line reproduction and evolution can be seen as providing a critical means for large and slowly reproducing organisms to survive in competition with smaller more rapidly evolving pathogens.

Humoral and Cellular Responses Are the Two Arms of the Adaptive Immune Response

The two arms of the adaptive immune response that permit rapid "evolutionary" responses to microbial infection are the humoral and cellular immune responses. Humoral responses are manifested by the development of antibodies — soluble proteins — that can exist in multiple forms (IgG, IgM, IgA, IgD or IgE). Antibodies are produced by B lymphocytes and their plasma cell progeny. Antibodies can bind to extracellular pathogens by recognition of three dimensional structures through unique hypervariable antigen binding domains and may block the infectivity of viruses (neutralization) through inhibiting key interactions between viruses and host cellular targets or occasionally through the activation of complement that may result in the enzymatic disruption of the integrity of the virus.

Intracellular pathogens may escape most humoral defenses by residing within host cells where antibodies generally do not penetrate. Cell mediated immune responses are manifested by the emergence of T lymphocytes that are capable of recognizing viral encoded peptides expressed on the surface of host cells bound by host major histocompatibility (MHC) antigens. Upon recognition of viral peptides in this setting, CD4+ T helper lymphocytes can be activated to express powerful helper cytokines that transmit activating and recruitment signals to other cells and CD8+ cytolytic T lymphocytes may be activated to lyse the infected host cell thereby destroying the cells that are responsible for viral propagation.

A diverse genetic repertoire that is capable of recombination underlies the evolutionary capabilities of the adaptive immune response. The diversity of recognition is "restricted" however by major histocompatibility (MHC) antigen structure [1].

It is the diversity of the families of genes encoding the variable regions of the antibody molecules and of the T cell receptor chains that permits evolutionary adaptation to diverse microbial pathogens. During the development of T and B lymphocytes, recombinations among these variable gene segments permit the development of a diverse repertoire of T cell receptor and immunoglobulin structures. It is the structure of these molecules that of course determines the nature of the antigens that these T cell receptors or antibodies can recognize. As noted above, antibody molecules recognize and bind to three dimensional structures whereas T cells bind to small linear segments of peptides, approximately 8 to 20 amino acids in length that are bound by host MHC antigens on the antigen presenting cell surface. The structure of the MHC antigen determines which peptides can be bound for antigen presentation. Thus there is a restriction on the structures of the peptide chains that can be presented for T cell recognition. Thus MHC or HLA "restriction" determines which peptides can be presented to T cells for recognition, stimulation and cellular expansion. In contrast, B cell recognition for generation of antibody is not directly MHC restricted. B cells however respond optimally when help is provided by CD4+ T helper lymphocytes. Thus the presence of a peptide that can be bound by host MHC antigens can enhance the B cell response to antigen by providing T cell help in proximity to the B cell – antigen interaction. Thus, conjugation of sugars (which generally do not stimulate T cell responses) to peptides which are recognized by T helper cells enhances the antibody response to the polysaccharide through proximate delivery of T cell help.

Upon first exposure to antigen a rare naïve B lymphocyte for humoral responses or a rare naïve T lymphocyte for cellular responses whose immunoglobulin or T cell receptor gene has been rearranged to result in the structure that will bind the antigen in question is activated to divide. These first exposures generally take place in lymphoid organs (lymph nodes, spleen or gut associated lymphoid tissue) to which antigens are transported or trapped by professional antigen presenting cells. Multiple rounds of cellular replication increase the magnitude of immune responsiveness to the newly encountered antigen. Some of the activated cells will become short lived effector cells or will die through a self-regulatory mechanism called programmed cell death or apoptosis, however a proportion of the newly divided cells will persist as memory cells and upon re-exposure to antigen, these cells are capable of a more rapid and greater magnitude anamnestic response.

Memory, Specificity and the Timing of Immune Responses

Immune responses that are capable of adaptation can be defined operationally as possessing two cardinal characteristics: memory and specificity.

Memory means that an immune competent host can "remember" prior exposures to the same pathogen or substance. Memory means that the subsequent or secondary immune response to a remembered pathogen or substance emerges more rapidly than the initial or primary immune response to that pathogen or substances. Operationally, subsequent exposures to pathogens are met with heightened immune responses that may protect against disease. This phenomenon is related to the prior expansion and persistence of memory cells as noted above and underlies the long-recognized "immunity" seen after a first bout of most viral diseases and is the underpinning of immunization strategies in the protection against infectious diseases.

Specificity means that secondary immune responses to one pathogen do not confer secondary or heightened immune responses to another pathogen. The extraordinary diversity and selectivity of immune responses confers enormous flexibility to immune-competent species that permits targeting host defense "energy" to the recognition of pathogens when these are most needed.

Thus the first exposure to a virus results in the development of a primary immune response. T cell-mediated immune responses are often detectable within days of infection. As this response is amplified by cellular expansion to achieve sufficient magnitude to actually mediate antiviral activity, intrinsic non-adaptive defenses are required to provide some degree of antiviral defense until host cell-mediated defenses are able to take over. Cell mediated responses are followed by the development of an IgM antibody response. IgM antibody levels generally decay within a few weeks of exposure and are replaced by the emergence of an IgG antibody response. These IgG molecules contain the same antigen binding domains as the earlier IgM response but now contain IgG constant regions. This "isotype switch" is mediated by the effects of "type-1" T helper cytokines elaborated by CD4+ T cells.

Humoral and Cellular Immune Responses Are Interconnected and Are Critically Dependent Upon the CD4+ T Cell

CD4+ T cells are key facilitators of immune responses both humoral and cellular. The production of critical T helper cytokines by CD4+ T cells can optimize the magnitude of both antibody responses and cell-mediated effector mechanisms. Thus CD4+ T cell dysfunction affects both cell-mediated and humoral immune competence as is seen in persons with the acquired immune deficiency syndrome.

Role of Humoral and Cellular Immune Systems in the Natural History of Viral Disease

Although there may be exceptions to this, as a general rule, antibody responses tend to protect against the acquisition of viral infections but also may participate in clearance of infection whereas cell-mediated immune responses most importantly determine the outcome of infection once it is established. This stated, cell-mediated immune responses also protect against clinical disease acquisition as children born with congenital inability to produce immunoglobulin are protected from recurrence of most viral infections after primary infection.

At the same time, it is important to recognize that some viral infections are characteristically self-limited whereas others are characterized by life-long infection, either chronic (eg HIV) or intermittent (eg HSV) once infection is established. As a general rule, infections with RNA viruses are characteristically self-limited whereas infections with DNA viruses or with RNA viruses that contain a DNA intermediate form are characteristically life-long. As exceptions to this general "rule", infection with the Hepatitis C virus can be transient or life-long despite the absence of a DNA intermediate form and infection with measles virus is rarely associated with long term persistence and chronic disease.

Innate Host Defences

Anatomic barriers protect against viral infection while innate non-adaptive host defenses provide early protection from viral infection and arm more specific adaptive immune defenses.

Anatomic barriers such as the skin provide effective protection against infection with viruses that can be breached when there are cuts or other forms of skin breakdown. Mucosal surfaces on the other hand are often sites of more effective virus penetration and require additional host protective mechanisms to prevent virus infection. In the respiratory tract, a moving mucociliary blanket can serve to move invading organisms upward until they and the particles with which they migrate can stimulate a cough reflex and expectoration. This can serve both as a mechanism for host defense but viruses also can capitalize on the cough reflex as a means for spread to other susceptible hosts. In the gastrointestinal tract, gastric acid and proteolytic enzymes can serve to inactivate ingested pathogens including enveloped viruses. Likewise, a number of host-derived molecules that can be found on mucosal surfaces are able to inactivate viruses *in vitro* and may contribute to intrinsic host defense against viral infection. Examples include small charged peptides: defensins, and proteolytic enzymes with antiviral activities such as secretory leukocyte protease inhibitor (SLPI) that may provide an intrinsic barrier to viral propagation and survival.

Viral density, route and mode of transmission determine the first line of host defense. Adenovirus, Epstein Barr Virus or Hepatitis A virus infect first the mucosal tissues of the respiratory or digestive tracts; Hepatitis B and C viruses and the Human Immunodeficiency Virus also are spread by body fluids. Mucosal epithelium serves as an efficient barrier against most viruses which must adhere specifically to epithelial cells to penetrate and cause infection; the rhinovirus for example will bind to an intercellular adhesion molecule (ICAM) in order to invade the mucosa and cause infection. Viruses, as intracellular pathogens will then spread from cell to cell either by direct transmission or by release into the extracellular fluids and re-infection of adjacent or distant cells. At this point, adaptive, immune host defenses become key protectors against infection.

Most virus particles are eliminated within hours by defense mechanisms that do not require expansion and differentiation of specific immune effectors. Such innate immunity acts immediately and is followed by early induced responses some hours later, helping to keep infection under control while antigen-specific immune responses are generated. The delay of 4-7 days observed after virus exposure and before adaptive immune responses take effect illustrates the importance of innate immunity during this window period. The innate immune system also plays a critical role in the initiation and subsequent direction of adaptive virus-specific immune responses. Indeed, cytokines produced during this early period will determine whether the subsequent T cell responses will develop as predominantly a type I helper (Th1) response or a type 2 helper (Th2) response.

Complement May Be Deposited on Virion Surfaces and May Inactivate Enveloped Viruses

Complement can be deposited on viral surfaces even in the absence of an adaptive immune response and at least *in vitro*, some enveloped viruses can be neutralized by the cascade of proteolytic events initiated by complement deposition. The importance of this defense against viruses is uncertain.

Phagocytic Cells: Two Edged Swords in Viral Pathogenesis

Innate (non-adaptive) defenses include both cellular and non-cellular defenses. Phagocytic cells, macrophages and neutrophils, are major effector cells of the innate defense system and bear surface receptors that have evolved to recognize and bind components of most pathogen surfaces. However viruses rarely express surface molecules that are recognized by cellular receptors that initiate phagocytosis. On the other hand, macrophages themselves may be targets for early viral infection. Thus the role of macrophages in viral disease pathogenesis is complex. On the one hand, because they can be infected early in the course of infection and can traffic to multiple compartments, macrophages have been accused of spreading virus throughout the body, particularly to the central nervous system. On the other hand, macrophages are potent producers of cytokines and other factors that may mediate antiviral defenses directly or can activate other cells to limit viral propagation. As an example, macrophages express nitric oxide synthase that catalyzes production of nitric oxide – a molecule that can react with oxygen to generate other reactive products capable of interfering with viral replication by reacting with and inactivating a number of key viral enzymes [2].

Natural Killer Cells: An Early Non-adaptive Defense Against Viruses

Natural killer or NK cells are large granular lymphocytes equipped with cytolytic machinery [3]. They spontaneously kill tumor cells and virus-infected cells *in vitro* without prior immunization or activation and may contribute to early antiviral defenses particularly against herpes viruses as a rare case of NK cell deficiency was associated with heightened susceptibility to herpesvirus infections [4]. In other settings however, the role of NK cells in host defense against viral infection has been difficult to demonstrate. This may be due to the presence of intricate mechanisms to prevent uninfected host cells from NK cell-mediated lysis.

NK cell cytolytic activity is increased by 20- to 100- fold by interferon alpha (IFN-α) and IFN-β induced early in viral infections. A cytokine produced by antigen-presenting cells, interleukin-12 (IL-12) can also elicit the production of large amounts of IFN-γ by NK cells. In turn, IFN-γ produced by NK cells can help to enhance the differentiation of virus-specific CD4 T cells toward the Th1 pathway that promotes the generation of cytotoxic CD8 T cells.

NK cells recognize host major histocompatibility complex I (MHC I) molecules as well as certain glycoproteins induced by viral infection. Some receptors provide an activation signal, including type-C lectins that recognize carbohydrate ligands found on cell surfaces. A second class of receptors inhibits NK cell activation and cytolysis of normal cells. These inhibitory receptors (KIRs) recognize poorly polymorphic regions of the MHC class I proteins [5]. Each NK cell expresses at least one KIR that can recognize at least one host MHC class I antigen: for instance, the human killer inhibitory receptors p58 and p70 bind HLA-B and HLA-C antigens resulting in inhibition of NK cytolysis and protection of uninfected cells. Some viruses inhibit all protein synthesis in host cells, including MHC class I protein synthesis. Others such as herpesviruses and the human immunodeficiency virus may selectively prevent the export of the MHC class I molecules that present viral antigens to CD8 cytotoxic T cells as a means to escape host immune defenses. These cells may be sensitive to NK cell killing. Once humoral immune responses are induced, NK cells can be activated to lyse cells expressing viral antigens on the cell surface by binding of virus specific IgG to NK cell type III Fc receptors (FcRIII) and reduction of antibody dependent cellular cytotoxicity (ADCC).

Gamma-delta T Cells – Intermediates Between Innate and Adaptive Host Defenses

Another lymphocyte type, the γδ T cell, also may participate in pre-adaptive host defenses. These are T cells of thymic origin but differ from the majority of T cells as their T cell receptors (TCR) are composed of γδ chains instead of αβ chains and they lack CD4 and CD8 cell surface expression. They represent a small fraction (<10%) of circulating T cells. Some γδ T cells are found in lymphoid tissues and display a diverse repertoire of TCR structures. Other γδ T cells are found in epithelial tissues, particularly in mice, and display a very limited diversity of TCR. These γδ T cells recognize "unconventional" ligands such heat-shock proteins, MHC class IB molecules, nucleotides and phospholipids, but do not generally recognize conventional viral peptides presented by MHC class I or class II molecules [6]. These properties place them in an intermediate position between innate and adaptive defenses.

Soluble Mediators of Innate (Non-Adaptive) Defenses Against Viruses

Type I Interferons

Virus infection of cells induces the production of interferons that interfere directly with the cycle of virus replication in infected cells and block the spread of viruses to uninfected cells. Interferons also facilitate the differentiation of cells that are critical in adaptive immune defenses against viruses [7, 8, 9].

The class-I interferons (IFN) α and β are produced by many infected cell types and thus differ from IFN-γ which is produced only by natural killer (NK) cells and effector T cells. IFN-α represents a family of several closely linked proteins while IFN-β comprises a single gene product. Synthesis of both is induced by double-stranded RNA which is not present in normal non-infected mammalian cells. Interferons induce a state of resistance to viral replication in all cells. IFN-α and IFN-β bind to a shared cellular interferon receptor, which induces synthesis of host-cell proteins that inhibit viral replication and degrade viral RNA. IFN-α and IFN-β also inactivate the eukaryotic protein synthesis initiation factor eIF-2, thereby inhibiting protein synthesis and viral replication.

Hundreds of host genes are activated by type I interferons and the roles of these interferon-inducible genes in viral defense and pathogenesis are under investigation. One of these interferon-inducible proteins called Mx is required for cellular resistance to influenza virus replication in mice. Interferons also increase the expression of MHC class I molecules, as well as other molecules involved in antigen processing through the MHC-class I pathway such as the TAP transporter proteins and the Lmp2 and Lmp7 components of the proteasome. This enhances the ability of host cells to present viral peptides to cytotoxic CD8 T cells and protects uninfected host cells against the promiscuous activities of natural killer cells (NK cells). Type I IFNs also promote NK cell function and the Th1 differentiation of CD4 T cells which in turn will allow the priming and generation of cytotoxic CD8 T cells.

Together these anti-viral and immune-enhancing effects of type I IFNs can be used for therapeutic purposes in hepatitis C virus infection where administration of IFN-α together with ribavirin can help clear virus from circulation.

Cytokines Serve as a Means of Intercellular Communication and Many Can Directly or Indirectly Affect Viral Propagation

Cytokines produced by phagocytic and inflammatory cells at sites of infection have long-range effects that contribute to host defense. Inflammatory cytokines such as tumor necrosis factor alpha (TNF-α), interleukin-1 (IL-1) and IL-6 have systemic effects. They initiate the synthesis of the acute-phase response proteins in the liver and increase body temperature thus limiting growth of many pathogens while increasing the efficacy of adaptive immune responses at raised temperatures. Inflammatory cytokines have also local effects at site of infection where they induce expression of adhesion molecules and facilitate extravasation of phagocytic cells, although the importance of this latter process might be somewhat limited in the case of viruses. Interferon-γ and TNFα may synergize with type I interferons in initiating intracellular antiviral activities as noted above. Interleukin-12, a macrophage product, is a powerful inducer of IFN-γ production and also may induce nitric oxide synthase. IL-2 and probably IL-15 are potent growth factors produced by virus-specific T cells to allow clonal amplification of virus-specific T cells but appear only once virus-specific T cells have been generated.

Viruses have developed "star wars technologies" against the immune system by encoding genes for cytokine-like molecules or receptors that can suborn the immune system for the purpose of promoting viral propagation [10, 11]. As examples, herpes viruses can encode Fc receptor-like molecules or complement receptor like molecules that can block antibodies from binding to viral epitopes or block the activation of complement respectively. Epstein-Barr virus and human herpes virus type 8 encode several immunologically relevant molecules such as an IL-6 homologue an IL-10 homologue, a bcl-2 homologue or an IL-8 receptor like molecule that may contribute to viral escape or pathogenesis [12].

Chemokines Recruit Immune Competent Cells to Sites of Infection

A family of closely related cytokines, the chemokines, are also released in response to early infection [13]. All are related in amino acid sequence and are chemoattractants for leukocytes: they recruit monocytes, neutrophils, and lymphocytes to sites of infection. Chemokine receptors are integral membrane proteins containing seven membrane-spanning loops. Many chemokine receptors are promiscuous and can bind several chemokines which in turn can bind several chemokine receptors. Chemokines are produced by various cell types in response to viruses. Chemokines direct leukocyte migration on endothelial cells along a gradient towards the site of infection. Chemokines may act on different cell types. For example, IL-8 promotes the migration of neutrophils and SDF-1 promotes T cell migration while macrophage chemoattractant protein-1 (MCP-1) promotes macrophage migration and RANTES is a chemoattractant for T lymphocytes [14].

Viruses may also use chemokine-receptors for their own ends. The human immunodeficiency virus-1 (HIV-1) utilizes beta chemokine receptors as coreceptors to promote membrane fusion and cellular entry. Although more than a dozen different chemokine co-receptors may be utilized for cellular entry *in vitro*, the two most important co-receptors are CCR-5 (utilized by M tropic strains) and CXCR4 (utilized by T tropic strains). Individuals who are homozygous for a 32 base-pair deletion in the CCR5 coding sequence that results in failed surface expression of the molecule are essentially resistant to infection with HIV-1. More recently pox-viruses have also been shown to use CCR-5 as a receptor for cellular entry which may account for the high prevalence of this mutant allele in the Caucasian population (approximately 15% are heterozygous for this polymorphism). High concentrations of beta chemokines — RANTES, MIP-1α and β, that bind to this receptor also can inhibit HIV-1 infection. In that sense, chemokines may also represent an early non-adaptive host defense that may block or limit the early steps of viral infection. In summary, early non-adaptative defenses against viruses are non-specific and often involve complex interactions among cells to protect uninfected cells from non-targeted defenses. Nonetheless, these defenses can both provide some "breathing room" while adaptive immune defenses are mobilized. Non-adaptive defenses also may participate in the recruitment and activation of adaptive immune-competent cells. Phagocytic cell activity and proinflammatory cytokine release may be less important during the early phase of viral infections (as opposed to early infection with other pathogens) and for this reason, the early phases of many viral infections remain clinically silent until the virus is spread systemically and adaptive immune responses are activated.

Immune Host Defences

Antibody-mediated Defenses Against Viral Infection

Antibodies are large glycoprotein products of B lymphocytes and plasma cells that are capable of recognizing and binding to microbes and other foreign structures. In contrast to T lymphocytes whose receptors recognize short linear peptides, antibodies recognize and bind to three dimensional structures from native unprocessed antigens and therefore are capable of binding soluble molecules and other extracellular microbial components.

Antibodies exist in 5 classes, IgA, IgG, IgM, IgD and IgE (Table 1). Each immunoglobulin molecule contains two identical heavy chains that each comprise a constant region that defines the class and a variable region that contains the antigen-binding domains. Two identical light chains, (either kappa or lambda) each with a constant region

Table 1. Immunoglobulin classes and subclasses

	IgM	IgG1	IgG2	IgG3	IgG4	IgA	IgD	IgE
Primary location	Membrane; plasma	Plasma	Plasma	Plasma	Plasma	Mucosa, plasma	Membrane	Cell bound
Form	Pentamer	Monomer	Monomer	Monomer	Monomer	Mono – Dimer	Monomer	Monomer
Complement activation	++	++	+	++		+		
Fc R binding		+		+		+		+
ADCC		++		++				
Placental transfer		++	+	++	+/-			
Plasma levels[1]	.7-1.7	3.3-8.5	0.5-5.5	.1-1.2	.7-1.2	1.5-2.6	.04	.0003

[1] expressed in mg/mL

and a variable region that also participates in antigen binding complete the structure of an antibody molecule. Thus the basic antibody structure (Figure 1) comprises two identical heavy chains, and two identical light chains that result in a molecule capable of binding two identical antigens. The constant region of certain heavy chains (Fc portions of IgG, IgA and IgE) can bind to specific leukocyte receptors (Fc receptors) and the Fc portions of IgM, IgA and IgG1, IgG2 and IgG3 can also bind and activate complement.

IgD is predominantly expressed on the surface of B lymphocytes and is present in very low concentrations in serum. Membrane IgD is important in B cell activation.

IgM is expressed on the surface of B lymphocytes where its binding by antigen can trigger B cell activation. In serum IgM is found as a pentameric molecule (with 10 antigen-binding sites). IgM is a predominant immunoglobulin in infancy and also is the first immunoglobulin to be synthesized in many infections. Thus, the presence of IgM of a particular specificity in serum can be used to provide evidence for recent infection by that agent. IgM can activate complement.

IgG is the most prevalent immunoglobulin class in serum comprising approximately 75% of all immunoglobulins. IgG exists in monomeric form and is comprised of four subclasses, IgG_1, IgG_2, IgG_3, and IgG_4. Both IgG_1 and IgG_3 can bind to leukocyte Fc receptors and IgG1, IgG2 and IgG3 can activate complement when aggregated or complexed to antigens.

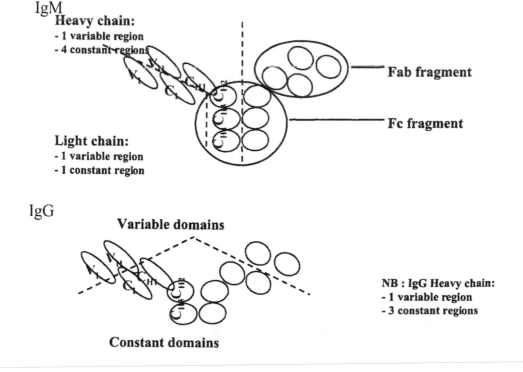

Figure 1.   Structure of prototypic antibody molecule.

IgA exists both in monomeric and dimeric form. IgA comprises only about 15% of serum immunoglobulins but is the predominant immunoglobulin class in mucosal surfaces and secretions. Thus this species of antibody often provides key defenses against microbial invasion. Dimeric IgA is transported to mucosal surfaces from the lamina propria through epithelial cells by a process of transcytosis.

IgE molecules can bind to specific Fc receptors on mast cells and basophils and mediate immediate-type hypersensitivity reactions through the induction of cellular degranulation and release of vasoactive products. IgE is found in very low levels in plasma and exists primarily bound to mast cells and basophil Fc receptors. Activated eosinophils also can bind IgE. In collaboration with eosinophils, IgE may play an important role in defense against multicellular parasites.

The variable regions of antibody molecules are capable of enormous diversity in structure and hence antigen recognition. An estimated 10^8 possible antigen-binding structures can be generated through rearrangement of the multiple variable (V), joining (J) genes for light chains and variable, joining and diversity (D) genes for heavy chains [15]. In addition, somatic mutation of these genes during B cell maturation may contribute to enhanced affinity of these molecules for antigen binding.

Although some antigens (particularly those with repetitive motifs such as bacterial polysaccharides) may elicit antibodies "independently" of T cell help, immunoglobulin responses to most antigens are enhanced when related peptides are recognized by CD4+ T cells after binding and presentation by class II MHC antigens on the B lymphocyte surface. Activation of T helper cells and binding of these cells to B lymphocytes results in the generation of helper cytokines and intercellular signals that enhance B cell proliferation, differentiation and immunoglobulin production. Exposure to these cytokines and cellular interactions determine the class of antibody that is produced in response to stimulation.

Antibody molecules may facilitate antiviral host defenses through several mechanisms:

1. Neutralization. Antibodies may bind to critical viral components, blocking their ability to interact with host elements needed for productive infection either directly or through induction of conformational changes.
2. Opsonization. Antibodies may bind to viruses and enhance phagocytosis through Fc-receptor mediated phagocytosis.
3. Complement activation . Antibodies bound to viral components may activate complement enzymes that neutralize or opsonize virus particles.
4. Agglutination. Antibodies may bind and agglutinate viruses thereby promoting their clearance.
5. Antibody-mediated cellular cytotoxicity (ADCC). Antibodies directed against viral antigens that are expressed on the surface of an infected cell when bound to Fc receptors on natural killer (NK) cells can activate the NK cell to lyse the virus infected target cell.

Antibodies also may facilitate viral replication by enhancing uptake of viruses into cells where they can replicate or they may enhance the morbidity of viral disease.

Generation of Antibody Responses

As is the case for T lymphocyte activation, generation of antibody responses generally takes place in lymphoid tissues: lymph nodes, spleen and gut-associated lymphoid tissue [16].

The B Lymphocyte Antigen Receptor Is an Immunoglobulin Molecule That Activates the B Cell When Bound By Antigen

Each B lymphocyte expresses surface immunoglobulin (IgM and IgD) with a shared antigen binding structure that is the consequence of genetic rearrangement (above). When antigen is recognized and bound to surface immunoglobulin, signals are transmitted to activate the cell and the antigen is then ingested. Even particles as large as viruses whose surface proteins can be bound by antibody can be ingested, degraded and peptides are then transported to the cell surface bound to class II MHC molecules.

By Presenting Class II MHC-bound Peptide Antigen to T Helper Cells, B Cell Activation Is Enhanced by the Action Of T Helper Cytokines and CD40:CD40 Ligand Interactions

At this point, the peptide: MHC complex can be recognized by a CD4+ T helper cell with the appropriate T cell receptor structure [17]. Activation of the T cell receptor by this interaction results in the elaboration of T helper cytokines that together with binding of B cell CD40 by T cell CD40 ligand result in enhanced B cell activation [18]. Directed release of the T helper cytokine interleukin-4 (IL-4) helps to drive clonal expansion of the activated B lymphocyte.

Differential Transcription of Heavy Chain Constant Region Genes Driven By Different Cytokines Results in "Isotype Switching" But Unchanged Antigen-combining Regions

Differential expression of cytokines can determine the predominant isotypes of secreted immunoglobulins. Antibody molecules secreted by a B lymphocyte and its progeny express only a single antigen binding region, however isotype switching as a result of exposure to different cytokines results in the maturation of B lymphocytes to express immunoglobulin molecules of specific isotypes. This relationship has been best studied in mouse systems where IL-4 enhances switching to IgG1 and IgE production, IL-5 induces expression of IgA molecules, interferon gamma induces expression of IgG2a and IgG3, and transforming growth factor beta (TGFb) induces expression of IgG2b and IgA. This is effected by cytokine-induced activation of transcription of messenger RNA for specific heavy chain constant regions resulting in the emergence of antibody molecules with the same variable regions and hence antigen-binding domains as were present in the founder B cell but with different heavy chain constant regions resulting in different immunoglobulin isotypes [19].

High Level B Lymphocyte Proliferation in Lymphoid Germinal Centers and High
Frequency Somatic Mutations Result in the Evolution of B Lymphocyte Clones With
Enhanced Affinity for Antigen

After naïve B lymphocytes are activated by T helper cells some will mature into IgM or IgG secreting plasma cells that provide the early serum antibody response while others move to primary follicles in the lymph nodes. Within the primary follicles are follicular dendritic cells that are capable of prolonged binding of intact antigens including whole viruses on the surface of long specialized tendrils. In this antigen-enriched environment, B lymphocytes are activated by antigen and by binding CD23 on the follicular dendritic cell surface to undergo many rounds of cell division resulting in the development of the germinal center. In this site, with each cellular division, immunoglobulin variable regions of the rapidly dividing B lymphocytes tend to accumulate mutations at a rate of approximately one per thousand bases (in contrast to an error rate of approximately one per 10^{12} bases in other somatic cells). As a result of this somatic hypermutation, B lymphocytes with higher affinity for antigen are more likely to expand resulting in the selective expansion of cell populations producing increasingly high affinity antibodies [20].

As Virus-reactive B Cells Multiply, Their Secreted Immunoglobulins Are Detected
in Serum

Within a week after exposure to viral antigens, antiviral antibodies can generally be detected. IgM antibodies are the first to appear in serum and these are later replaced by IgG antiviral antibodies (Figure 2). The delay in the appearance of a measurable antibody response is related to the time needed to amplify the mass of antigen-reactive immunoglobulin secreting B cells and plasma cells. Likewise, T cell responses to primary viral infection can be first detected within the first week after infection. These delays underscore the importance of innate host defenses (above) that are needed to contain viral infection before more targeted adaptive immune responses are generated.

After expansion and maturation, B cells differentiate into effector plasma cells (short-lived antibody factories) or memory B cells that can be activated upon later exposure to antigen to divide and result in a rapid and high level (secondary) immune response.

Plasma cells with a rich rough endoplasmic reticulum are highly specialized cells designed to constitutively secrete high levels of antibody. As terminally differentiated cells, plasma cells eventually die thereby regulating the duration of antibody production after primary exposure. Memory B cells on the other hand, retain the ability to be activated after antigen exposure. Upon later re-exposure to antigen, memory B cells can quickly divide and differentiate, providing a rapid and amplified response to antigen. This **anamnestic** (memory) response protects persons from many second rounds of infection with viruses and also is the underpinning for the effectiveness of immunization strategies.

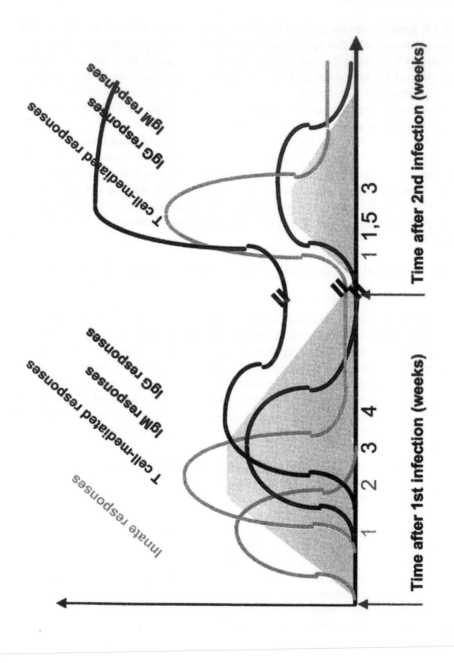

Figure 2. Timing of immune response.

Certain B Cell Antigens Can Activate B Cells to Produce Antibody in the Absence of Cognate T Cell Help But These Responses are in Part T Cell Dependant Responses to these T Cell "Independent" Antigens Can Be Amplified If the T Cell Independent Antigen is Complexed with an Immunodominant peptide

Some microbial antigens – particularly repetitive polysaccharides may activate B cells directly by cross linking multiple immunoglobulin receptors to produce antibody in the absence of T cell help. In the instance of repetitive polysaccharides, primarily mature B cells are activated and although antibody can be synthesized the absence of help, T helper cytokines augment the magnitude of antibody production by these cells. Thus, persons with T cell immunodeficiency (eg HIV infection) tend to have poor responses to immunization with T cell "independent" polysaccharide vaccines. Cognate T cell help can be provided by conjugating the polysaccharide antigen to an immunogenic peptide. B cell ingestion of the peptide/polysaccharide complex results in presentation of the peptide to T helper cells by MHC class II antigens. The cognate T cell help provided by this interaction as outlined above results in an amplified B cell response. Thus, B cell epitopes that are targets for antibody recognition need not contain peptide epitopes for T helper activation as long as they are present in the same ingested molecule or particle. Thus, conjugation of bacterial polysaccharides to immunodominant peptides can provide a more effective vaccine for antibody generation than polysaccharide vaccines alone and such conjugate vaccines have been used to generate high level antibody responses to conjugated bacterial polysaccharides even in young children..

Cell Mediated Immune Defenses

Cellular immune defenses are mediated primarily by T lymphocytes. CD4+ T lymphocytes provide helper cytokines that may augment the activity of numerous effector cells including cytotoxic T lymphocytes (CTL) that are the main mediators of antiviral activity.

Cytotoxic T Lymphocytes (CTL) Exquisitely Recognize Virus-infected Cells

Cytotoxic CD8 T cells are the major cellular component of adaptive host immune defenses against viruses. Viruses multiply in the cytoplasm of infected cells where they are not accessible to antibodies and can be eliminated only by the destruction of their infected niche. The elimination of infected cells requires specific recognition and the powerful and accurately targeted cytotoxic machinery of CD8 T cells. CD8+ cytotoxic T lymphocytes (CTL) recognize antigens derived from replicating virus on the surface of infected cells and kill the cell before viral replication is complete. The critical role of CTL in limiting virus infection is suggested by increased susceptibility of animals depleted of CD8 T cells, or of individuals who lack MHC class I molecules that are needed to present viral antigens to T cells [21].

CD4+ and CD8+ T lymphocytes are cells of thymic origin that display αβ TCR and when matured, either the CD4 or CDD8 cell surface molecule. T cells recognize short amino acid sequences called epitopes that are often buried in the native protein, only when bound to the appropriate host cell MHC molecule. Viral peptides first undergo degradation or "processing" within specific intra-cellular compartments. MHC class I and MHC class II molecules have a distinct distribution among cells: MHC class I molecules present to CD8 cytotoxic T cells, peptides from intra-cellular pathogens that are synthetized in the cytosol whereas MHC class II molecules present ingested peptides that are generally synthesized outside the ingesting cell and degraded within phagosomes and present these digested peptides to CD4+ T cells. Thus, the CD8 molecule binds a non polymorphic region of the MHC class I molecule while CD4 binds homologous regions on MHC class II molecules.

Whereas class II MHC molecules are expressed primarily on specialized antigen presenting cells such as skin Langerhans cells, macrophages, thymic epithelial cells, B lymphocytes and activated T cells, all nucleated cells express MHC class I molecules and thus viruses infecting these cells can be recognized by CTL once viral peptides are synthesized, bound by class I MHC molecules and expressed on the cell surface [22] (Figure 3). Non-nucleated cells, such as red blood cells, express little or no MHC class I, and can, in principle, be a sanctuary for viruses such as the equine infectious anemia virus of horses. As viral proteins are synthesized using cellular machinery, polypeptide precursors enter the proteasome, where they are cleaved into small peptides 8-10 amino-acids in length. These peptides are collected and transported into the endoplasmic reticulum by specific transporter TAP proteins that are encoded in the MHC locus. MHC class I molecules bind newly synthesized peptide as an integral part of the MHC molecular structure; thus a foreign or non-host derived peptide in this cell-surface groove indicates that the cell is "infected" by an exogenous agent that is synthesizing protein.

Most peptides that bind to MHC molecules have anchor residues that bind to specific amino acid residues within the MHC locus; a single amino acid change at any anchor site can prevent the peptide from binding. In order to adapt to multiple antigenic sequences the class I and the class II MHC molecules contain regions that are highly variable. The MHC locus encodes for three sorts of class I MHC molecules: A, B and C. The MHC class II locus comprises three kinds of class II molecules: DR, DP and DQ (the TAP peptide transporter genes and the LMP genes that encode the proteasomes are also within this locus). The DR cluster may encode another chain that may pair with the chain resulting in three class I antigen presenting molecules and as many as four class II antigen presenting molecules per haplotype. In the human population, these genes are highly polymorphous, with more than 200 alleles for the class I B locus and the class II DR locus. With chromosomal contributions from each parent, heterozygosity at each locus is common. Thus although these loci can restrict the peptides that can be bound at these sites, in any individual, there is a substantial diversity of peptide binding MHC antigens and within the human population, the diversity of antigen binding potential is enormous. This enormous diversity may permit a species to recognize a great diversity of foreign peptides; however the structure of the MHC molecule in any individual limits or "restricts" any individual's ability to recognize a specific peptide.

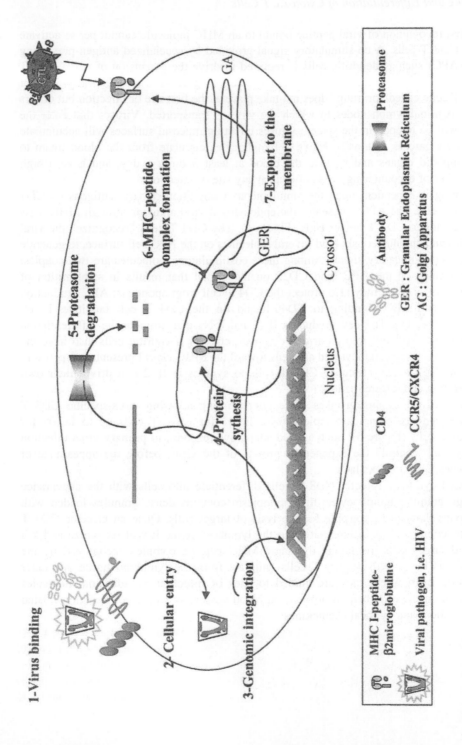

Figure 3. Antigen processing in an HIV-infected cell and presentation to MHC-I restricted CTL.

Priming and Differentiation of Cytotoxic T Cells

The first recognition of viral peptide bound to an MHC molecule cannot per se activate naive CD8 T cells. A co-stimulatory signal provided by specialized antigen-presenting cells (APC) such as dendritic cells is required to drive the expansion of naive CD8 T cells and their differentiation into armed effectors (Figure 4). This initial activation of naive T cells called "priming" does not take place at the first site of infection but occurs in the regional lymph nodes to which the virus is transported. Viruses that enter the blood will be trapped in the spleen; viruses infecting mucosal surfaces will accumulate in Peyer's patches or tonsils. Naive T lymphocytes circulate from the bloodstream to the lymphoid organs and back to the blood at least 3 times a day, and have a high probability of encountering viral antigens at any site of infection.

Priming is dependent upon the simultaneous recognition of viral antigens by CD4 T helper cells. The APC "presents" the endocytosed viral antigens through MHC class II molecules to CD4 T helper cells (Figure 4). The CD4 T cells "recognize" the viral peptides and simultaneously bind several molecules on the APC cell surface, to generate a potent co-stimulatory signal. Among these costimulatory molecules are two couples: B7 molecules on the APC bind CD28 on the T cell that results in stabilization of cytokine mRNA and may also protect the CD4 T cell from apoptosis; APC production of IL-12 and CD40 binding to CD40-ligand on the CD4 T cell facilitate T cell differentiation to a Th1 cell producing IL-2 and IFNγ that promote the differentiation of the naïve CD8 cell into an armed cytotoxic effector. Dendritic cells also have the capacity to re-direct endocytosed antigens toward the MHC-class I presentation pathway and can also directly stimulate CD8 T cells to synthesize IL-2 that drives their own proliferation and differentiation.

Major clonal expansion takes place after priming allowing virus-specific CD8 T cells frequencies to increase rapidly from $1x10^{-6}$ for naïve T cells up to $1x10^{-1}$ for effector T cells (Figure 5). Such a rapid adaptative response to primary virus infection usually can "control" the exponential growth of the virus, before the appearance of antibodies, 2 or 3 weeks later.

Armed cytotoxic effector CD8 T cells differentiate into cells with the appearance of large granular lymphocytes; their cytoplasm contains dense granules loaded with cytotoxins that are responsible for the lysis of target cells. Once an effector CD8 T cell has completed its differentiation in the lymphoid tissue it will recognize and kill infected target cells displaying the same MHC peptide complex recognized by the T cell's TCR. Armed effector T cells emigrate from the lymphoid tissue and enter the blood from where they are guided to sites of infection by adhesion molecules expressed on the endothelium of the local blood vessels as a result of infection-related inflammation, and by local chemokines.

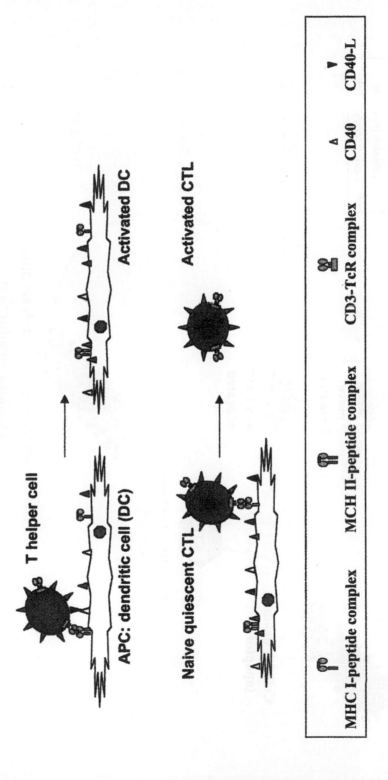

After a first contact and through CD40-CD40L interaction, the APC is activated and can further transform a naive quiescent CTL into a potential killer CTL

T helper cell

APC: dendritic cell (DC)

Activated DC

Naive quiescent CTL

Activated CTL

MHC I-peptide complex   MCH II-peptide complex   CD3-TcR complex   CD40   CD40-L

Figure 4. Priming of naive CTL: role of CD4+ helper lymphocytes (Th) and antigen presenting cells (APC).

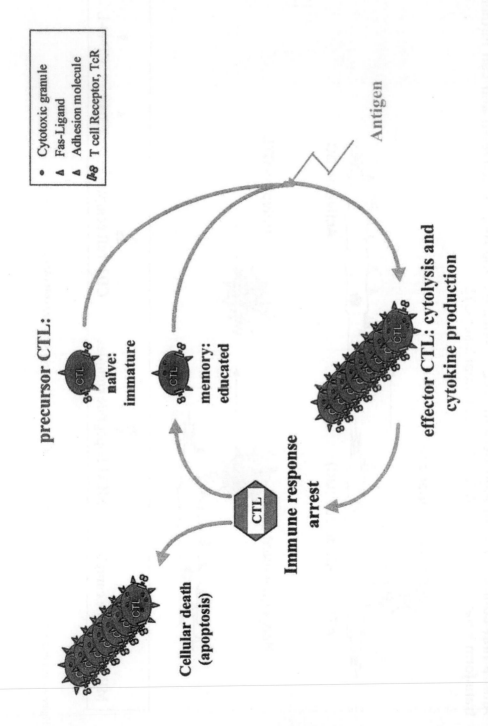

Figure 5.   Different activation stages of a cytotoxic T lymphocyte.

T Cell Mediated Cytotoxicity Mediates Killing of Host Cells Expressing Foreign (Viral) Peptides

The Lethal Kiss

To kill virus-infected cells the TCR of the CD8 effector CTL must first recognize and bind the peptide/MHC complex. Ligation of The antigen-specific TCR and of various adhesion molecules induce stable binding of CD8 effector cells to target cells. These molecules concentrate at the binding region and create a very narrow space resembling a synapse. This process - called "The lethal kiss" - results in the formation of a "conjugate" between The killer cell and its target. TCR ligation will then activate the cell To release effector molecules and will focus their delivery at the site of contact. Effector T-cell activity is thus highly selective for target cells that express antigenic peptides, although the effector molecules themselves are not antigen-specific.

Cytotoxic T Lymphocytes are Serial Killers

CD8 cytotoxic T cells kill by releasing specialized lytic granules upon recognition of antigen on the surface of the target cell. These granules are modified liposomes that contain at least two distinct classes of cytotoxins. **Perforin** polymerizes To generate transmembrane pores in the target cell through which serine proteases called **granzymes** can enter and induce target cell apoptosis [23].

A single cytotoxic T cells acts as a serial killer and can rapidly kill many targets in succession. Indeed lytic granules store inactive forms of cytotoxins which are synthesized on the first encounter of a naive cytotoxic precursor T cell with specific antigen. Ligation of the T–cell receptor similarly induces de novo synthesis of perforin and granzymes in armed effector CD8 cells, so that the supply of lytic granules is replenished.

The release of granule content accounts for most the cytotoxic activity of CD8 effector T cells, as shown by the loss of most killing activity in perforin gene knock-out mice [24]. Some CD4 T cells are also capable of killing other cells, yet do not contain granules and make neither perforin nor granzymes. Membrane proteins of activated CD8T cells and some CD4 effector T cells can also activate apoptosis. A membrane-bound molecule, **Fas ligand**, expressed by activated CD8 and CD4 T cells is also capable of inducing apoptosis by binding to **Fas** on target cells. The nucleases activated by this mechanism can degrade viral DNA as well as cellular DNA. This prevents the assembly of virions and thus the release of virus and infection of nearby cells. Cytotoxic CD8 T cells also produce IFN-γ, which is an inhibitor of viral replication and an important inducer of MHC class I expression and macrophage activation.

Cytotoxic T cells thus can kill virus infected targets with great precision, sparing normal cells and minimizing tissue damage, while allowing the eradication of infected cells. Viruses responsible for acute cytolytic infections are rapidly cleared after primary infection. In contrast infection with HIV generates an adaptive CD8 T cell response that contains the virus at time of primary infection but cannot eradicate infection. Evidence for destruction of HIV-infected cells by CTLs comes from infected individuals in whom cytotoxic T cells specific for HIV peptides can directly kill infected cells *in vitro*. The CD8 T cell clones specific for various HIV peptides can comprise a sufficient proportion of the CD8 cell population to result in a biased TCR repertoire, and have been shown to infiltrate infected lymphoïd tissues where replication of HIV takes place. In addition CD8 T cells producing large amounts of IFN-γ are also detected at the site of virus production in lymphoïd tissues, suggesting that elimination of infected cells by cytotoxic CD8 T cells occurs concurrently with viral replication.

Once viral infection is cleared, lack of antigenic stimulation provokes the death of the vast majority of effector CD8 T cells, while some survive and return to a semi-quiescent status of memory T cells. Such memory T cells will rapidly reexpand in a few days during next exposure to virus-infected cells; together with memory B cells, thus ensure protection against viral recurrences [25, 26].

Potent Immune Defenses Have Imposed On Viruses the Need To Escape Immune Surveillance in Order To Survive

Immune Escape by Antigenic Variation

A virus can evade immune surveillance by altering its antigen sequences. Viral escape by mutation is typical of the **influenza** virus: a single virus type, responsible for worldwide epidemics to which the human population has developed protective immunity, is at risk for a shortage of susceptible hosts. Antigenic drift caused by point mutations in the genes encoding hemagglutinin and neuraminidase affect epitopes recognized by T cells. Antigenic shift occurs as a result of reassortment of the segmented RNA genome of the influenza virus in an animal host, leading to major changes in hemagglutinin protein structure. The resulting virus is recognized poorly by antibodies and memory T cells directed at the previous variant, so that most people are highly susceptible to the new virus.

In **hepatitis B** virus infection and in **HIV** infection, certain viruses express mutant peptides that can compete with the binding of wild type peptide thus antagonizing the antiviral activities of CTL [28]. Similar mutant peptides may contribute to the persistence of viral infections where the immune response is dominated by T cells specific for a particular immunodominant epitope.

Some Viruses Can Escape Immune Defenses by Latency

Some viruses such as Herpes viruses can enter a state of latency in which virus is not transcriptionally active. These non replicating latent viruses do not produce viral proteins and peptides and are therefore not detected by T cells. In these latent states, the virus does not cause disease but cannot be eliminated. A quiescent CD4+ T cell infected by HIV harbars a transcriplicnally inactive inactive prouval DNA that behaves as a "Trojan horse" and cannot be eliminated until the T cell becomes activated. Such latent infections can be reactivated, thus resulting in recurrent illness in the case of herpes viruses and may provide a "reservoir" of infected cells that are unaffected by antiviral drugs as in the case of HIV.

After an effective immune response controls epithelial infection, **Herpes simplex virus** persists in a latent state in sensory neurons. Neurons display very low levels of MHC class I molecules making them less susceptible to CD8 T cell recognition. Physical stresses, sun exposure or bacterial infections can reactivate the virus which re-infects epithelial tissues and reactivates the immune response which in turn kills the epithelial cells, producing a new sore. **Varicella zoster** also remains latent in dorsal root ganglia after acute illness. Stress or immunosuppression can reactivate the virus which spreads down the nerve and infects the regional skin, creating the characteristic dermatomal vesicular rash.

Some Viruses Have Developed Multiple Mechanisms to Escape Host Defenses

HIV is an example of a virus that has developed numerous other mechanisms: high mutation rate, and immunosuppression, that may permit escape from host immune defenses. First replication of the HIV genome depends upon the transcription of viral genomic RNA into DNA by an error-prone reverse transcriptase. This enzyme's high mutation rate rapidly results in infection with numerous quasispecies within any infected individual. Thus in response to selection pressures of host defenses, HIV is capable of emerging new epitopes that are not recognized by pre-existing cytotoxic T cells. Most of these mutant peptides however are still immunogenic and induce a new generation of specific CD8 T cells that in turn may control these new variants [29]. Adaptation of immune defenses to virus variability more likely occurs during asymptomatic infection when sufficient functional CD4 T helper cells are present to support immune defenses. The selective pressure mediated by CD8 T cells in non progressors shapes the quasi-species emerging in a single individual. This constant race between viral variation may in time exhaust the CD8 T cell repertoire and in most persons immune defenses fail in time to contain infection. As HIV induces progressive decreases in circulating CD4+ T lymphocyte numbers and function, virus-induced immune deficiency also contributes to the success of HIV replication. In this regard both HIV-induced cytolysis and the immunosuppressive effects of viral proteins such as Tat that induces programmed cell death and Nef that decreases expression of class I MHC antigens may contribute to impaired host defenses in HIV disease.

Laboratory Methods for Diagnosis and Management of Viral Diseases

Basic Principles Of Antibody Measurement And the Utility Of Antibodies in the Diagnosis And Management Of Viral Diseases

Laboratory assays can be designed to measure specific antibody levels by capitalizing on the specificity of antibody antigen binding. The detection of specific antibodies to viral constituents can both be used to establish a diagnosis of infection and also may confirm immunity to infection if protective antibody types and levels can be identified.

Enzyme linked immunosorbent assay (ELISA or EIA) for measurement of antiviral antibodies. In a simple form of this assay, viral antigen is bound to a plastic well and antibody binding to antigen is detected after washing non-bound antibodies from the well by the addition of antibodies that recognize human immunoglobulin band to the antigen-antibody complex. Covalent attachment of an enzyme such as alkaline phosphatase to the antihuman antibody permits identification of wells containing human antibodies by placing in the well a substrate of the enzyme whose colored product can be measured by light absorption. In the related **radioimmunoassay** (RIA), a radioisotope substitutes for the enzyme and bound antibody is detected by measuring radioactivity. Similar techniques also can be used to measure antigen molecules. Using the **sandwich** technique, antibodies are bound to the solid plastic support and sample containing antigen is incubated in the wells. After unbound molecules are washed off, an enzyme-linked or radioactive labeled developing antibody to the antigen is then placed in the well and binding of the antibody is measured as above. This technique assumes that the antigen is multivalent and works best if the two sandwich antibodies recognize different non-overlapping epitopes. **Competition** assays whereby the binding to antibody of labeled antigen can be displaced by antigen within an unknown sample can be used to quantitate viral antigens.

Western blotting can be used to identify antibodies reactive with viral antigens of different size. Using this technique, preparations containing disrupted viral antigens are incubated in the ionic detergent sodium dodecyl sulfate (SDS) and are permitted to migrate through a polyacrylamide gel through which an electric current is run. Proteins are separated on this gel by size and are then transferred to nitrocellulose paper. Incubation of the paper strips with test serum and then with enzyme-linked anti-human antibodies results in the visual detection of bands that represent viral proteins bound by the human antibodies in the test serum. Western blotting is routinely used to confirm a diagnosis of HIV infection.

Neutralization assays measure the ability of human serum containing antibodies to block the ability of viruses to infect susceptible cells. These more complex biologic assays are performed by incubating virus stocks with varying dilutions of serum and identifying those dilutions of serum that block the ability of virus to propagate in the test cells. Although these assays measure a biologic activity of antibody as opposed to simple antigen binding that is measured in the ELISA and Western Blot, these assays are difficult to standardize and are performed only for research purposes.

Serologic Assays for Diagnosis of Infection

Measurement of serum antibodies is often used clinically to diagnose or to determine susceptibility or resistance to infection. The presence of IgM antibodies or a rising or falling titer of IgG antibodies generally indicates recent infection. (Use of an isotype specific secondary antibody in the ELISA can be used to identify antibody isotypes). High levels of antibodies are generally detectable in serum within 2 to 6 weeks after infection with most viruses. For some viral infections such as Hepatitis C infection, antibodies to viral antigens are indicative of ongoing infection and antiviral antibodies are generally not detectable after viral infection is resolved. For other viral infections such as Hepatitis B virus, sufficient levels of antibodies to certain viral antigens (surface antigen) are suggestive of immunity to infection whereas antibodies to other antigens (core antigen) develop after infection is acquired and persist during acute and chronic infection and after infection is resolved (Figure 2).

Methods for Measuring Virus-specific Cytotoxic CD8 T Lymphocytes

The ⁵¹chromium release assay (CRA) is the traditional functional method which permits evaluation of virus-specific CTL activity . Target cells, loaded with ⁵¹Cr, are incubated with effector cells to permit binding and conjugate formation. The lysed target cell releases the radioactive chromium into the culture supernatant where its measurement reflects effector CTL lytic potential. To increase the sensitivity of these assays, it is usually necessary to expand the eCTL population *in vitro* prior to the CRA. Thus enumeration of eCTL is not possible unless cells are expanded in a limiting dilution assay (LDA). The LDA method, which is technically demanding and notoriously gives variable results, is based on the assumption that eCTL can divide and will not die by apoptosis as most activated cell do. Nevertheless, this test has been the standard to estimate virus-specific memory CTL numbers.

Three recent major technical advances have provided novel insights into CD8+ T cell responses to viruses (Figure 6). The **"tetramer"-staining** technique, developed by Altman et al. allows direct enumeration of peptide-specific CD8+ T lymphocytes by binding the peptide-reactive TCR with a fluorochrome-coupled complex composed of four MHC class I molecules, each loaded with an antigenic peptide. Tetramer binding to the CTL does not require *in vitro* pre-stimulation and is evaluated by flow cytometry (Figure 6), thereby allowing multiparametric characterization of the phenotype of antigen-specific lymphocytes as well as purification by cell-sorting. Two other methods measure CD8 T cell cytokine production after antigenic stimulation. The first technique, called **ELISPOT** (Enzyme-Linked Immuno-Spot) assay, enumerates cells that secrete a cytokine (usually IFN-γ) after an 6 to 24 hour *in vitro* stimulation: the IFN-γ produced is immobilized on a filter and spots representing cytokine producing effector cells are identified using a capture system similar to the one used in ELISA assays (see above). The other technique measures **intracellular cytokine production** (usually FN-γ) after a 6-18 hour antigenic stimulation and pharmacologic blockade of extracellular secretion. After cell permeabilization and staining with fluorochrome labeled antibodies to the cytokine, cells are analyzed by FACS. Analysis using multicolor flow cytometry also permits the simultaneous characterization of the phenotype of the antigen-specific cytokine producing cell. MHC-peptide tetramer staining accurately estimates the size of effector/ activated memory CTL population expanded *in vivo*, which is often higher, than the numbers of functional T cells measured by the two other methods.

Using these 3 new methods, experiments with lymphocytic choriomeningitis virus (LCMV) or influenza virus in mice have shown that the eCTL compartment size is 10 to 50-fold larger than results of LDA had previously suggested. Thus up to 70% of splenic CD8 T cells are LCMV-specific during acute infection, these numbers decrease after control of virus replication. In humans, similar ranges of effector cell frequencies were reported during acute EBV infection, while in chronic HIV infection as many as 0.1 to 5% of CD8 cells may bind a single HIV peptide. These revolutionary

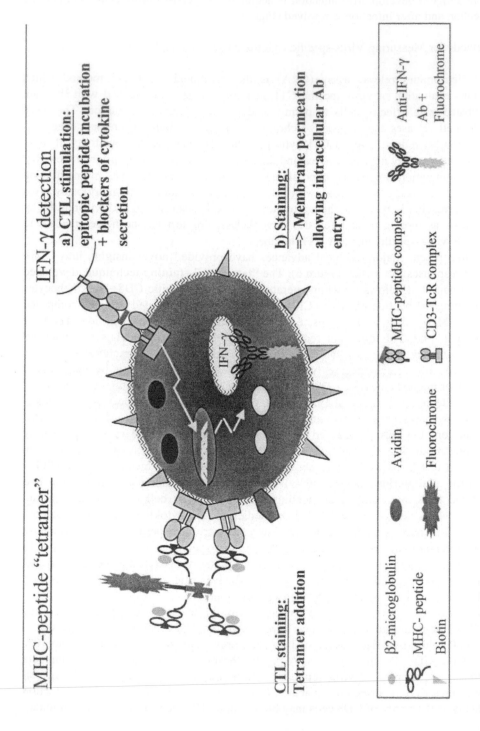

Figure 6.   CTL enumeration by flow cytometry.

methods have thus demonstrated that most of the CD8 cell bursts observed during virus infection are due to *in vivo* expansion of virus-specific CD8 cells.

Methods to Measure CD4+ T Cell Responses to Viral Infection

As CD4+ T cells can respond to exogenously expressed viral antigens taken up by and presented by class II MHC antigens in phagocytic cells, assays of **lymphocyte proliferation** in response to exogenously added viral proteins have been used to detect CD4+ T cell recognition of viral peptides. In these assays, preparations of peripheral blood mononuclear cells containing responder CD4+ T cells and monocytes as antigen presenting cells are incubated in microwells to which are added whole inactivated virus or virus-derived proteins. Five to six days of incubation with antigen result in multiple rounds of cellular division and expansion resulting in sufficient numbers of dividing cells to generate a signal by incorporation of radioactive thymidine into the DNA of proliferating cells. This assay does not permit enumeration of the frequency of reactive cells but high levels of thymidine incorporation reflect the presence of memory cells reactive with viral antigens. **ELISPOT** assays and flow cytometric assays for **intracellular cytokine** expression also can be used to enumerate the frequency of CD4 cells reactive to viral antigens as discussed above.

References

1. Janeway CA. The immune system evolved to discriminate between infectious monself from non infectious self. Immunol. Today 1992; 13: 11-16.
2. MacMicking J, Xie QW, and Nathan C, Nitric oxide and macrophage function. Annu Rev Immunol 1997; 15: 323-50.
3. Lanier LL, Phillips JH. Evidence for three types of human cytotoxic lymphocytes. Immunol Today 1986; 7: 132
4. Biron, CA, Byron KS and Sullivan JL, Severe herpesvirus infections in an adolescent without natural killer cells. N Engl J Med 1989; 320(26): 1731-5.
5. Lanier LL. NK receptors. Ann Rev Immunol 1998; 16: 359-393.
6. Haas W, Pereira P, Tonegawa S. γδ cells. Annu Rev Immunol 1993; 11: 637-685.
7. Muller U, et al., Functional role of type I and type II interferons in antiviral defense. Science 1994; 264(5167): 1918-21.
8. Biron CA. Role of early cytokines including α and β interferons in innate and adaptive immune responses to viral infections. Semin Immunol 1998; 10: 383-390.
9. Fearon DT, Locksley RM. The instructive role of innate immunity in the acquired immune response. Science 1996; 272: 50-53.
10. Baringa M. Virus launch their own "star wars" by stealing genes and turning key immune-system proteins against the host, viral invaders have learned to elude the body's attacks. Science 1992; 258: 1730-31.
11. Smith GL, Virus proteins that bind cytokines, chemokines or interferons. Curr Opin Immunol 1996; 8(4): 467-71.
12. Moore KW, Vieira P, Fiorentino DF, Trounstine ML, Kahn TA, Mosmann TR. Homology of cytokine

synthesis inhibitory factor (IL10) to the Epstein-Barr virus gene BCRF1. Science 1990; 248: 1230-34.

13. Nelson PJ, Krensky AM. Chemokines, lymphocytes and viruses: what goes around comes around. Curr Opin Immunol 1998; 19: 265-70.

14. Cocchi, F, et al., Identification of RANTES, MIP-1 alpha, and MIP-1 beta as the major HIV-suppressive factors produced by CD8+ T cells. Science 1995; 270(5243): 1811-5.

15. Fanning, LJ, Connor AM, Wu GE. Development of the immunoglobulin repertoire. Clin Immunol Immunopathol 1996; 790: 1-14.

16. Szakal AK, Kosco MH and Tew JG. Microanatomy of lymphoid tissue during humoral immune responses: structure function relationships. Annu Rev Immunol 1989; 7: 91-109.

17. Parker DC. T-cell dependent B-cell activation. Annu Rev Immunol 1993; 11: 331-340.

18. Foy TM, Aruffo A, Bajorath J, Buhlmann JE, Noelle RJ. Immune regulation by CD40 and its ligand gp39. Annu Rev Immunol 1996; 14: 591-617.

19. Stavnezer J. Immunoglobulin class switching. Curr Opin Immunol 1996; 8: 199-205.

20. Neuberger MS, Milstein C. Somatic hypermutation. Curr Opin Immunol 1995; 7: 248-254.

21. Zinkernagel RM and Doherty PC. H-2 compatibility requirement for T-cell mediated lysis of target cells infected with lymphocytic choriomeningitis virus. J Exp Med 1975; 141: 1427-36.

22. Townsend ARM, Gotch FM and Davey J. Cytotoxic T cells recognize fragments of influenza nucleoprotein. Cell 1985; 42: 457-67.

23. Berke G. The functions and mechanisms of action of cytolytic lymphocytes. In Fundamental Immunology. Ed WE Paul, p. 965-1015.

24. Zinkernagel RM. Immunity to viruses. In Fundamental Immunology. Ed WE Paul 1999; 1211-51.

25. Sprent J and B memory cells. Cell 1994; 76: 315-322.

26. Ahmed R, Biron CA. Immunity to viruses. Fundamental Immunology. Ed. WE Paul, p 1295-1334.

27. Zinkernagel RM. Immunology taught by viruses. Science 1996; 271: 173-78.

28. Chisari FV, Ferrari C. Hepatitis B virus immunopathogenesis. Annu Rev Immunol 1995; 13: 29-60.

29. Autran B, Hadida F, Haas G. Evolution and plasticity of CTL responses against HIV. Current Opinion Immunol 1996; 8: 546-53.

Janeway CA, Travers P, Walport M, Capra JD. Immunobiology: The immune system in health and disease. Fourth Edition. Current Biology.

Mandel B. Neitralization of polio virus: a hypothesis to explain the mechanism and one hit character of the neutralization reaction. Virology 1976; 69: 500-510.

Paul WE. Fundamental Immunology. Fourth Edition. Lippincott Raven, Philadelphia 1999.

Rinaldo, CR Jr., Modulation of major histocompatibility complex antigen expression by viral infection. Am J Pathol 1994; 144(4): 637-50.

Whitton JL and Oldstone MB. Immune response to viruses. Fields Virology. Third Edition. 1996; 345-374.

Zinkernagel RM and Hengartner H. Antiviral immunity. Immunol Today 1997; (18)6: 258-60.

CHAPTER 5

HUMAN IMMUNODEFICIENCY VIRUS

MARK HOLODNIY and VERONICA MILLER

Table of Contents

Introduction

Human Immunodeficiency Virus type 1 (HIV-1) causes progressive immunologic dysfunction through the destruction of T helper cells, leading to the development of opportunistic infections (OI), malignancies and death. HIV-1 is transmitted through sexual contact, parenteral exposure to infected blood, bodily fluids or blood products, and from mother to child (vertical transmission). Over 36 million people are infected with HIV around the world, with the greatest concentration in Sub-Saharan Africa. Over 16,000 new cases of HIV infection occur globally on a daily basis [1]. In the U.S.,

Practical Guidelines in Antiviral Therapy Ed. by Charles A.B. Boucher and George J. Galasso. 95 — 125
© 2002 *Elsevier Science. Printed in the Netherlands.*

an estimated 50,000 new cases of HIV infection occur per year, primarily in gay youth, women and people of color.

HIV is an enveloped RNA virus that is a member of the lentivirus subfamily of retroviruses. HIV RNA strands are10kb in length, and contain nine genes. These genes encode structural (*env* and *gag*), functional (*pol* including the protease, reverse transcriptase, and integrase enzymes), and regulatory (*rev, tat, nef, vif, vpr* and *vpu*) proteins. HIV-1 is divided into three major genetic types, which includes the M (Major), O (outlier) and the newly described N type [2, 3]. The M type includes several subtypes or clades (A-J, with subtype B being the most common in the US) with distinct geographical distribution patterns. The O type also includes 2 subtypes. Whether these strains are pathogenically different is the subject of much research, however, most data on HIV-1 is derived from M, subtype B viruses, which currently predominant in the U.S. and Europe.

The virus initiates infection through envelope glycoprotein (gp120) binding to CD4 and one or more chemokine co-receptor molecules (CXCR4, CCR5) on T lymphocytes, monocytes, macrophages or dendritic cells [4]. After internalization, HIV uses a viral reverse transcriptase (RT) and cellular polymerase to convert negative strand viral RNA to double stranded DNA, followed by integration into host cell DNA. These cells carry infection to lymphoid tissues where viral replication and amplification leads to viremia and dissemination throughout the body. Studies of the dynamics of HIV replication indicate that the rate is extremely high [5]. The error prone function of HIV-1 RT allows the generation of viral variants, which may be present in lymphoid tissues, the brain and body fluids including blood, semen, vaginal and cervical secretions, and breast milk. Variants may differ in drug sensitivity if specific protease or RT codon changes associated with altered drug susceptibility have taken place.

Infection is followed by an initial high level of viral replication, which decreases after 2-3 months associated with HIV specific CD8+ cytotoxic T cell (CTL) responses and B cell production of HIV specific antibodies [6]. CTL responses play a key role in control of HIV replication [7] and may determine the steady state of viral replication or "set point", which correlates directly with the rate of progression of disease to AIDS and death [8]. Recent studies have determined that despite clinical latency, viral replication is highly dynamic and continuous [9] and CD4 cell destruction occurs continuously in the absence of therapy. This ultimately results in the development of the acquired immunodeficiency syndrome (AIDS) and/or death.

As a preventive vaccine is not yet available, antiretroviral medications are of critical importance for prevention (as post exposure prophylaxis) as well as treatment of HIV infection. Despite the advent of highly active antiretroviral therapy (HAART), newly described findings suggest that viral eradication is not achievable with current treatment strategies. Although HAART is highly effective in lowering plasma HIV RNA levels (viral load) to undetectable levels (<50 copies/ml) and decreasing or discontinuing viral replication in lymphoid tissue within a few weeks of treatment initiation, HIV infected cells capable of producing replication competent virus that can subsequently infect T cells remain [10-12].

HAART also results in marked increases in CD4 count. Acute increases in memory T (CD45RO+) cells are observed within a few weeks of therapy, whereas naïve T cells

(CD45RA+), begin increasing slowly after several weeks [13]. The former is the result of redistribution of CD4 cells from lymphoid tissue into the periphery and the latter is the result of renewed thymic processing of new T cells. Immune reconstitution (as measured by proliferative or CTL responses) has been demonstrated primarily to recall antigens [14].

Clinical Diagnosis

Diagnosis of HIV infection can be challenging. The spectrum of presentation ranges from acutely or chronically infected adults to infants in the neonatal period. Diagnosis of HIV infection requires an assessment of risk factors, clinical presentation and the use of appropriate diagnostic tests. A few days to weeks after infection, fever, fatigue, lymphadenopathy, apthous oral ulcers, a macular truncal rash and other flu-like symptoms develop. Some patients may present with aseptic meningitis. This syndrome is known as the Acute Retroviral Syndrome (ARS) or Primary HIV Infection (PHI) [15]. Although some patients may be asymptomatic, the majority, experience a constellation of mild to moderate symptoms, requiring hospitalization in a few. The symptoms of 'acute HIV infection may be confused with other febrile illnesses or viral infections. Typical laboratory abnormalities may include: transient pancytopenia, (including CD4+ lymphopenia) and elevated serum transaminases. Symptoms may last for days to several weeks.

Most patients experience relatively good health during the next several months to few years. However, during this period of clinical latency, profound reductions in CD4 counts become evident. Minor diseases related to immune deficiency such as oral candidiasis, oral hairy leucoplakia, and constitutional symptoms such as fever and malaise can develop. This constellation of signs and symptoms has historically been referred to as the AIDS related complex (ARC). Continued viral replication and destruction of CD4 cells (below 200 cells/mm^3), leads to further loss of immune regulatory control, resulting in OIs such as Pneumocystis pneumonia (PCP), cytomegalovirus (CMV) retinitis, and malignancies including non-Hodgkin's lymphoma.

In the absence of treatment the median time of onset of clinical AIDS and death is 7 and 10 years respectively from infection. Specific HLA and chemokine receptor alleles are associated with progression rates. (I.e. CCR5 deletion mutations and MIP-1 levels), level of CTL response, or cytopathogenicity of the transmitted viral strain [i.e. syncytia-inducing (SI) or nonsyncytia (NSI) inducing phenotype, *nef* deletional mutants or drug resistant strain]. Patients with high levels of viral replication progress more quickly than those patients in whom viral replication is contained perhaps due to a more effective immune response.

Laboratory Diagnosis

Pre-test counseling and informed consent are required by law in many states and countries prior to testing for HIV. Results should be provided with appropriate post-test counseling. Pretest counseling should include education about HIV disease, information about the specific test, and an assessment of HIV risk factors. Other provider responsibilities may include spousal or partner notification, governmental reporting of HIV infection and education about risk reduction. Post-test counseling should include a discussion of the test results, an assessment of the patient's understanding of the results, psychological status, a discussion of behavioral modification, and the need for follow up medical or psychological care [16]. Counseling and testing pregnant women and their infants may require considerations of additional factors such as the interaction between pregnancy and HIV infection, the risk of perinatal HIV transmission and prognosis for infants who are subsequently infected.

Humoral and cellular immune responses develop within days to weeks of HIV infection. Although IgM antibodies develop first, most commercial antibody assays detect IgG antibodies *gag* protein (p55, p24, p18) and envelop protein (gp160, gp120, gp41), which appear first during acute seroconversion [17]. These are followed in days to weeks by antibodies against HIV viral enzyme proteins (p66, p55, p51). A complete IgG response to HIV may take weeks to a few months to develop. In very rare cases, patients may not manifest seroconversion, or may have a prolonged period of seroconversion. Newer generation EIA tests have a sensitivity and specificity of >99.9% in serum from subjects with known HIV infection [18]. However, during PHI when antibodies against HIV may not yet be present, these assays have much lower sensitivity [17].

Diagnosis of HIV infection usually requires a two stage testing procedure. A screening serum HIV-1 antibody test is performed with an enzyme immunoassay (EIA). Positive tests are confirmed by the more specific Western blot test. Most EIA tests also look for specific HIV-2 antibodies. Criteria have been established which define positive or indeterminate Western blots. An indeterminate Western blot may be the result of incomplete seroconversion during primary HIV infection, a rare false positive reaction or possibly abortive HIV infection [19, 20]. In cases where EIA assays or western blots are found to be negative or indeterminate in high risk patients or in those with symptoms suggestive of ARS, repeat testing is recommended 8-12 weeks later. Absence of bands on the western blot at this time point is interpreted as negative.

Viral proteins, such as p24 (gag) antigen, or infectious HIV virus, either from peripheral blood mononuclear cells (PBMC) or in cell free plasma, can be readily detected prior to seroconversion [17]. Plasma associated infectious virus and p24 antigen, and to a lesser degree PBMC associated infectious virus levels, drop precipitously in the first few days to weeks after infection. Plasma virus and p24 antigen become undetectable for months to years in most patients. As a diagnostic test, serum p24 antigen is only moderately useful before and during the seroconversion period. Modifications introduced for greater sensitivity, including acid dissociation of antigen-antibody complexes have only marginally improved its sensitivity.

Virion associated HIV RNA in plasma (viral load) or PBMC associated proviral HIV DNA can be detected throughout the entire course of infection. Although not US FDA approved for this indication, viral load testing is useful in the diagnosis of patients with PHI when serum p24 antigen may be negative and HIV serology is not yet positive or is indeterminate. Viral load tests have little value, as a diagnostic test in chronic infection, as HIV serology is expected to be positive. PCR methods are also used to detect proviral HIV DNA in PBMCs for the diagnosis of HIV infection. Both viral load and PBMC DNA tests are expected to be positive within 2-4 weeks of infection [17]. Finally, practitioners should be aware that serologic and molecular diagnostic tests might not detect all subtypes of HIV-1 equally. Only some EIA assays have been modified to allow detection of genetically diverse group M and group O isolates [21].

Other serologic screening and confirmatory assays include rapid agglutination assays, dipsticks, and recombinant immunoblot assays for HIV-1/2. These screening tests have comparable sensitivities to that of EIA assays in chronically infected and most sero-converting patients [22]. Immunoblot testing is another confirmatory test and has significantly reduced the number of indeterminate western blot results and can discriminate HIV-1 from HIV-2 in one blot [23].

HIV-1 antibody testing can also be accomplished at home using the Home Access System (Home Access Health Corporation). After blood is collected at home, it is mailed to a reference laboratory where standard EIA and confirmatory western blot technology are performed. The patient receives the result via telephone. This system has reported 100% concordance with standard results from an EIA obtained from blood after venipuncture [24]. It should be noted all of these assays are sensitive and specific for subtype B infection. Newer versions of tests are now being, or have been developed which will detect non-subtype B viruses and Group O.

Oral fluids and urine also contain antibodies against HIV. Antibodies in saliva are primarily of the IgG isotype and in some instances are in greater concentration than concomitant serum levels. Recently, commercially available tests using oral mucosal transudate (OMT) (Orasure, Epitope, Inc) and urine (Calypte, Berkeley, CA) have been developed for HIV antibody detection. The OMT sample is sent to a referral laboratory for standard EIA and western blot confirmation. Sensitivity of OMT EIA in true HIV+ subjects was 99.99% and specificity of 99.99% when compared to standard western blot confirmation [25]. Urine antibody testing, which must also be confirmed by Western blot, has been reported to be more sensitive than serum testing in some studies [26].

Quantification of cell free viral load in plasma has now become an important marker in assessing the risk of disease progression and monitoring antiretroviral therapy [27]. Three commercial assays are currently available to detect and quantitate plasma viral load utilizing reverse transcription-polymerase chain reaction (RT-PCR, HIV Monitor™, Roche Diagnostics), nucleic acid sequence based amplification (NASBA, Nuclisens™, Organon-Teknika) and branched DNA signal amplification (bDNA, Quantiplex 3.0™, Bayer Diagnostics) [28]. Current generation assays have a lower limit of detection of between 50-80 copies/ml. Although they all measure the same HIV RNA template, the copy numbers derived from each of these assays are not equivalent because of the differences in assay methodologies and efficiencies of sample preparation.

Recent studies demonstrate that viral load levels during PHI are extremely high, ranging from 10^5 to $>2 \times 10^7$/ml and are detectable before seroconversion [29]. Levels drop precipitously within the first 4-8 weeks after infection [15]. Thus, viral load levels during early chronic infection range from <1000 to >100,000/ml (a 2 to 4 $\log_{10}$, or 100 to 10,000 fold reduction/ml). Viral load levels during seroconversion are not significantly different between those patients who have symptoms and those who are asymptomatic [30]. However, symptoms during seroconversion are associated with significantly higher levels 6-12 months after seroconversion [31]. During clinical latency, levels remain relatively stable, but increase gradually over time. Thus, viral load levels are detectable throughout the course of infection in the absence of effective antiretroviral therapy. In a recent study utilizing subjects from the multi-center AIDS cohort study (MACS), less than 2% of patients within 6 months of seroconversion had viral load levels <500 copies/ml [8]. Recent data suggest that women may have lower HIV plasma RNA levels and higher CD4 cell numbers early in infection, although their rate of clinical progression is similar compared to men [27, 32].

Serologic diagnosis of HIV infection in newborns may be problematic because maternal anti-HIV IgG antibodies cross the placenta into fetal/neonatal circulation. Thus, routine serology does not offer useful information about infection until at least 12-15 months of age. Vertical transmission is defined as intrauterine if HIV viral culture or DNA PCR is positive within the first 48 hours of birth and intrapartum if these studies are negative within the first week of life. Culture and serum p24 antigen are not sufficiently sensitive for diagnosis of infection in infants [33]. Plasma viral load appears to be more sensitive than PBMC DNA PCR within the first four weeks of life [34, 35].

When to Treat

Since HIV eradication has not been achievable with current highly active antiretroviral therapy (HAART), the goal of antiretroviral therapy in HIV disease is to maximally suppress viral replication for as long as possible, improve immune function, and thereby decrease the incidence of AIDS associated complications. Current treatment strategies require a combination of three or more agents, in combinations with non-overlapping toxicity profiles and different resistance patterns. This improves antiviral potency, limits drug-related toxicity and maintains activity in the setting of emerging resistance to a single agent. Less than 5% of HIV infected patients have sufficient immunologic responses to HIV infection, or transmitted viral strains with low cytopathogenicity as manifested by very low or undetectable viral loads, and no CD4 cell decline in the absence of HAART. Indeed these long-term nonprogressors (LTNP) do not progress to AIDS, despite the lack of antiretroviral therapy [36]. Thus, antiretroviral therapy in this setting may be of questionable benefit and may expose the patient to unnecessary drug toxicities. However, > 95% of infected patients will require initiation and maintenance of HAART treatment.

The complexity, toxicities, drug/drug interactions, cost, and long-term side effects of HAART, as well as the impact on co-morbid conditions, will determine the optimal time for initiation of treatment. Some experts recommend the initiation of treatment during seroconversion. This appears to present the greatest opportunity for stabilization and preservation of immunologic (CD4) function. However, patients with ARS are difficult to identify as they very rarely present during this period. Updated guidelines support treatment of patients identified with primary infection in the context of clinical trials designed to assess the impact of therapy. In terms of overall patient well-being, short-term benefit with respect to surrogate markers may be offset by the complications of antiretroviral therapy such as the development of toxicities and drug resistance. The overwhelming majority of patients, present in early or late chronic phases of infection with declining CD4 cell numbers with subsequent development of ARC or AIDS symptoms. HAART is strongly recommended for all HIV infected patients with less than 300-500 CD4 cells/mm^3, or with high HIV RNA levels, or clinical symptoms.

Treatment Algorithms

Antiretroviral choices should consider the needs of each individual patient. With the availability of new effective medications, this tenet is easier to achieve. However, treatment decisions have become more complex; no single combination of medications can be recommended to the exclusion of all others. Various factors must be considered when choosing an initial regimen and when altering therapy for virologic failure or tolerability problems. The process of selection must include a review of the background medical conditions (i.e. a history of or active hepatitis, neuropathy, or anemia), psychosocial issues (depression, post traumatic stress disorder (PTSD) and other forms of chronic mental illness), ethno cultural issues (i.e. perceived lack of clinical benefit from certain HIV drugs) and patient lifestyle and habits (i.e. employment, homelessness or incarceration). These issues need to be considered within the context of other limiting factors, including pill burden, frequency of doses, coordination of dose administration with or without food, predicted side effect profile (i.e., diarrhea in someone who travels for a living) and patient preference.

Tailoring a treatment regimen to the individual will help achieve increased adherence and the desired therapeutic goals. Most importantly, a regimen must have adequate potency to achieve an undetectable viral load by an ultra sensitive assay (<50 copies/ml) and should be tolerable with respect to side effects and complexity. It should be chosen with a view towards maximizing adherence and minimizing significant drug-drug interactions and overlap of side effect profiles. Long-term adherence to the initial highly active regimen will minimize development of resistant viral mutants and hopefully preclude the need to use more complex regimens.

There are currently 15 antiretroviral agents in three different classes approved for use by the US FDA in managing HIV-1 infection. Nucleoside reverse transcriptase inhibitors (NRTI) are nucleoside analogues or chain terminators of reverse transcription and include zidovudine (ZDV, or azidothymidine, AZT), didanosine (ddI), zalcitabine (ddC), stavudine (d4T), lamivudine (3TC), and abacavir (ABC). The nonnucleoside reverse transcriptase inhibitors (NNRTI) are non-competitive inhibitors (binding away from the active site) of the reverse transcriptase enzyme and include nevirapine (NVP), delavirdine (DLV) and efavirenz (EFV). The HIV-1 protease inhibitors (PI) inhibit cleavage of *gag* and *gag-pol* polyprotein precursors, preventing the packaging of mature infectious virions. Currently US FDA approved PIs include saquinavir (SQV), ritonavir (RTV), indinavir (IDV), nelfinavir (NFV), amprenavir (AMP), and lopinavir (LPV, in combination with RTV known as Kaletra). Two additional combination pills are also available, Combivir (AZT and 3TC) and Trizivir (AZT, 3TC and Abacavir). Additional drugs are also available through expanded access programs. Current daily doses and pill burden are at (http: //hiv.medscape.com/updates/quickguide).

First Line. IAS-USA, DHHS/Kaiser Family Foundation, British HIV Association and other agencies have developed treatment guidelines. These guidelines are the result of expert panels that reviewed the evidence for treatment effect of various regimens. These recommendations are based on studies with clinical or virologic endpoints, or in the absence of specific data, expert opinion [37, 38] (http: //www.bhiva.org/trtgdlns.htm; jama.ama-assn.org/issues/v283n3/ffull/jst90023.htm; www.hivatis.org/guidelines.html). These guidelines recommend that at least three antiretroviral agents should be given when treatment is initiated in drug naïve patients. This usually includes a combination of two NRTI and a PI, or two NRTI and a NNRTI. Recent studies have shown that a single or double NRTI regimen is virologically and immunologically inferior compared to a HAART regimen [39]. NNRTI (efavirenz) or PI (indinavir) containing regimens appears equally effective [40]. Triple NRTI have also been found to have potencies similar to those of the aforementioned combinations [41]. Due to the recent availability of drugs in each class with higher potency, the concept of class (generally PI) sparing therapy may be considered at the outset. The possibility of 3 NRTI such as AZT/3TC/Abacavir or 2 NRTI/NNRTI (nevirapine, or efavirenz) as an initial regimen might be entertained in those patients requiring a <2-3 $\log_{10}$/ml decrease in viral load and in whom adherence may be a problem. In any case, it is prudent to preserve options for the future whenever clinically feasible. This may help prevent the dilemma that many patients face who have developed viral strains with broad class resistance to currently available drugs.

Therapy should be instituted in patients with established infection who have detectable viral load (>5000-10,000/ml) and/or CD4+ T cell count <500/mm^3. Treatment is optional with higher CD4 counts and this level of viral load. Patients with a VL > 10,000/ml and CD4 count >500 are considered at higher risk for clinical progression (CD4 decline) and therefore HAART should be recommended. It has recently been shown that decreasing viral load to undetectable levels (by an ultra sensitive assay) is associated with a more durable response [42]. However, standard HAART consisting of three drugs may not be sufficient to achieve this goal in patients with viral load in the higher range (>250,000/ml) at the start of treatment. Thus, four or more drugs may be necessary in this clinical situation to achieve undetectable (<50 copies/ml) viral loads [43]. Another strategy to achieve this goal is intensification of therapy. That is, the early addition of medications to a regimen after observing lack of complete suppression (i.e. detectable virus load), but prior to the development of significant resistance. For example, addition of abacavir to either ZDV/3TC or to stable background therapy (>12 weeks) improved virologic suppression and durability of response [44, 45]. However the sequential addition of agents may result in less viral load reductions, than when three drugs are started simultaneously [46].

Simplification of therapeutic regimen following successful maximal viral suppression by a more highly active (complex) regimen has been proposed as a means to improve adherence, at the same time decreasing medication cost and risk of toxicity. Recent results of AIDS Clinical Trials Group (ACTG) 343 and other studies, have been disappointing in that regard. In ACTG 343, viral suppression was achieved with ZDV/3TC/indinavir but was subsequently lost if therapy was simplified/reduced to ZDV/3TC or indinavir monotherapy [47]. In contrast, the recently presented "Maintavir" study showed that substitution of an NNRTI (in 17 NNRTI naïve patients) for a PI when viral loads were undetectable, resulted in persistent viral suppression in all patients at 8 weeks and in all 9 patients after 4 months in whom data was available [48]. Thus, substitution of one agent for another, when viral load is very low or undetectable, may well be a valid option to allow preservation of PI containing regimens for future use, simplify medication regimens, reduce patient perceived side effects, or prevent PI associated lipodystrophy (see below).

When to Change

Current therapies may not achieve total suppression of viral replication. A complex "library" of mutant virus is likely present in each HIV infected person. In untreated patients, these mutants are kept in the minority by the superior replicative ability of the "wild type" virus. However, no matter how effectively a drug suppresses replication of wild-type virus, the overall effectiveness of treatment is limited by the frequency of drug resistant mutants present at the start of treatment and by the ability of these strains to replicate in the presence of drug. Although combination therapy is more likely to suppress replication of more genetic variants than monotherapy, resistant variants will emerge. Resistant viruses may also accumulate more mutations to increase their relative fitness, and these more "fit" viruses will emerge as the predominant variant. In addition, other specific mutations or insertion mutants have been found to confer broad resistance to an entire class of antiretroviral agents. *In vitro* studies have been predictive of the nature and pattern of clinical phenotypic resistance. For most drugs, specific, primary (canonical) mutations in the HIV-1 viral genome have been identified that are associated with reduced antiretroviral activity (http: //hiv.medscape.com/updates/quickguide [49]. The analysis of HIV strains from patients treated with specific drugs or drug combinations has led to the recognition of specific genotypes, which confer phenotypic resistance leading to clinical resistance.

The prevalence of drug resistant variants in drug naïve patients ranges from 1-20% depending on the drug [50, 51]. Transmission of antiretroviral resistant variants has also been reported, which may make first line HAART choices ineffective [52].

Preliminary data indicate that drug specific resistance and cross-resistance within a drug class markedly reduces the effectiveness of antiretroviral combinations in patients previously exposed to antiretroviral therapy (clinical resistance). Current studies indicate that emergence of antiretroviral resistance occurs in more than 50% of patients treated with HAART [53].

The first sign that a HAART regimen is no longer effective for a patient is an increase in viral load of 0.5 $\log_{10}$ copy/ml or greater above the level of detection or above a stable background level on two occasions in the absence of concurrent infection or recent vaccination. Absolute CD4 count or percentage decreases may lag behind virologic changes. A rebound in VL should prompt an assessment of adherence to the current regimen and consideration for modification of the current medication regimen. Modification of the regimen should be based on the considerations for improved adherence, limiting toxicity and limiting potential for resistance development as discussed above.

Secondary Options

Patients who are HIV drug experienced present with difficult treatment challenges. When selecting a second, third, or fourth HAART regimen, it is imperative to collect a thorough drug dosing history. The extent of previous drug exposure, in addition to past intolerance or toxicity will help guide the selection of the next regimen. What has been learned in the past few years is that most, if not all of the medications in a given regimen need to be changed in virologic failure. Various regimens have been utilized for patients with extensive antiretroviral experience who are failing their current therapy and as for first line HAART, it is not possible to recommend specific drug combinations, but rather, these regimens have an even greater requirement for individualization. If a regimen appears to be failing (as defined above) a new regimen should be chosen using at least 2 medications to which the person has not been previously exposed. These should be chosen based on the susceptibility of their virus and a low likelihood of cross-resistance. In the case of a class-sparing regimen the not-yet-used class of drugs presents a good option for starting to design a new regimen. But this will be applicable primarily to patients with first-line failure. Designing follow-up regimens does require a high level of background knowledge regarding antiretroviral resistance and cross-resistance potential in order to effectively change regimens. Depending on the clinical status of the patient and options still available, one may consider the use of aggressive salvage regimens, continuation of the current regimen until new drugs become available, or treatment discontinuation [54] (http: //www.bhiva.org/guidelines.htm) (jama.ama-assn.org/issues/v283n3/full/jst90023.html) (www.hivatis.org/trtgdlns.html). Other current salvage strategies include "mega-HAART" therapy. This involves utilizing more than six antiretrovirals, including agents that patients may have received previously and/or have demonstrated resistance to. Moderate success has been achieved, whereby a third of heavily pretreated patients demonstrated undetectable viral loads (<400 copies/ml). However, many subjects required discontinuation of the regimen because of severe toxicities [55].

Scheduled treatment interruptions, previously often referred to as "drug holidays" are being used increasingly in patients with limited options available. In the salvage setting, the effects of this strategy has been evaluated in patients with multi-drug resistant virus who have limited or no new treatment options available, or in whom medication toxicities have greatly affected their quality of life. The previously multi-drug resistant plasma virus population has been shown to shift to a predominantly wild type population in a relative short period of time, but only in a subpopulation of patients [56]. In very preliminary studies, reinitiation of HAART or mega-HAART was associated with improved virologic response in patients who displayed the shift to wild-type phenomenon, with a higher proportion of these achieving plasma viral load levels <500 copies/ml [57]. However, it must be stressed that the CD4 counts decreased dramatically in the majority of patients who stopped all medication, and this may put them at unacceptable clinical risk for progression. Thus, it can currently not be recommended to use treatment interruptions as a strategy in the population as a whole. Patients who have absolutely no other choice, due to toxicities or "medication fatigue" should be counseled and monitored very extensively during the interruption period. The effects of treatment interruptions in the salvage patient population should not be confused with the effects in patients with complete virus suppression. Treatment interruptions have also been analyzed in a very small number of patients who were treated early in infection and whose treatment regimen had achieved full suppression of virus replication. In an anecdotal few, viral replication continued to be suppressed after treatment interruptions, and this has been associated with HIV specific immune responses [58]. It should also be noted that stopping one or two drugs from a regimen is TREATMENT REDUCTION not interruption, and this will expose the patient to the potential of viral drug resistance development. Studies of treatment reduction as a strategy did not yield positive results, as discussed above (maintenance/simplification section). Thus, it remains necessary to counsel and inform the patient about the requirements of adherence to a prescribed treatment regimen.

Hydroxyurea (HU) is a cytoreductive agent that inhibits the ribonucleotide reductase enzyme of cells leading to decreased intracellular concentrations of deoxynucleotide triphosphates (dNTP) for DNA synthesis. This leads to a relative increase in incorporation of adenosine analogs such as ddI and the acyclic nucleotide analogs PMEA (adefovir) and PMPA. HU is active in resting T lymphocytes, and may compensate for HIV drug resistance, which could offer an advantage in improving virologic control [59]. HU does not currently have a label indication for treatment of HIV disease. However, HU containing regimens have been used across the spectrum of HIV disease. The optimal dose and when HU should be initiated remains to be determined. Current dosing strategies suggest a dose of 500 mg twice daily may result in additive effects for ddI. However HU can result in mild to moderate cytopenias, and fatal pancreatitis after concomitant use with ddI has recently been reported.

Immunomodulatory agents such as interleukin-2 (IL-2) may have a beneficial effect on the course of HIV infection. IL-2 has been extensively studied in clinical trials. As IL-2 activates T cells, it may increase viral replication. In the presence of HAART however, IL-2 infusion or subcutaneous injection leads to significant improvement in CD4 counts with no significant increase in viral load [60]. Activation of latently infected resting T cells in the presence of effective antiretroviral therapy might lead to elimination of that reservoir of infected cells. Many patients are able to sustain CD4 counts in the normal range (800-1200/mm^3) for several years with intermittent subcutaneous dosing strategies. IL-2 is not US FDA approved for use in HIV infection. The optimal dose, frequency, and when during HIV infection IL-2 should be administered, remains to be determined. Whether IL-2 should be used in early chronic infection as an adjunct to HAART, also needs to be determined. Furthermore, clinical benefit sufficient to merit the cost and risk of significant side effects has not been shown.

Finally, many new anti-HIV medications are currently under investigation. These include additional agents within existing classes and new target agents such as HIV-1 integrase inhibitors; fusion and entry inhibitors such as co-receptor blockers; or new viral replication inhibitor strategies using anti-sense molecules or gene therapy.

Evaluation of Treatment Effect

CD4 count and percentage as well as plasma viral load quantification, are the current standard tests for evaluation of treatment effect. In drug naïve patients, HAART should result in a prompt decrease in plasma viral load within 2-4 weeks reaching goal levels of <500 copies/ml within 4-12 weeks and < 50 copies/ml in up to 24 weeks [61]. There does not appear to be gender or racial differences in viral load response after initiation of HAART. Viral load should be monitored by the same ultra sensitive method at least every 3-4 months. Upon abrupt discontinuation of HAART, viral load will rebound to pretreatment levels within days to weeks in the majority of patients. If all drugs are withdrawn, the likelihood of resistance is low, and patients can have the same regimen reinitiated and expect the same virologic response [62]. However, this should not be considered a recommended therapeutic strategy.

CD4 count should increase by a minimum of 50 cells/mm^3 or 3% after HAART initiation. CD4 count increases are somewhat contingent on the baseline value. Absolute increases will be much greater in those patients with CD4 counts of > 200/mm^3 than in those patients with CD4 counts of <50/mm^3. After an initial robust increase in the first 3 to 4 months, CD4 counts can continue to increase modestly in some patients for months [63]. It has recently been found that baseline CD4 count and relative change following treatment initiation, are highly predictive of the duration of viral load response, and that the previously experienced CD4 count nadir is significantly correlated with the relative hazard of progression in spite of CD4 cell count recovery to levels >200 cells/mm^3 [64, 65].

A small subset of patients, experience a lack of virologic response or virologic rebound after an initial, or subsequent responses to HAART, concurrent with preserved improvement in CD4 T cell counts [66, 67]. As the morbidity and mortality from HIV disease is predominantly related to immune dysfunction as measured by CD4 T cell count, it is concerning to change therapy in this setting and there is no clear correct course of action. On one hand, a detectable viral load may herald the emergence of resistance to current therapy while on the other, one might prefer to expose the patient to as few medications as possible to preserve future options. Such discordant CD4+ responses in persons receiving protease inhibitors have been accompanied by substantial clinical benefit. In a cohort of over 2500 patients, the incidence of new AIDS-defining diagnoses or death in patients who maintained a viral load of less than 500 copies/ml has been reported as being no different than that of patients who achieved, but failed to sustain such viral suppression [68].

HIV treatment guidelines call for the prompt alteration of anti-retroviral regimen upon the confirmed detection of a viral load of greater than 50 – 500 copies/ml but less than 10,000 copies/ml, reflect the perspective that the risk of continued therapy pending demonstration of greater amounts of viral replication is unacceptable. This stance, which is largely based on expert opinion, affects the management of many HIV-infected patients. According to data recently announced by HCSUS, of HIV-infected persons in the United States who are currently on 3 or more antiretrovirals, 29% have viral loads below 50 copies/mL, while 58% have viral loads above 10,000 copies/mL. Thus, the viral load threshold at which the rate of resistance development becomes unacceptable and mandates alterations in HAART remains to be determined. This may also be different for different drugs. In particular, it is not known at what point the demerits of changing anti-retroviral therapy (and thus exposing the patient to an increased number of drugs, with the possibility of cross-resistance and increased drug toxicity) outweigh the benefits (suppressing viral replication, preventing immunological deterioration, and promoting immune reconstitution). The rates of immune reconstitution are greater in persons with viral loads less than 50 – 400 copies/ml than in persons with less complete suppression of HIV replication. Nonetheless, persons with partial suppression have demonstrated dramatic and sustained increases in their total and naïve CD4+ cell counts. Again, decision making in this setting is multifactorial and must take into account issues such as patient preference, adherence, and psychosocial factors among others.

Recently HIV drug resistance testing has been applied successfully in clinical practice. Drug resistance can be measured phenotypically, which is a direct measurement of virus growth and susceptibility to an antiretroviral drug. Alternatively, genotypic changes at positions known to be associated with drug resistance can be assessed and resistance thus inferred. Which assays are better suited in specific situations is a subject of much current research. It should be noted that these two approaches deliver complimentary information in many cases.

Most routinely available phenotypic assays are based on a recombinant virus assays (RVA). The patient's viral strain reverse transcriptase and protease enzymes are amplified using PCR technology and incorporated into a laboratory strain. Phenotypic assays are by nature more complex to perform than sequencing (see below). Thus, their availability may be more restricted; costs are generally higher than genotypic resistance assays and turn-around time longer. Clinically significant inhibitory concentration cut-off values remain to be determined for most drugs.

Genotypic resistance testing also uses PCR for amplification of relevant genes and subsequent probe hybridization or nucleic acid sequencing to demonstrate mutations in HIV-1 reverse transcriptase and protease genes. Since this technology is somewhat less complex than phenotyping, genotypic assays are generally more widely available, have the potential for delivering results more rapidly (although the long turnaround times of many laboratories negate this advantage) and reduced costing. However, genotypic assays are only an indirect measure of susceptibility and may not always correlate with phenotype. Since HIV can exist in blood as multiple strains, genotyping cannot distinguish whether different mutations are co-aggregated within a single strain or exist singly in multiple strains. The lack of a particular resistance mutation unfortunately may not predict success, as current genotypic tests often do not reliably detect low frequency variants (<25%), which may be selected in response to a new regimen. A minimum of 500-1000 HIV RNA copies/ml of plasma is required for both genotypic and phenotypic assays. There are no US FDA approved standard procedures (kits). Thus, most laboratories have incorporated "home brew" assays. As expected, this leads to problems in reproducibility, validity and quality assurance for the results obtained. Furthermore, these assays are technically demanding and require experienced operators, expert interpretation of test results for clinical correlation. Knowledge of which mutations constitute primary or secondary drug mutations or drug class is required.

Research in the area of resistance and treatment outcome has proceeded at a very rapid rate and generally the impression has been that drug susceptibility is indeed associated with response. It was demonstrated that drug susceptibility status is predictive of response, independent of virus load, CD4 cell count and previous treatment history [69, 70]. However, results have frequently been based on retrospective studies with small patient populations, often with significant differences in previous drug exposures. Methods of assessing resistance (diverse genotypic or phenotypic assays) as well as definitions of resistance (phenotypic cut-offs, which mutations are counted for genotypic assays) and treatment response have not been uniform. A recent U.S. FDA advisory hearing addressed several issues regarding resistance testing in the clinical and drug-development setting. For this purpose, an international resistance collaborative group designed a common analysis plan for the re-evaluation of published studies. Using a common set of definitions for treatment response and resistance, the association between baseline drug susceptibility and treatment outcome was established (http: //www.fda.gov/ohrms/dockets/ ac/99/backgrd/3541b1d.pdf) [71]. Further information on the association of mutations and specific drug resistance can be found at http: //hivdb.stanford.edu.

Several recently completed clinical studies have prospectively demonstrated utility of genotyping resistance testing in clinical practice. In the genotypic antiretroviral resistance testing (GART) and Viradapt studies, there was a significantly greater reduction in viral load after 12 weeks and 6 months respectively after a regimen change in those patients in whom resistance information was provided to the treating physician than in those patients whose physicians made changes in there antiretroviral regimen based solely on clinical history and judgment [72, 73]. Phenotypic resistance testing may have the same predictive value [74]. These studies suggest that there is at least short-term viral load benefit to using genotypic or phenotypic resistance testing after failure of a first HAART regimen. Two additional studies in heavily pretreated patients did not find a significant virologic advantage of using resistance testing when compared to standard of care [75, 76]. The HAVANNA trial found that expert interpretation of resistance testing results was found to be independently important over the resistance test results and standard of care alone [77]. Because of the complexity of information provided, these tests may be difficult to interpret for the uninitiated. Long-term virologic and clinical benefit however, remain to be determined.

Guidelines on the use of resistance testing were recently published by the U.S. Department of Health and Human Services (DHHS) and International AIDS Society-USA (IAS-USA) (www.hivatis.org/trtgdlns.html) [49]. These guidelines suggest that it may be appropriate to perform resistance testing in patients who are newly infected prior to initiating antiretroviral therapy, or to rule out resistance in patients whose viral load becomes detectable, or never became undetectable after starting HAART. Resistance testing is currently not recommended prior to treatment initiation in chronically infected patients. The role of resistance testing in post-exposure prophylaxis has not been defined.

Dosing Schemes, Drug Interactions

Adherence to antiretroviral regimens is of critical importance in the success of antiretroviral therapy. Studies have shown a correlation between estimates of adherence and virologic response to therapy [78]. Regimens with less frequent dosing requirements are under investigation and should be increasingly available. However, less frequent dosing does not always improve adherence to therapy [79]. Due to the risk of resistant viral variant selection in patients with erratic drug levels, it may be prudent to withhold therapy in these patients until these and other issues that may adversely affect adherence can be addressed.

Once Daily Dosing/Simplified Regimens

Adherence to antiretroviral regimens is often difficult due to complexity of the regimen and pill burden. Assessing the efficacy of simplified regimens is therefore an important area of investigation. Twice daily dosing of nelfinavir and once daily dosing of ddI (in regular tablets and EC forms) are now US FDA approved. Nevirapine has been similarly evaluated and results demonstrate that a single 400 mg daily dose has similar efficacy [80].

Once daily dosing of a highly active antiretroviral medication regimen would be expected to significantly improve adherence. Nevirapine, 3TC and ddI have favorable pharmocokinetics for once daily dosing. A pilot study in an IVDU population demonstrated that this combination led to undetectable viral loads in over 90% of patients at 24 weeks [81].

Drug Interactions

Members of both the NNRTI and PI classes of drugs undergo extensive metabolism through the hepatic cytochrome p450 system. In addition, these medications can inhibit or induce some of these isoenzymes, thereby impacting the metabolism of other medications. This is important not only for the other anti-HIV medications, but with any concomitant medications that share the same metabolic pathway. With respect to enzyme inhibition, the following medications produce mild to potent inhibitory effects on particular p450 isoenzymes; saquinavir, amprenavir, indinavir, nelfinavir, delavirdine, and ritonavir. Drugs with narrow therapeutic windows, such as cisapride, calcium channel blockers, and some tricyclic antidepressants, may reach toxic levels in the presence of potent inhibitors [82]. Co-administration of these drugs should be closely monitored or avoided if possible.

There are cases, though, where the use of an inhibitor can be beneficial to the patient. For instance, the strong inhibitory properties of ritonavir can decrease metabolism of other, co-metabolized, anti-HIV drugs. The inhibition of the hepatic cytochrome p450 isoenzyme 3A4 by ritonavir allows lower doses of other drugs (i.e. SQV, IDV) to be given at decreased frequency. Ritonavir and saquinavir or indinavir have been used in combination with NRTIs in this fashion. This interaction has resulted in more favorable pharmacokinetic profiles including twice a day and even once-a-day regimens [83].

Different combinations and dosing regimens are currently under investigation but this strategy may improve cost, adherence and side effect profile while maintaining potent antiviral effect. Note, none of these regimens are approved by the US FDA.

For those anti-HIV medications that, in general, induce these metabolic systems (i.e. efavirenz and nevirapine), the provider may need to increase dosages of concomitant medications to compensate for potentially sub-therapeutic drug concentrations. An example is the combination of efavirenz and indinavir, where indinavir dosages are increased by 25% to offset higher indinavir hepatic clearance rates [84]. Current anti-HIV drug interactions and concomitant changes in serum concentration are listed at hiv.medscape.com/updates/quickguide. The same holds true for non-HIV medications, such as rifampin, which may increase the metabolism of the HIV drugs (and therefore decrease efficacy). To maximize patient safety, providers should check first with a primary drug reference, pharmacist, or drug information resource prior to adding any suspect drug to a person receiving anti-HIV therapy. Additional drug combinations may be contraindicated. A drug-drug interaction calculator is located at hiv.medscape.com/Medscape/HIV/druginteractions/index.cfm; to determine whether certain drugs can or should be combined. Also, as patients age and require other medications, drug-drug interactions may be increasingly problematic.

Finally, some HIV medications should not be combined because their efficacies may be limited by intracellular metabolic interactions. D4T should not be used in combination with ZDV as both compete for activation by thymidine kinase, and thus may be antagonistic for that reason. This was reflected in clinical experience as well. In ZDV naïve or experienced patients, ZDV/d4T was inferior to ZDV/ddI, ZDV/3TC or d4T or ddI monotherapies [85].

Side Effects

Depending on the regimen prescribed (see side effects below), routine safety labs (e.g. CBC, serum transaminases, serum lipid profiles, etc) and scheduled visits should be used to guide HIV therapy. Toxicities to the anti-HIV medications can appear during the initial days of therapy and/or in the months to years of chronic exposure. The most common side effects are listed at hiv.medscape.com/updates/quickguide. Since many of these toxicities do not manifest themselves for months to years, the actual long-term toxicity profiles of the newer agents are unknown. Hypersensitivity to abacavir bares special mention. This is a syndrome, which develops after several days or within the first weeks of treatment and is manifested by fever, abdominal pain and rash. Symptoms can get worse with subsequent dosing. Rechallenge with abacavir has resulted in death [86]. Lactic acidosis and concomitant symptoms including fatigue, muscle aches, gastrointestinal complaints, and hepatomegaly has been recognized increasingly with NRTI containing regimens [87]. It is thought to be due to mitochondrial dysfunction secondary to NRTI inhibition of mitochondrial enzymes [88].

Lipodystrophy characterized by peripheral fat wasting (face, arms buttocks) and central adiposity, dyslipidemias (elevated triglycerides and cholesterol), and hyperglycemia (insulin tolerance) was first recognized in conjunction with PI treatment [89, 90].

They may contribute to morbidity and mortality due to cardiovascular disease. These conditions can appear within the first month of therapy (hyperglycemia and lipid abnormalities) or may take months to develop (lipodystrophy). To date, the mechanism(s) behind these conditions are unknown. However, the abnormalities are usually (partially) reversible following discontinuation of the suspect agent(s). A recent article reviews the current understanding of adverse effects of HAART [91].

Dietary modification and medical therapy of dyslipidemia should be considered as well as treatment interventions for cardiac risk factors such as smoking and hypertension should be undertaken. Guidelines for the management of dyslipidemias have recently been published [92]. Rarely, this syndrome has been noted in HIV infected patients treated only with NRTI and NNRTI agents [93, 94]. Substitution of a PI with efavirenz may be effective in improving the condition while maintaining viral suppression [95]. As the number of treatment options for HIV infection increases, avoidance of the long term complications of specific medications may become a more important factor in the choice of a regimen.

Special Considerations

Pregnancy

Antiretroviral therapy including ZDV should be administered during pregnancy to decrease risk of vertical transmission to the neonate. ACTG 076 showed that ZDV therapy antepartum (initiated at 14-34 weeks gestation) and intra-partum to the mother and post-partum to the infant for six weeks decreased the incidence of transmission by approximately two thirds (25.5% in the placebo group vs. 8.3% in the ZDV group) [96]. However, a more recent study found that ZDV started at 35 weeks of pregnancy, with 3 days of treatment for infants, did not result in a reduced incidence of HIV transmission [97]. The HIVNET 012 study compared single dose zidovudine *versus* single dose nevirapine given to the mother at the time of birth, and to the newborn immediately afterward. Nevirapine was significantly better in reducing fetal transmission when compared to ZDV or placebo [98]. Additionally, elective cesarean section may decrease transmission rates to 2% in patients receiving standard ZDV prophylaxis [99].

Although the maternal plasma viral load level has not been well correlated with HIV transmission, in general, viral loads of >10,000 copies/ml, have been associated with higher rates of transmission. Since HAART regimens will decrease viral load to undetectable levels, it is likely that combination therapy would decrease transmission further still. Due to the strength of the above findings, current guidelines suggest that for those women already receiving HAART therapy at the time of pregnancy, the regimen should be continued but that ZDV should be added to (or substituted in) an existing regimen if not present; and that women not on any treatment, should have ZDV, at a minimum, initiated in the second trimester. Retrospective HIV/pregnancy registry information has found HAART regimens to be generally well tolerated during pregnancy. However, efavirenz is contraindicated during pregnancy because of the risk of teratogenicity, which has been documented in primates [84]. Further guidance on antiretroviral management during pregnancy can be obtained at http: //hivatis.org/guidelines/perinatal/ Nov_00/text/PerinatalNov00.pdf.

Pediatric

Antiretroviral therapy in infants and children involves certain unique considerations. As absolute CD4+ T cell count may vary with age, CD4 T cell percentage should be followed for disease progression. HIV-RNA levels are also more variable in infants and may be less predictive of disease progression than in adults [100]. As most children acquire infection perinatally, early identification and intervention is possible and may lead to more complete preservation of immune function. Medication regimens and their concomitant toxicities are similar to those used and seen in adults. Thus, HAART regimens should be employed whenever possible regardless of age or symptoms [101]. Adherence is particularly difficult for children and adolescents and may lead to development of resistance resulting in decreased therapeutic options in these patients who will likely require lifelong therapy. Further information on pediatric HIV treatment can be obtained at http: //www.hivatis.org/trtgdlns.html.

Hepatitis C Virus (HCV) Co-infection

Recent epidemiology studies indicate that HCV co-infection with HIV, leads to faster clinical progression to AIDS, and that HIV co-infection can hasten the development of cirrhosis [102]. Although increased HIV viral load is associated with HIV disease progression, increased HCV viral load does not appear to be associated with HCV progression. HCV viral load is higher in co-infected patients and is unrelated to HCV genotype [103]. HAART therapy can also affect HCV viral load [104].

It is unclear whether HAART will impact HCV associated liver disease. Acute elevations of serum transaminases have been reported in co-infected patients initiating HAART therapy. HCV treatment with interferon and ribavirin has resulted in marked reductions in HCV viral load and improvement in hepatic architecture in those patients previously unresponsive to interferon monotherapy. Preliminary data suggests that HIV co-infected patients can tolerate and respond to this regimen as well. HIV viral load and CD4 count is not affected by interferon and ribavirin treatment. However, significant anemia can result from ribavirin use [105]. Whether the responses are as robust and sustained in dually infected patients when compared to those in HCV only infected patients, and whether there is any deleterious effects on HIV infection are the subject of several ongoing studies.

Prophylaxis and Vaccination Strategies

Prophylaxis for HIV Infection

Occupational exposure should be assessed for risk and therapy instituted for exposures judged to be of significant risk. A risk assessment algorithm is provided in the US Public

Health Service Guidelines which includes step 1: determination of an exposure code based on the source material (blood, other potentially infectious material) and the type of exposure (intact skin, mucous membrane, or percutaneous exposure); step 2: determination of HIV status of the source patient (serostatus as well as clinical status based on viral load, CD4 count, primary infection or advanced disease) and step 3: choice of a prophylactic regimen [106]. While guidelines suggest the use of a "basic regimen" using standard doses of ZDV and 3TC in lower risk cases and the use of an "expanded regimen" using the basic regimen plus a PI (nelfinavir 750 mg TID or indinavir 800 mg po q8 hours), many clinicians choose to utilize the more highly active regimen in any case judged of sufficient risk to merit chemoprophylaxis. In selected cases (i.e. a source patient with poorly controlled viral load on antiretroviral therapy), genotypic testing of the source patient and appropriate adjustment of prophylactic regimen may be indicated. Since prophylactic treatment should not be delayed beyond a couple of hours after exposure, do not wait for resistance test results before initiating treatment. Further information can be obtained at http: //www.hivatis.org/trtgdlns.html.

HIV transmission risk varies with sexual practices. The highest per contact risk is for unprotected receptive anal intercourse (0.24%) followed by protected anal intercourse (0.10%) likely due to frequent condom failure, unprotected insertive anal (0.03%) and receptive oral intercourse (0.03%) [107]. Post sexual exposure prophylaxis with a HAART regimen for a 30-day duration may be offered to those individuals reporting such exposure within 72 hours. Efficacy data are lacking in humans and animal data suggest most of the potential benefit in prevention is gained within the first 4-24 hours [108]. Further information can be obtained at http: //hivatis.org/trtgdlns.html, or through the Post Exposure Prophylaxis (PEP) network at http: //pepline.ucsf.edu/PEP/pepnet.html.

Prophylaxis for OI

Patients with CD4 counts <200/mm3 are at great risk for the development of OI. Current guidelines for OI antimicrobial prophylaxis have recently been updated and published [109] and are available at http: //www.hivatis.org/guidelines/opport899.pdf. Emerging data suggests that some OI prophylaxis may be discontinued when sufficient CD4 cell recovery following HAART has been achieved. Several studies have now concluded that PCP prophylaxis may be discontinued in those patients who have not had PCP before and in whom the CD4 count has risen above 300/mm^3 following HAART [110]. There is also evidence for discontinuation of other primary OI prophylaxis (i.e. mycobacterium avium complex (MAC) and toxoplasmosis) [111-114]. In addition, if patients have had an OI, and are receiving secondary prophylaxis, it is prudent for them to continue receiving prophylaxis until further data regarding discontinuation of secondary prophylaxis is obtained. Practitioners should also be aware that atypical inflammatory syndromes with various OIs have been described following immune reconstitution after initiation of HAART therapy [115, 116].

Vaccination Strategies in Development

Several treatment and preventative vaccines are currently in development. These include DNA vaccines, using various vector delivery systems such as the canary poxvirus, which encode for various HIV immunogenic peptides (see above) including gp120. Candidates currently in clinical trials include an inactivated, gp120-depleted HIV-1 immunogen (Remune, Immune Response Corp.); and recombinant gp 120 vaccines (AIDSVAX, VaxGen). A recently published study found that Remune had no significant virologic effect compared to placebo, although HIV specific responses could be demonstrated in some vaccine recipients [117]. Likewise AIDSVAX was found to elicit specific HIV immune responses to a clade B virus, although 2/22 vaccine recipients became HIV infected with clade E virus [118]. Other envelop vaccine candidates have been shown to induce HIV specific responses. However responsiveness is correlated with CD4 count [119]. Due to structural changes of the gp120 envelope protein upon fusion with the cell membrane, a DNA based method of gp120 delivery may be superior to a subunit vaccine. At this time, no HIV specific preventative or therapeutic vaccine is available except under the auspices of clinical trials.

References

1.   Report on the global HIV/AIDS epidemic. Geneva: UNAIDS, June 1998
2.   Hu DJ, Donder TJ, Rayfield MA, et al. The emerging genetic diversity of HIV. JAMA 1996; 275: 210-6.
3.   Simon F, et al.: Identification of a new human immunodeficiency virus type 1 distinct from group M and group O. Nat Med 1998; 4(9): 1032-1037.
4.   Stauber RH, Rulong S, Palm G, Tarasova NI. Direct visualization of HIV-1 entry: mechanisms and role of cell surface receptors. Biochem Biophys Res Commun 1999; 258: 695-702.
5.   Ho D, Newmann AU, Perelson AS, et al. Rapid turnover of plasma virions and CD4 lymphocytes in HIV-1 infection. Nature 1995; 373: 644-651.
6.   Daar ES. Virology and immunology of acute HIV type 1 infection. AIDS Res Hum Retroviruses 1998; 14 suppl 3: S229-34.
7.   Musey L, Hughes J, Schacker T, et al. Cytotoxic T-cell responses, viral load, and disease progression in early human immunodeficiency virus type 1 infection. N Engl J Med 1997; 337: 1267-1274.
8.   Mellors JW, et al.: Plasma viral load and CD4+ lymphocytes as prognostic markers of HIV-1 infection. Ann Intern Med 1997; 126(12): 946-954.
9.   Pantaleo G, Graziosi C, Demarest JF, et al. HIV Infection is active and progressive in lymphoid tissue during the clinically latent stage of disease. Nature 1993; 362: 355-8
10. Finzi D, Blankson J, Siliciano JD, et al. Latent infection of CD4+ T cells provides a mechanism for lifelong persistence of HIV-1, even in patients on effective combination therapy. Nature Med 1999; 5: 512-7.
11. Zhang L, Ramratnam B, Tenner-Racz K, et al. Quantifying residual HIV-1 replication in patients receiving combination antiretroviral therapy. N Engl J Med 1999; 340: 1605-13.
12. Furtado MR, Callaway DS, Phair JP, et al. Persistence of HIV-1 transcription in peripheral-blood mononuclear cells in patients receiving potent antiretroviral therapy. N Engl J Med 1999; 340: 1614-22.

13. Bart PA, Rizzardi GP, Tambussi G, et al. Immunological and virological responses in HIV-1-infected adults at early stage of established infection treated with highly active antiretroviral therapy. AIDS 2000; 14: 1887-97.

14. Dalod M, Harzic M, Pellegrin I, et al. Evolution of cytotoxic T lymphocyte responses to human immunodeficiency virus type 1 in patients with symptomatic primary infection receiving antiretroviral triple therapy. J Infect Dis 1998; 178: 61-69.

15. Schacker T, Collier AC, Hughes J, Shea T, Corey L. Clinical and Epidemiologic Features of Primary HIV Infection. Ann Intern Med 1996; 125: 257-64.

16. CDC. Public Health Service guidelines for counseling and antibody testing to prevent HIV infection and AIDS. MMWR 1987; 36: 509-15.

17. Niu MT, Bethel J, Holodniy M, et al. Zidovudine treatment in patients with primary (acute) human immunodeficiency virus type 1 infection: a randomized, double-blind placebo-controlled trial. DATRI 002 Study Group. Division of AIDS Treatment Research Initiative. J Infect Dis 1998; 178: 80-91.

18. Sloand E, Pitt E, Chiarello RJ, Nemo GJ. HIV testing state of the art. JAMA 1991; 266: 2861-6.

19. Sayre KR, Dodd RY, Tegtmeier G, Layug L. Alexander SS, Busch MP. False-positive human immunodeficiency virus type 1 western blot tests in noninfected blood donors. Transfusion 1996; 36: 45-52.

20. Georgoulias VA, Malliaraki NE, Theodoropoulou M, et al. Indeterminate human immunodeficiency virus type 1 western blot may indicate an abortive infection in some low-risk donors. Transfusion 1997; 37: 65-72.

21. van Binsbergen J, de Rijk D, Peels H, et al. Evaluation of a new third generation anti-HIV-1/anti-HIV-2 assay with increased sensitivity for HIV-1 group O. J Virol Methods 1996; 60: 131-7.

22. Kuun E, Brashaw M, Heyns AD. Sensitivity and specificity of standard and rapid HIV antibody tests evaluated by seroconversion and non-seroconversion low-titre panels. Vox Sanguinis 1997; 72: 11-5.

23. Kline RL, McNairn D, Holodniy M, et al. Evaluation of Chiron HIV-1/HIV-2 recombinant immunoblot assay. J Clin Micro 1996; 34: 2650-3.

24. Frank AP, Wandell MG, Headings MD, Conant MA, Woody GE, Michel C. Anonymous HIV testing using home collection and telemedicine counseling. A multicenter evaluation. Archives of Int Med 1997; 157: 309-14.

25. Gallo D, George JR, Fitchen JH, Goldstein AS, Hindahl MS, (USA OraSure HIV Clinical Trials Group). Evaluation of a system using oral mucosal transudate for HIV-1 antibody screening and confirmatory testing. JAMA 1997; 277: 254-8.

26. Urnovitz HB, Sturge JC, Gottfried TD, Murphy WH. Urine antibody tests: new insights into the dynamics of HIV-1 infection. Clin Chem 1999; 45(9): 1602-13.

27. Katzenstein, DA, et al.: The relation of virologic and immunologic markers to clinical outcomes after nucleoside therapy in HIV-infected adults with 200 to 500 CD4 cells per cubic millimeter. AIDS Clinical Trials Group Study 175 Virology Study Team. N Engl J Med 1996, 335(15): 1091-1098.

28. Rivets H, Marissens D, De Wit S, et al. Comparative Evaluation of NASBA HIV-1 RNA QT, AMPLICOR-HIV Monitor, and QUANTIPLEX HIV RNA Assay, Three Methods for Quantification of Human Immunodeficiency Virus Type 1 RNA in Plasma. J Clin Micro 1996; 34: 1058-1064.

29. Piatak M, Saag MS, Yang LC, et al. High levels of HIV-1 in plasma during all stages of infection determined by competitive PCR. Science 1993; 259: 1749-54.

30. Henrard DR, Daar E, Farzadegan H, et al. Virologic and immunologic characterizations of symptomatic and asymptomatic primary HIV-1 infection. J Acq Imm Def Synd Hum Retro1995; 9: 305-10.

31. Katzenstein TL, Pederson C, Nielsen C, et al. Longitudinal serum HIV RNA quantification: correlation

to viral phenotype at seroconversion and clinical outcome. AIDS 1996; 10: 167-73.

32. Farzadegan H, et al. Sex differences in HIV-1 viral load and progression to AIDS. Lancet 1998; 352: 1510-14.

33. Burgard M, Mayaux MJ, Blanche S, et al. The use of viral culture and p24 antigen testing to diagnose human immunodeficiency virus infection in neonates. N Engl J Med 1992; 327: 192-7.

34. Dunn DT, Brandt CD, Krivine A, et al. The sensitivity of HIV-1 DNA polymerase chain reaction in the neonatal period and the relative contributions of intra-uterine and intra-partum transmission. AIDS1995; 9: 7-11.

35. Steketee RW, Abrams EJ, Thea DM, et al. Early Detection of perinatal human immunodeficiency virus (HIV) type 1 infection using HIV RNA amplification and detection. New York City Perinatal HIV Transmission Collaborative Study. J Infect Diseases 1997; 175: 707-11.

36. Pantaleo G, Menzo S, Vaccarezza M, et al. Studies in subjects with long-term nonprogressive HIV infection. N Engl J Med 1995; 332: 209-16.

37. Carpenter CCJ, Cooper DA, Fischl MA, et al. Antiretroviral therapy in Adults: Updated recommendations of the International AIDS Society - USA panel. JAMA 2000; 283: 381-390.

38. Guidelines for the use of antiretroviral agents in HIV-infected adults and adolescents. Department of Health and Human Services and Henry J. Kaiser Family Foundation [published erratum appears in MMWR Morb Mortal Wkly Rep 1998 Jul 31; 47(29): 619]. MMWR Morb Mortal Wkly Rep 1998. 47(RR-5): p. 43-82.

39. Gulick RM, Mellors JW, Havlir D, et al. Treatment with indinavir, zidovudine, and lamivudine in adults with human immunodeficiency virus infection and prior antiretroviral therapy. N Engl J Med 1997; 337: 734-9.

40. Staszewski S, Morales-Ramirez J, Tashima KT, et al. Efavirenz plus zidovudine and lamivudine, efavirenz plus indinavir, and indinavir plus zidovudine and lamivudine in the treatment of HIV-1 infection in adults. Study 006 Team. N Engl J Med 1999; 341: 1865-73.

41. Fischl MA. Antiretroviral therapy in 1999 for antiretroviral-naïve individuals with HIV infection. AIDS 1999; 13: S49-59.

42. Raboud JM, Rae S, Hogg RS, et al. Suppression of plasma virus load below the detection limit of a human immunodeficiency virus kit is associated with longer virologic response than suppression below the limit of quantitation. J Infect Dis 1999; 180: 1347-50.

43. Hogg R, Montaner JSG, Yip B et al. Are three drugs enough? Baseline plasma viral load as a predictor of virologic response to triple therapy. Presented at: 12th International Conference on AIDS, Geneva, Switzerland 1998 (Abstract 22359).

44. Rozenbaum W, Delphin N, and Katlama C. et al. Treatment Intensification with Ziagen in HIV Infected Patients with Previous 3TC/ZDV Antiretroviral Treatment-CNAB3009. Presented at: 6th Conference on Retroviruses and Opportunistic Infections; February 1999; Chicago Ill. Abstract 377.

45. Katlama C, Clotet B, Plettenberg A, et al. The role of abacavir (ABC, 1592) in antiretroviral therapy-experienced patients: results from a randomized, double blind, trial. CNA3002 European Study Team. AIDS 2000; 14: 781-9.

46. Gulick RM, Mellors, Havlir D, et al. Simultaneous vs sequential initiation of therapy with indinavir, zidovudine, and lamivudine for HIV-1 infection: 100 week follow-up. JAMA 1998; 280: 35-41.

47. Havlir, D.V., et al.: Maintenance antiretroviral therapies in HIV infected patients with undetectable plasma HIV RNA after triple-drug therapy. AIDS Clinical Trials Group Study 343 Team [see comments]. N Engl J Med 1998, 339(18): 1261-1268.

48. Raffi F, Bonnet B, Ferre V, et al. Substitution of NNRTI for Protease Inhibitor in the treatment of

Patients with Undetectable Plasma Human Immunodeficiency Virus Type 1 RNA. Clin Infect Dis 2000; 31: 1274-1278.

49. Hirsch MS, Brun-Vezinet F, D'Aquila RT, et al. Antiretroviral drug resistance testing in adult HIV-1 infection: recommendations of an International AIDS Society-USA Panel. JAMA 2000; 283: 2417-26.

50. Boden D, Hurley A, Zhang L, et al. HIV-1 Drug Resistance in Newly Infected Individuals. JAMA 1999; 282: 1135-41.

51. Little S, Daar ES, D'Aquila RT, et al. Reduced Antiretroviral Drug Susceptibility Among Patients With Primary HIV Infection. JAMA 1999; 282: 1142-49.

52. Hecht FM, Grant RM, Petropoulos CJ, et al. Sexual Transmission of an HIV-1 Variant Resistant to Multiple Reverse Transcriptase and Protease Inhibitors. New Engl J Med 1998; 339: 307-311.

53. Gulick R. Integrating New agents into Second-line Therapy: When do you switch and why. AIDS Reader 1999; 9: suppl 1: 12-18.

54. Collier AC, Schwartz MA. Strategies for second-line antiretroviral therapy in adults with HIV infection. Adv Exp Med Biol 1999; 458: 239-66.

55. Miller V, Cozzi-Lepri A, Hertogs K, et al. HIV drug susceptibility and treatment response to mega-HAART regimen in patients from Frankfurt HIV cohort. Antiviral therapy 2000; 5;49-55.

56. Devereux HL, Youle M, Johnson MA, Loveday C. Rapid decline in detectability of HIV-1 drug resistance mutations after stopping therapy. AIDS 1999; 13: F123-7.

57. Miller V, Sabin C, Hertogs K, Larder B, Bloor S, Martinez-Picado J, D'Aquila R, Larder B, Lutz T, Gute P, Weidmann E, Rabenau H, Phillips A, Staszewski S. Virological and immunological effects of treatment Interruptions in HIV-1 infected patients with treatment failure. AIDS 2000; 14 (18): 2857-2867.

58. Lisziewicz J, Rosenberg E, Lieberman J, et al. Control of HIV despite the discontinuation of therapy. N Engl J Med 1999; 340: 1683-1684.

59. Lori F. Hydroxyurea and HIV: 5 years later—from antiviral to immune-modulating effects. AIDS 1999; 13: 1433-42.

60. Kovacs JA, et al. Controlled trial of interleukin-2 infusions in patients infected with the human immunodeficiency virus. N Engl J Med 1996, 335(18): 1350-1356.

61. Cohen SJW, Schuurman R, Burger DM, et al. Randomized trial comparing saquinavir soft gelatin capsules *versus* indinavir as part of triple therapy (CHEESE study). AIDS 1999; 13(7); F53-8.

62. Neumann AU, Tubiana R, Calvez V, et al. HIV-1 rebound during interruption of highly active antiretroviral therapy has no deleterious effect on reinitiated treatment. Comet Study Group. AIDS 1999; 13: 677-83.

63. Staszewski S, Miller V, Sabin C, et al. Determinants of sustainable CD4 lymphocyte count increases in response to antiretroviral therapy. AIDS 1999; 13: 951-6.

64. Miller V, Mocroft A, Reiss P, et al. Relations among CD4 lymphocyte count nadir, antiretroviral therapy, and HIV-1 disease progression: results from the EuroSIDA study. Ann Intern Med 1999; 130: 570-7.

65. Miller V, Staszewski S, Sabin C, et al. CD4 lymphocyte count as a predictor of the duration of highly active antiretroviral therapy-induced suppression of human immunodeficiency virus load. J Infect Dis 1999; 180: 530-3.

66. Kaufmann D, Pantaleo G, Sudre P, Telenti A. for the Swiss HIV Cohort Study. CD4-cell count in HIV-1-infected individuals remaining viraemic with highly active antiretroviral therapy (HAART). Lancet 1998; 351: 723-4.

67. Kaufmann D, Munoz M, Bleiber G. et al. Virological and immunological characteristics of HIV

treatment failure. AIDS 2000; 14;1767-74.

68. Mezzaroma I, Carlesimo M, Pinter E, et al. Clinical and Immunologic Response without Decrease in Virus Load in Patients with AIDS after 24 months of Highly active Antiretroviral Therapy. Clin Infect Dis 1999; 29: 1423-30.

69. Harrigan PR, Hertogs K, Verbiest W, et al. Baseline HIV drug resistance profile predicts response to ritonavir-saquinavir protease inhibitor therapy in a community setting. AIDS 1999; 13: 1863-71.

70. Zolopa A, Shafer RW, Warford A, et al. HIV-1 genotypic resistance patterns predict response to saquinavir-ritonavir therapy in patients in whom previous protease inhibitor therapy had failed. Ann Intern Med 1999; 131: 813-21.

71. DeGruttola V, Dix L, D'Aquila R, et al. The relation between baseline HIV drug resistance and response to antiretroviral therapy: re-analysis of retrospective and prospective studies using a standardized data analysis plan. Antivir Ther 2000; 5: 41-8.

72. Baxter JD, Mayers DL, Wentworth DN, et al. A randomized study of antiretroviral management based on plasma genotypic antiretroviral resistance testing in patients failing therapy. CPCRA 046 Study Team for the Terry Beirn Community Programs for Clinical Research on AIDS. AIDS 2000 Jun 16; 14(9): F83-93.

73. Durant J, Clevenburgh P, Halfon et al. Drug-resistance genotyping in HIV-1 therapy: the VIRADAPT randomized controlled trial. Lancet 1999 353: 2195-2199.

74. Cohen C, Hunt S, Sension S, et al. Phenotypic resistance testing significantly improves responses to therapy: a randomized trial. 7th Conference on Retroviruses and Opportunistic Infections, January 2000, San Francisco, CA., Abstract 237.

75. Melnick D, Rosenthal J, Cameron M, et al. Impact of Phenotypic Antiretroviral Drug Resistance Testing on the Response to Salvage Antiretroviral Therapy (ART) in Heavily Experienced Patients. 7th Conference on Retroviruses and Opportunistic Infections, San Francisco, CA, 1/30-2/2/2000 (abstract 786).

76. Meynard JL, Vray M, Morand-Joubert L, et al. Impact of Treatment guided by phenotypic or genotypic resistance tests on the response to antiretroviral therapy (ART): A randomized Trial (NARVAL, ANRS 088). 40th Interscience Conference on Antimicrobial Agents and Chemotherapy, 9/17-20/2000, Toronto, Canada (abstract 698).

77. Tural C, Ruiz L, Holtzer C, et al. The Potential role of Resistance Decision support software with or without Expert Advice in a Trial of HIV genotyping *versus* standard of care. 40th Interscience Conference on Antimicrobial Agents and Chemotherapy, 9/17-20/2000, Toronto, Canada (abstract L-10).

78. Montaner JSG, Raboud JM, Rae S, et al. Adherence to Treatment Increases Duration of Virologic Suppression Regardless of pVL Nadir. Program and abstracts of the 38th Interscience Conference on Antimicrobial Agents and Chemotherapy; September 24-27 1998; San Diego, CA. Abstract LB 10.

79. Paterson DL, Swindels S, Mohr JA, et al. Adherence to protease inhibitor therapy and outcomes in patients with HIV infection. Ann Intern Med 2000; 133(1): 21-30.

80. Raffi F, Reliquet V, Ferre V, et al. The VIRGO study: nevirapine, didanosine and stavudine combination therapy in antiretroviral-naïve HIV-1-infected adults. Antiviral Therapy 2000; 5;267-72.

81. Staszewski S, Haberl A, Gute P, Nisius G, Miller V, Carlebach A et al. Nevirapine/Didanosine/ Lamivudine once daily in HIV-1 infected intravenous drug users. Antivir Ther 1998; 3 suppl 4: 55-6.

82. Malaty LI, Kuper JJ. Drug interactions of HIV protease inhibitors. Drug Saf 1999; 20(2): 147-69.

83. Kilby M, Sfakianos G, Gizzi N, et al. Safety and pharmacokinetics of once-daily regimens of soft-Gel capsule Saquinavir plus minidose Ritonavir in human immunodeficiency virus-negative adults. Antimicrob Agents Chemother 2000; 44: 2672-8.

84. Adkins JC, Noble S. Efavirenz. Drugs 1998; 56(6): 1055-64.

85. Havlir DV, Tierney C, Friedland G, et al. *In Vivo* antagonism with Zidovudine plus Stavudine combination therapy. J Infect Dis 2000; 182: 321-5.

86. Walensky RP, Goldberg JH, Daily JP. Anaphylaxis after rechallenge with abacavir. AIDS 1999; 3: 999-1000.

87. Marra A, Lewi D, Lanzoni V. Lactic acidosis and antiretroviral therapy: A case report and literature review. Braz J Infect Dis 2000 Jun; 4(3): 151-5.

88. Moyle G. Clinical manifestations and management of antiretroviral nucleoside analog-related mitochondrial toxicity. Clin Ther 2000 Aug; 22(8): 911-36; discussion 898.

89. Vigouroux C, Gharakhanian S, Salhi Y, et al. Adverse metabolic disorders during highly active antiretroviral treatments (HAART) of HIV disease. Diabetes Metab 1999; 25: 383-92.

90. Carr A, Samaras K, Thorisdottir A, Kaufmann GR, Chisholm DJ, Cooper DA. Diagnosis, prediction, and natural course of HIV-1 protease-inhibitor-associated lipodystrophy, hyperlipidemia, and diabetes mellitus: a cohort study. Lancet 1999; 353: 2093-99.

91. Carr A, Cooper DA. Adverse effects of antiretroviral therapy. Lancet 2000; 356: 1423-30.

92. Dube MP, Sprecher D, Henry WK, et al. Preliminary Guidelines for the Evaluation and Management of Dyslipidemia in Adults Infected with Human immunodeficiency virus and Receiving Antiretroviral Therapy: Recommendations of the Adult AIDS Clinical Trial Group Cardiovascular Disease Focus Group. Clin Infect Dis 2000; 31: 1216-1224.

93. Madge S, Kinloch-De Loes, Tyrer M, et al. Lypodystrophy Syndrome (LS) In Patients On Reverse Transcriptase Inhibitors. Presented at: 6th Conference on Retroviruses and Opportunistic Infections; February 1999; Chicago Ill. Abstract 654.

94. Saint-Marc T, Partisani M, Poizot-Martin I, et al. A Syndrome of peripheral fat wasting (Lipodystrophy) in Patients Receiving long-term Stable Nucleoside-Analogue Therapy. AIDS 1999; 13: 1659-67.

95. Moyle G, Baldwin C. Switching from a PI-based to a PI-sparing regimen for management of metabolic or clinical fat redistribution. AIDS Read 2000 Aug; 10(8): 479-85.

96. Connor, EM., et al.: Reduction of maternal-infant transmission of human immunodeficiency virus type 1 with zidovudine treatment. Pediatric AIDS Clinical Trials Group Protocol 076 Study Group. N Engl J Med 1994, 331(18): 1173-80.

97. Lallemant M, Jourdain G, Le Coeur S, et al. A trial of shortened Zidovudine regimens to prevent mother-to-child transmission of human immunodeficiency virus type 1. Perinatal HIV Prevention Trial (Thailand) Investigators. N Engl J Med 2000; 343: 982-91.

98. Guay LA, Musoke P, Fleming T, et al. Intrapartum and neonatal single dose nevirapine compared with zidovudine for prevention of mother-to-child transmission of HIV-1 in Kampla, Uganda: HIVNET 012 randomized trial. Lancet 1999; 354: 795-802.

99. The International Perinatal HIV Group. The Mode of Delivery and the Risk of Vertical Transmission of Human Immunodeficiency Virus Type 1--A Meta-Analysis of 15 Prospective Cohort Studies. N Engl J Med 1999; 340: 977-87.

100. Shearer WT, Quinn TC, LaRussa P, et al. Viral Load and Disease Progression in infants infected with human immunodeficiency virus type 1. N Engl J Med 1997; 336: 1337-42.

101. Guidelines for the use of antiretroviral agents in pediatric HIV infection. Center for Disease Control and Prevention. MMWR Morb Mortal Wkly Rep 1998, 47(RR-4): 1-43.

102. Lesens O, et al. Hepatitis C virus is related to progressive liver disease in human immunodeficiency virus-positive hemophiliacs and should be treated as an opportunistic infection. J Infect Dis 1998; 26: 16-19.

103. Zylberberg H, Benhamou Y, Lagneaux JL, et al. Safety and efficacy of interferon-ribavirin combination therapy in HCV-HIV confected subjects: an early report. Gut 2000; 47: 694-7.

104. Ragni MV, Bontempo FA. Increase in hepatitis C virus load in hemophiliacs during treatment with highly active antiretroviral therapy. J Infect Dis 1999; 180: 2027-9.

105. Causse X, Payen JL, Izopet J, Babany G, Girardin MF. Does HIV-infection influence the response of chronic hepatitis C to interferon treatment? A French multicenter prospective study. French Multicenter Study Group. J Hepatol 2000; 32: 1003-10.

106. Public Health Service guidelines for the management of health-care worker exposures to HIV and recommendations for Postexposure prophylaxis. Centers for Disease Control and Prevention. MMWR Morb Mortal Wkly Rep 1998, 47(RR-7): 1-33.

107. Vittinghoff E, Douglas J, Judson F, et al. Per-contact Risk of HIV transmission between male sexual partners. Am J Epidemiol 1999; 150: 306-11.

108. Management of possible sexual, injecting-drug-use, or other non-occupational exposure to HIV, including considerations related to antiretroviral therapy. Public Health Service statement. Centers for Disease Control and Prevention. MMWR Morb Mortal Wkly Rep 1998. 47(RR-17): 1-14.

109. 1999 USPHS/IDSA Guidelines for the prevention of opportunistic Infections in Persons Infected with Human Immunodeficiency virus. MMWR Morb Mortal Wkly Rep 1999. 48 (RR10): 1-59.

110. Furrer H, Egger M, Opravil M, et al. Discontinuation of primary prophylaxis against Pneumocystis carinii pneumonia in HIV-1 infected adults treated with combination antiretroviral therapy. Swiss HIV cohort study. N Engl J Med 1999; 340: 1301-6.

111. Currier JS, Willams PL, Koletar SL, et al. Discontinuation of Mycobacterium avium complex prophylaxis in patients with antiretroviral therapy-induced increases in CD4+ cell count. A randomized, double blind, placebo-controlled trial. AIDS Clinical Trials Group 362 Study Team. Ann Intern Med 2000; 133: 493-503.

112. Furrer H, Telenti A, Rossi M, Ledergerber B. Discontinuing or withholding primary prophylaxis against Mycobacterium avium in patients on successful antiretroviral combination therapy. The Swiss HIV Cohort Study. AIDS 2000; 14: 1409-12.

113. Furrer H, Opravil M, Bernasconi E, Telenti A, Effer M. Stopping primary prophylaxis in HIV-1 infected patients at high risk of toxoplasma encephalitis. Swiss HIV Cohort Study. Lancet 2000; 355: 2217-8.

114. Jubault V, Pacanowski J, Rabian C, Viard JP. Interruption of prophylaxis for major opportunistic infections in HIV-infected patients receiving triple combination antiretroviral therapy. Ann Med Interne (Paris) 2000; 151: 163-8.

115. French MAH. Immune restoration Disease in HIV-infected patients on HAART. AIDS Reader 1999; 9: 548-562.

116. Behrens GM, Meyer D, Toll M, Schmidt RE. Immune reconstitution syndromes in human immunodeficiency virus infection following effective antiretroviral therapy. Immunobiology 2000; 202: 186-93.

117. Kahn JO, Cherng DW, Mayer K, Murray H, Lagakos S. Evalution of HIV-1 immunogen, an immunologic modifier administered to patients infected with HIV having 330 to 549 x 10^6/L CD4 cell counts: A randomized controlled trial. JAMA 2000; 284: 2193-202.

118. Migasena S, Suntharasamai P, Pitisuttithum P, et al. AIDSVAX (MN) in Bangkok injecting drug users: a report on safety and immunogenicity, including macrophage-tropic virus neutralization. AIDS Res Hum Retroviruses 2000; 16: 655-63.

119. Schooley RT, Spino C, Kuritzkes D, et al. Two double-blinded, randomized comparative trials of 4 human immunodeficiency virus type 1 (HIV-1) envelope vaccines in HIV-1 infected individuals

across a spectrum of disease severity: AIDS clinical trials groups 209 and 214. J Infect Dis 2000; 182: 1357-64.

Table 1. Clinical diagnoses and disease processes caused by human immunodeficiency virus infection

Patients/Presentation	Frequency of Symptomatic Disease
Congenital and Perinatal Infection	15-30% of infants born to HIV+ women Become infected and most develop an immunodeficiency syndrome over 5 yrs.
Acute, Primary Infection	>50% of patients have a moderate to severe Primary acute viral syndrome within weeks of infection
Chronic Infection	Infection leads to progressive immunodeficiency characterized by declining CD4+ (helper) Cell numbers, with increasing risk for opportunistic infection and malignancy.
Relapse/recurrence	Cessation or resistance to antiviral therapy may be associated with increased viremia immunodeficiency and recurrent symptoms.
Transplant and Chemotherapy	Limited experience suggests that transplantation or aggressive chemotherapy leads to rapid progression of AIDS.

Table 2.   Laboratory diagnosis of infection

Diagnostic Methods	Interpretation
Serologic tests:	
ELISA assays	Sensitive and specific for infection within 4 weeks. Recombinant peptide or whole virus lysate assays developed for IgG antibodies to multiple epitopes.
Western Blot	Whole virus lysate or recombinant proteins used primarily to confirm ELISA tests
Antigen detection: p24 antigen assays	Structural (gag) protein in plasma can be quantified in serum or plasma in up to 50% of chronic infection. May be detected prior to antibodies in primary infection. Increased sensitivity with heat or alkaline denaturation of competing anti-p24 antibodies.
Nucleic Acid amplification assays:	HIV plasma RNA measured by commercial RT-PCR, b-DNA, and NASBA assays to quantify circulating viremia. Currently, to determine the need for therapy and used as a surrogate marker for drug activity.
Cell Culture Assays	Requires PHA stimulated PBMC and assays for p24 or reverse transcriptase to detect infection. Used primarily for research rather than clinical assessment

Table 3. Indications for antiretroviral (ARV) therapy (A) and opportunistic infection prophylaxis (B)

A			
CD4 count (/mm^3)	Viral Load Copies/ml	Symptoms (AIDS, thrush, fever, etc)	Initiate ARV Therapy
Any	Any	Yes	Yes
< 200	< Any	No	Yes
> 200, < 350	> Any	No	Yes
> 350	< 30-50,000	No	No
> 350	> 30-50,000	No	Yes

B	
Disease	CD4 count Threshold for prophylaxis
TB	Any and PPD > 5 mm
Pneumocystis carinii	< 200
Toxoplasmosis gondii	< 100 (with positive IgG serology)
Mycobacterium avium complex	< 50

Prophylaxis generally not recommended for CMV, candida, cryptococcal, and other fungal diseases

Table 4. Antiretroviral medication dosages and major toxicities

Nucleoside Reverse Transcriptase Inhibitors (NRTI)	Dosage (pill #/dose)	Toxicities
Zidovudine (AZT)	300 mg BID (1)	nausea, headache, fatigue, anemia
Lamivudine (3TC)	150 mg BID (1)	GI intolerance (mild)
Didanosine (ddI)	400 mg qd (1)	pancreatitis, peripheral neuropathy
Stavudine (d4T)	40 mg BID (1)	peripheral neuropathy
Zalcitabine (ddC)	0.75 mg TID (1)	peripheral neuropathy, stomatitis
Abacavir (ABC)	300 mg BID (1)	Hypersensitivity Reaction (Fever, vomiting, cough, rash) **DO NOT Rechallenge**
Combination Pills		
AZT/3TC	300/150 mg BID (1)	
AZT/3TC/ABC	300/150/300 mg BID (1)	
Nonnucleoside Reverse Transcriptase Inhibitors (NNRTI)		
Efavirenz (EFV)	600 mg qhs (3)	sleep disturbances, hallucinations Bad dreams, rash **DO NOT Use in Pregnancy**
Nevirapine (NVP)	200 mg BID (1) 400 mg qd (2)	Rash (20-30%) (Alternative dosing)
Delavirdine (DLV)	400 mg TID (2)	Rash, headaches
Protease Inhibitors (PI)		
Indinavir (IDV)	800 mg q 8h (2)	GI symptoms, kidney stones, ↑bilirubin
Ritonavir (RTV)	600 mg BID (6)	GI symptoms, circumoral paraesthesias
Saquinavir (SQV)	1200 mg TID (6)	GI symptoms
Nelfinavir (NFV)	1250 mg BID (5)	Diarrhea (20-30%)
Amprenavir (AMP)	1200 mg BID (8)	GI symptoms
Combination Pills		
Lopinavir/ritonavir	300/100 mg BID (3)	GI symptoms
Other PI Combinations Currently in Use		
Ritonavir/Saquinavir	400/400 mg BID (6)	
Ritonavir/Saquinavir	100/1600 mg qd (9)	
Ritonavir/Indinavir	200/800 mg BID (4)	
Ritonavir/Amprenavir	200/600 mg BID (6)	

Table 5. Recommendations for therapy/post exposure prophylaxis (PEP)

Initial Treatment
Preferred Regimens

	Column A	**Column B**
	Efavirenz	d4T/3TC
	Indinavir	AZT/ddI
	Nelfinavir	AZT/3TC
	Ritonavir/Saquinavir	d4T/ddI

Alternative Regimens

	Abacavir	ddI/3TC
	Amprenavir	AZT/ddC
	Delavirdine	
	Nevirapine	
	Ritonavir	
	Saquinavir (Fortovase)	
	Nelfinavir/Saquinavir	
	Ritonavir/Indinavir	

Not Recommended

	Saquinavir (Invirase)	ddI/ddC
		d4T/ddC
		ddC/3TC
		AZT/d4T

From DHHS Guidelines (1 from Column A and 2 from column B)

Salvage Treatment
Depends somewhat on the prior regimen and resistance profile

Prior Regimen	Salvage Regimen
2NRTI + PI	2 new NRTI + NNRTI
	2 new NRTI + 2 new PI (without cross resistance)
2NRTI + NNRTI	2 new NRTI + 1 or 2 PI

Post Exposure Prophylaxis (PEP)

Exposure Category	**Treatment**
No to low risk of exposure	Consider AZT/3TC
Low to moderate risk	AZT/3TC
High Risk	AZT/3TC + Indinavir or nelfinavir

MMWR 1998, 47: RR-7

CHAPTER 6

HERPESVIRUSES: AN INTRODUCTION WITH A FOCUS OF HERPES SIMPLEX VIRUS

RICHARD J. WHITLEY and PAUL D. GRIFFITHS

Table of Contents

Practical Guidelines in Antiviral Therapy Ed. by Charles A.B. Boucher and George J. Galasso. 127 — 149
© 2002 *Elsevier Science. Printed in the Netherlands.*

Introduction To Herpesvirus

In nature, herpesviruses infect both vertebrate and non-vertebrate species, and over a hundred have been at least partially characterized [1]. Only eight of these have been isolated routinely from humans, including herpes simplex virus type 1 (HSV-1), herpes simplex virus type 2 (HSV-2), varicella-zoster virus (VZV), cytomegalovirus (CMV), Epstein-Barr virus (EBV), human herpesvirus 6 (HHV-6), human herpesvirus 7 (HHV-7) and, most recently, Kaposi's Sarcoma herpesvirus or human herpesvirus 8 (HHV-8). A primate herpesvirus, namely B virus, is an uncommon human pathogen that may cause life-threatening disease. This chapter will serve as the introduction to the family of herpesviruses. The principal focus will be HSV but it will also include EBV, HHV-6, HHV-7, HHV-8 and B virus. The following chapters deal with CMV and VZV as separate entities. Of note, for the purpose of this book, treatment of HSV infections provides a model for the development of antiviral therapeutics.

Biologic Properties

The human herpesviruses share four significant biologic properties [1]. First, all of the herpesviruses code for unique enzymes which process nucleic acids. These enzymes are structurally diverse and, parenthetically, provide unique sites for inhibition by antiviral agents. The best examples are HSV thymidine kinase and DNA polymerase. Secondly, the synthesis and assembly of viral DNA is initiated in the nucleus. Assembly of the capsid also begins in the nucleus. Envelopment with associated glycosylation events occurs in the Golgi. Third, release of progeny virions from infected cells is accompanied by cell death. Finally, all herpesviruses establish latent infection within tissues that are characteristic for each virus, reflecting the unique tissue tropism of each member of this family.

Membership in the family *Herpesviridae* is based on the structure of the virion. These viruses contain double-stranded DNA which is located at the central core. The precise arrangement of the DNA within the core is not known. Herpesvirus DNA varies in molecular weight from approximately 80 to 150 million, or 120 to 250 kilobase pairs, depending on the virus. This DNA core is surrounded by a capsid that consists of 162 capsomers, arranged in icosapentahedral symmetry. The capsid is approximately 100 to 110 nanometers in diameter. Tightly adherent to the capsid is the tegument, which appears to consist of amorphous material. Loosely surrounding the capsid and tegument is a lipid bilayer envelope derived from host cell plasma membranes. The envelope consists of polyamines, lipids, and glycoproteins. These glycoproteins confer distinctive properties to each virus and provide unique antigens to which the host is capable of responding [1].

A feature of herpesvirus DNA is its genomic sequence arrangement. Herpesviruses can be divided into six groups arbitrarily classified A to F [1]. For those herpesviruses which infect humans (group C, group D, and group E) unique structures are demonstrable. In the group C genomes, as exemplified by EBV and the newly identified Kaposi's Sarcoma Herpesvirus, the number of terminal reiterations divides the genome into several well delineated domains. The group D genomes, such as VZV, have sequences from one terminus repeated in an inverted orientation internally. Thus, the DNA extracted from these virions consist of two equal molar populations. For group E viral genomes, such as HSV and CMV, the genomes are divided into internal unique sequences whereby both termini are repeated in an inverted orientation. Thus, the genomes can form four equimolar populations that differ in relative orientation of the two segments.

The grouping of herpesviruses into sub-families serves the purpose of identifying evolutionary relatedness as well as summarizing unique properties of each member [1]. These subfamilies are relevant for the development of antiviral therapeutics.

Alpha herpesviruses. The members of the alpha herpesvirus sub-family — HSV-1, HSV-2, VZV and B virus — are characterized by an extremely short reproductive cycle (hours), prompt destruction of the host cell, and the ability to replicate in a wide variety of host tissues. They characteristically establish latent infection in sensory nerve ganglia. Antiviral therapy for this subfamily is directed toward the treatment of acute infection (both HSV and VZV) or suppression of recurrent infection (i.e. genital HSV) [2].

Beta herpesviruses. In contrast to the alpha herpesviruses, beta herpesviruses — CMV, HHV-6, HHV-7 — have a restricted host range. While their reproductive life cycle is shorter than historically appreciated, cytopathic evidence of infection progresses slowly in cell culture systems. A characteristic of these viruses is their ability to form enlarged cells, as exemplified by human CMV infection. These viruses can establish latent infection in secretory glands, cells of the reticuloendothelial system, and the kidneys. While a separate chapter addresses therapeutic successes achieved for CMV disease, a brief note will be made about the potential treatment of HHV-6 and HHV-7.

Gamma herpesviruses. Finally, the gamma herpesviruses — EBV and Kaposi's sarcoma herpesvirus — have the most limited host range. They replicate in lymphoblastoid cells *in vitro* and can cause lytic infections in certain targeted cells. Latent virus has been demonstrated in lymphoid tissue. Successful therapies for diseases caused by these viruses have not been established in controlled clinical trials.

Replication of all herpesviruses is a multi-step process [2]. Following the onset of infection, DNA is uncoated and transported to the nucleus of the host cell. This is followed by transcription of immediate-early genes, also known as alpha genes, which encode for the regulatory proteins. Expression of immediate-early gene products is followed by the expression of proteins encoded by early (beta) genes and, then, late (gamma) genes. Successful therapy is best illustrated by drugs directed against HSV [3]. In this model, drugs such as acyclovir act at the level of early gene expression. The activity of acyclovir and similar drugs is discussed below.

Assembly of the viral core and capsid takes place within the nucleus. This is followed by envelopment at the nuclear membrane and transport out of the nucleus through the endoplasmic reticulum and the Golgi apparatus. Glycosylation of the viral membrane occurs in the Golgi apparatus. Mature virions are transported to the outer membrane of the host cell inside vesicles. Release of progeny virus is accompanied by cell death. Replication for all herpesviruses is considered inefficient, with a high ratio of non-infectious to infectious viral particles. No drugs have yet proven successful in clinical trials for events of the inhibition of assembly through release of progeny virions.

A unique characteristic of the herpesviruses is their ability to establish latent infection [2]. Each virus within the family has the potential to establish latency in specific host cells, and the latent viral genome may be either extra-chromosomal or integrated into host cell DNA. Herpes simplex virus 1 and 2, and VZV all establish latency in the dorsal root ganglia. Epstein-Barr virus can maintain latency within B lymphocytes and salivary glands. Cytomegalovirus can be latently detected in lymphocytes, platelets and endothelial cells. Human herpesvirus 6 and HHV-7, Kaposi's sarcoma, and B virus have unknown sites of latency. No drugs prevent the establishment of latency.

Latent virus may be reactivated and enter a replicative cycle at any point in time. The reactivation of latent virus is a well-recognized biologic phenomenon, but not one that is understood from a biochemical or genetic standpoint. Stimuli that have been observed to be associated with the reactivation of latent HSV have included stress, menstruation, and exposure to ultraviolet light. Precisely how these factors interact at the level of the ganglia remains to be defined. Reactivation of herpesviruses may be clinically asymptomatic, or it may produce life-threatening disease. With the recent development of polymerase chain reaction (PCR) as an assay to detect viral DNA, it is possible to demonstrate evidence of infection three to five times as many days as by virus culture.

Diagnosis

With the exception of CMV retinitis, the definitive diagnosis of a herpesvirus infection requires either isolation of virus or detection of viral gene products. For virus isolation, swabs of clinical specimens (vesicles, throat, conjunctiva, etc.) or other body fluids can be inoculated into susceptible cell lines and observed for the development of characteristic cytopathic effects. This technique is most useful for the diagnosis of infection due to HSV-1 and -2 or VZV because of their relatively short replicative cycles. Similarly, B virus can be isolated in cell culture. Epstein-Barr virus does not induce cytopathic changes in cell culture systems and, therefore, can only be identified in culture by transformation of cord blood lymphocytes. Similarly, HHV-6 and -7 have unique growth characteristics that make identification in cell culture systems difficult.

Newer and more rapid diagnostic techniques involve the detection of viral gene products. This can be done by applying fluorescence antibody directed against immediate-early or late gene products to tissue cultures after 24 to 72 hours of incubation. A positive result is the appearance of intranuclear fluorescence. Alternatively, fluorescence antibodies may be applied directly to cell monolayers or scrapings of clinical lesions, with intranuclear fluorescence again indicating a positive result.

Recently developed diagnostic techniques that have clinical utility include *in situ* and dot-blot hybridization and, importantly, PCR DNA amplification. This latter technique has proved most successful in the diagnosis of HSV infections of the central nervous system, particularly when applied to cerebrospinal fluid. Importantly, this tool has been utilized to study the natural history of genital HSV infections. For viruses such as HHV-6 and HHV-7, detection by PCR is the diagnostic approach most frequently utilized. Blood specimens provide biologic material for detection of viral DNA.

In addition to new tests for virus gene products and viral DNA, improved serologic assays are also becoming available, particularly the application of immunoblot technology to distinguish HSV-1 from HSV-2 infections. However, these tests are only useful for making a diagnosis in retrospect.

Herpes Simplex Viruses

Introduction

Of all the herpesviruses, HSV-1 and HSV-2 are the most closely related, with nearly 70 per cent genomic homology. These two viruses can be distinguished most reliably by DNA composition; however, differences in antigen expression and biologic properties also serve as methods for differentiation.

Transmission of HSV, regardless of virus type, is dependent upon intimate contact between a person who is shedding virus and a susceptible host, as reviewed [4]. After inoculation onto the skin or mucous membrane and an incubation period of four to six days, HSV replicates in epithelial cells. As replication continues, cell lysis and local inflammation ensue, resulting in characteristic vesicles on an erythematous base. Regional lymphatics and lymph nodes become involved: viremia and visceral dissemination may develop depending upon the immunologic competence of the host. In all hosts, the virus generally ascends the peripheral sensory nerves to reach the dorsal root ganglia. Replication of HSV within neural tissue is followed by retrograde axonal spread of the virus back to other mucosal and skin surfaces via the peripheral sensory nerves. Virus replicates further in epithelial cells, reproducing the lesions of the initial infection, until infection is contained through both host systemic and mucosal immunity. Latency is established when HSV reaches the dorsal root ganglia after anterograde transmission via sensory nerve pathways. In its latent form, intracellular HSV DNA cannot be detected routinely unless specific molecular probes are utilized. Herpes simplex virus DNA is maintained in a circularized and episomal state. Therapy of HSV disease is directed toward accelerating the resolution of acute disease or chronic suppressive therapy for individuals with frequently recurrent infections. Of note, however, studies are in progress to determine if therapy prevents person-to-person transmission.

Clinical Diagnosis

Diseases caused by HSV span a broad spectrum, as defined below. With cutaneous evidence of HSV disease, i.e. a vesicular eruption, the diagnosis can be suspected clinically. However, with some cutaneous eruptions, the manifestations are not typical of HSV, resulting in fissures or cracks in the skin, particularly in the genital tract. In the immunocompromised host, cutaneous manifestations are always more severe and of longer duration. Additionally, involvement of the central nervous system with HSV can be suspected because of age (newborn) or focality (temporal lobe) of presentation. However, the diagnosis can only be confirmed utilizing laboratory tests.

Antiviral therapies are available for diseases caused by HSV. They will be discussed accordingly (Table 1). Acyclovir (9-{2-hydroxyethoxymethyl} guanine), a synthetic acyclic purine nucleoside analogue has become the standard of therapy of HSV infections [5]. It is the most widely prescribed and clinically effective antiviral drug available to date. The prodrug valaciclovir (converted to acyclovir) and famciclovir (converted to penciclovir) have recently been licensed and provide enhanced oral bioavailability compared to acyclovir and penciclovir, respectively. These drugs have been described in detail in chapter 1 and 2 and are recently reviewed [3].

Mucocutaneous Infections (Table 2)

Gingivostomatitis

Mucocutaneous infections are the most common clinical manifestations of HSV-1 and -2. Gingivostomatitis, which is usually caused by HSV-1, occurs most frequently in children less than five years of age. Gingivostomatitis is characterized by fever, sore throat, pharyngeal edema and erythema, followed by the development of vesicular or ulcerative lesions on the oral and pharyngeal mucosa. Recurrent HSV-1 infections of the oropharynx are most frequently manifest as herpes simplex labialis (cold sores), and usually appear on the vermillion border of the lip. Intraoral lesions as a manifestation of recurrent disease are uncommon in the normal host but do occur frequently in immunocomporomised individuals.

Therapy of HSV gingivostomatitis has only been evaluated with acyclovir. Early intervention will accelerate cutaneous healing [6].

Herpes Labialis (Table 2)

Topical therapy with penciclovir (Denavir) will accelerate clinical healing by approximately one day [7]. Orally-administered acyclovir (at a dose of 200 mg 5 times daily for 5 days) reduces the length of time to the loss of crusts by approximately one day (7 *versus* 8 days), but does not alter the duration of pain or the length of time to complete healing. Oral administration of acyclovir can alter the severity of sun-induced labial reactivation of labial HSV infections [8]. The administration of 200 mg 5 times daily to skiers did not decrease the frequency of recurrent labial infections as compared with placebo, but significantly fewer lesions formed on days 5-7 among acyclovir recipients. Short-term prophylactic therapy with acyclovir may benefit some patients with recurrent herpes labialis who anticipate engaging in a high-risk activity (e.g., intense exposure to sunlight). The intermittent administration of acyclovir does not alter the frequency of subsequent recurrences. No data support the use of long-term treatment with any of these drugs for the prevention of herpes labialis.

Table 1. Therapeutic Options for Herpes Simplex Virus Infections[a]

Type of infection	Drug	Route and Dosage[b]	Comments
Genital HSV Initial episode	Acyclovir	200 mg po 5 times/d x 10 d	Preferred route in normal host
		5 mg/kg IV q 8 h x 5-7 d	Reserved for severe cases
	Valaciclovir	1 gm po bid x 5-10 d	
	Famciclovir	250 mg po tid x 5-10 d	
Recurrent oral or genital	Acyclovir	200 mg po 5 times/d x 5 d	
	Valaciclovir	400 mg po tid x 5 d	
		500 mg po bid x 5-7 d	
	Famciclovir	250 mg po bid x 5-7 d	
Suppresion (genital)	Acyclovir	400 mg po bid	Titrate dosage as required
	Valaciclovir	500 mg po bid or 1 g qd	
	Famciclovir	125 or 250 mg po bid	
Mucocutaneous HSV (immunocompromised)	Acyclovir	200-400 mg po 5 times/d x 10 d	
		5 mg/kg IV q 8 h x 7-10[c]	
	Valaciclovir	500 mg bid po	
	Famciclovir	500 mg tid po	
HSV encephalitis	Acyclovir	10 mg/kg IV q 8 h x 14-21 d	
Neonatal HSV	Acyclovir	20 mg/kg IV q 8 h x 14-21 d	
Herpetic conjunctivitis	Trifluridine	1 drop q 2h while awake x 7-14 d	Alternative: vidarabine ointment
Recurrent	Acyclovir	400 mg bid x 7-10 d	

[a] Adapted from Whitley R, Gnann J. N Engl J Med. 1992; 327: 782-789.
[b] The doses are for adults with normal renal function unless otherwise noted.
[c] A dose of 250 mg/m² should be given to children <12 years of age.

Genital Herpes (Table 2)

Genital herpes is most frequently caused by HSV-2 but an ever increasing number of cases are attributed to HSV 1. Primary infection in women usually involves the vulva, vagina, and cervix. In men, initial infection is most often associated with lesions on the glans penis, prepuce or penile shaft. In individuals of either sex, primary disease is associated with fever, malaise, anorexia, and bilateral inguinal adenopathy. Women frequently have dysuria and urinary retention due to urethral involvement. As many as 10 per cent of individuals will develop an aseptic meningitis with primary infection. Sacral radiculomyelitis may occur in both men and women, resulting in neuralgias, urinary retention, or constipation. The complete healing of primary infection may take several weeks. First episode of genital infection is less severe in individuals who have had previous HSV infections at other sites, such as HSV labialis.

Recurrent genital infections in either men or women can be particularly distressing. The frequency of recurrence varies significantly from one individual to another. It has been estimated that one-third of individuals with genital herpes have virtually no recurrences, one-third have approximately three recurrences per year and another third greater than three per year. Recent seroepidemiologic studies have found that between 25 per cent – 65 per cent of individuals in the United States had antibodies to HSV-2, and that seroprevalence is dependent upon the number of sexual partners [9]. Applying PCR to genital swabs from women with a history of recurrent genital herpes, virus DNA can be detected in the absence of culture proof of infection [10]. This finding suggests the chronicity of genital herpes as opposed to a recurrent infection. This finding suggests the chronicity or more frequent recurrences than previously appreciated of genital herpes.

Initial genital HSV infection can be treated with topical, oral, or intravenous acyclovir. While topical application of acyclovir reduces the duration of viral shedding and the length of time before all lesions become crusted, it is less effective than oral or intravenous therapy. In fact, it should not be a choice for the management of this form of disease. Intravenous acyclovir is the most effective treatment for first-episode genital herpes, and results in a significant reduction in the median duration of viral shedding, pain, and length of time to complete healing (8 *versus* 14 days). Since intravenous acyclovir therapy usually requires hospitalization, it should be reserved for patients with severe local disease or systemic complications. Oral therapy (200 mg 5 times daily or 400 mg tid) is nearly as effective as intravenous acyclovir for initial genital herpes, and has become the standard treatment, as reviewed [5]. Both valaciclovir and famciclovir offer similar degrees of therapeutic benefit as acyclovir but can be dosed less frequently [3]. Neither intravenous nor oral acyclovir treatment of acute HSV infection reduces the frequency of recurrences.

Recurrent genital herpes is less severe and resolves more rapidly than primary infection; thus, there is less time to successfully introduce antiviral chemotherapy. Oral acyclovir therapy (same dosing as above) shortens both the duration of viral shedding and the length of time to healing (6 *versus* 7 days) when initiated early (within 24 hours of onset), but the duration of symptoms and length of time to recurrence

Table 2.   Diagnosis of Herpes Simplex Virus

Syndrome	Diagnosis	
	Clinical Diagnosis*	Laboratory
Gingivostomatitis	Usually asymptomatic; extensive intra-oral vesiculo-ulcerative lesions	Culture Seroconversion
Herpes Labialis	Vermillion border lip lesions	Culture
Genital Herpes		
Primary	Usual asymptomatic	Culture and virus typing
	Extensive genital vesiculo-ulcerative lesions	PCR Culture
Recurrent	Limited genital vesicular lesions	Type-specific serology
Herpetic Whitlow	Apparent paronychia	Culture
Herpes Gladiatorum	Cutaneous Vesicular Lesion	Culture
Herpes Keratitis	Fluorescein staining of dendritic lesions of cornea	Culture PCR
Neonatal Herpes	Cutaneous lesions Meningoencephalitis Shock-syndrome	Culture PCR
Herpes Simplex Encephalitis	Focal encephalopathy Focal CT/MRI	PCR of CSF
Meningitis	Meningisms — usually young female adults	PCR of CSF
Immunocompromised HSV	Disseminated cutaneous lesions Esophagitis	Culture Endoscopic culture

* History is mandatory

are not affected. Valaciclovir (500 mg bid or 1 gm qd) [11] and famciclovir (250 mg bid) [12] likely provide a similar degree of benefit but are dosed less frequently.

Long-term oral administration of acyclovir, valaciclovir, or famciclovir effectively suppresses genital herpes in patients who have frequent recurrences both in the normal as well as immunocompromised [13-15]. Daily administration of acyclovir reduces the frequency of recurrences by up to 80 per cent, and 25-30 per cent of patients have no further recurrences while taking acyclovir. Successful suppression for as long as 6 years has been reported, with no evidence of significant adverse effects. Titration of the dose of acyclovir (400 mg twice daily, or 200 mg two to five times daily) may be required to establish the minimal dose that is most effective and economical. Valaciclovir and famciclovir can be administered as above. Treatment should be interrupted every 12 months to reassess the need for continued suppression. The emergence of acyclovir-resistant strains of HSV appears to be infrequent in immunologically normal individuals. Importantly, asymptomatic shedding of virus can continue despite clinically effective suppression with acyclovir, so that the possibility of person-to-person transmission persists.

Herpes Simplex Keratitis (Table 2)

Herpes simplex keratitis is usually caused by HSV-1 and is accompanied by conjunctivitis in many cases. It is the most common infectious cause of blindness in the United States. The characteristic lesions of herpes simplex keratoconjunctivitis are dendritic ulcers best detected by fluorescein staining. Deep stromal involvement has also been reported and may result in visual impairment. Acute disease is treated topically with trifluorothymidine drops applied q 2 hour while awake. Likely, the concomitant use of oral acyclovir at dosages employed for the treatment of recurrent genital herpes is of clinical benefit at the same dosages employed for the treatment of recurrent genital herpes. For individuals with recurrent herpes simplex keratitis, chronic suppressive acyclovir is of value [16]. Valaciclovir and famciclovir have not been studied for this indication.

Other Skin Manifestations

Herpes simplex virus infections can manifest at any skin site. Common among health care workers are lesions on abraded skin of the fingers, known as herpetic whitlows. Similarly, wrestlers, because of physical contact may develop disseminated cutaneous lesions known as herpes gladiatorum. Treatment with acyclovir (genital herpes doses) will accelerate healing. Likely, but not evaluated, valaciclovir and famciclovir would also prove efficacious.

Neonatal HSV Infection (Table 2)

Neonatal HSV infection is estimated to occur in approximately one in 3000 deliveries in the United States annually. Approximately 70 per cent of cases are caused by HSV-2 and usually result from contact of the fetus with infected maternal genital secretions at the time of delivery. Manifestations of neonatal HSV infection can be divided into three categories: 1) skin, eye and mouth disease, 2) encephalitis, and 3) disseminated infection. As the name implies, skin, eye and mouth disease consists of cutaneous lesions and does not involve other organ systems. Involvement of the central nervous system may occur with encephalitis or disseminated infection, and generally results in diffuse encephalitis. The cerebrospinal fluid formula characteristically reveals an elevated protein and a mononuclear pleocytosis. Disseminated infection involves multiple organ systems and can produce disseminated intravascular coagulation, hemorrhagic pneumonitis, encephalitis, and cutaneous lesions. Diagnosis can be particularly difficult in the absence of skin lesions. The mortality rate for each disease classification varies from zero for skin, eye and mouth disease to 15 per cent for encephalitis and 60 per cent for neonates with disseminated infection. In addition to the high mortality associated with these infections, morbidity is significant in that children with encephalitis or disseminated disease develop normally in only approximately 40 per cent of cases, even with the administration of appropriate antiviral therapy.

In a comparative study, acyclovir was as effective as (but not superior to) vidarabine in neonates with HSV infections. No baby with disease localized to the skin, eye, or mouth died, whereas 18 per cent of babies with CNS infection and 55 per cent of those with disseminated infection died. Among babies with HSV infections of the skin, eye and mouth, 90 per cent of those treated with vidarabine and 98 per cent of those treated with acyclovir were developing normally 2 years after infection. The comparable values were 50 per cent and 43 per cent among babies surviving encephalitis and 62 per cent and 57 per cent among babies surviving disseminated infection [17].

Recently, studies of high dose acyclovir have been completed in babies with either encephalitis or disseminated disease. At a dosage of 20 mg/kg given every 8 hours for 21 days, mortality from encephalitis was decreased to five per cent and for disseminated disease to 25 per cent [18]. These dosages are recommended for treatment of babies with neonatal herpes simplex virus in the American Academy of Pediatrics 2000 Red Book.

Thus, unlike the results of therapy in older patients with herpes simplex encephalitis, there were no significant differences in either morbidity or mortality among infants treated with acyclovir or vidarabine. Clearance of virus was slower in babies who received acyclovir than in immunocompromised adults, implying a requirement for host defense as well. The safety and ease of administration of acyclovir make it the treatment of choice for neonatal HSV infections. The currently recommended intravenous dose is 20 mg/kg every eight hours for 14-21 days. Long term oral suppressive therapy may be of value and warrants further study.

Herpes Simplex Encephalitis (Table 2)

Herpes simplex encephalitis is characterized by hemorrhagic necrosis of the inferio-medial portion of the temporal lobe. Disease begins unilaterally but can progress to involve the, contralateral temporal lobe. It is the most common cause of focal, sporadic encephalitis in the United States today, and occurs in approximately 1 in 150,000 individuals. Most cases are caused by HSV-1. The actual pathogenesis of herpes simplex encephalitis requires further clarification, although it has been speculated that primary or recurrent virus can reach the temporal lobe by ascending neural pathways, such as the trigeminal tracts or the olfactory nerves.

Clinical manifestations of herpes simplex encephalitis include headache, fever, altered consciousness, and abnormalities of speech and behavior. Focal seizures may also occur. The cerebrospinal fluid formula for these patients is variable, but usually consists of a pleocytosis with both polymorphonuclear leukocytes and monocytes present. The protein concentration is characteristically elevated and glucose is usually normal. Historically, a definitive diagnosis could only be achieved by brain biopsy, since other pathogens may produce a clinically similar illness. However, the application of PCR for detection of virus DNA has replaced brain biopsy as the standard for diagnosis.

Herpes simplex encephalitis is associated with substantial morbidity and mortality despite the use of antiviral therapy. The administration of acyclovir in a dose of 10 mg/kg every 8 hours for 14 to 21 days reduces mortality at three months to 19 per cent, as compared with approximately 50 per cent among patients treated with vidarabine [19]. Furthermore, 38 per cent of the patients treated with acyclovir regain normal function. Patients with a Glasgow coma score of less than 6, those over 30 years of age, and those with encephalitis longer than four days have a poor outcome. For the most favorable outcome, therapy must be instituted before semicoma or coma develops.

HSV Infections In The Immunocompromised Host (Table 2)

Herpes simplex virus infections in the immunocompromised host are clinically more severe, may be progressive, and require more time for healing. Manifestations of HSV infections in this patient population include pneumonitis, esophagitis, hepatitis, colitis, and disseminated cutaneous disease. Individuals suffering from human immunodeficiency virus infection may have extensive perineal or oro-facial ulcerations. Herpes simplex virus infections are also noted to be of increased severity in individuals who are burned.

Intravenous acyclovir therapy of HSV disease in the immunocompromised host is clinically beneficial. Immunocompromised patients receiving acyclovir had a shorter duration of viral shedding and more rapid healing of lesions than do patients receiving placebo [20]. Oral acyclovir therapy is also very effective in immunocompromised patients [21]. Acyclovir prophylaxis of HSV infections is of clinical value in immunocompromised patients, especially those undergoing induction chemotherapy or transplantation. Intravenous or oral administration of acyclovir reduces the incidence of symptomatic HSV infection from about 70 per cent to 5-20 per cent. A sequential regimen of intravenous acyclovir followed by oral acyclovir for 3 to 6 months can virtually eliminate symptomatic HSV infections in organ transplant recipients. A variety of oral dosing regimens, ranging from 200 mg 3 times daily to 800 mg twice daily, have been used successfully. Similar data exist for famciclovir and valaciclovir in patients with AIDS. Among bone marrow transplant recipients and patients with AIDS, acyclovir-resistant HSV isolates have been identified more frequently after therapeutic acyclovir administration than during prophylaxis. Notably, acyclovir-resistant HSV isolates usually are cross resistant to famciclovir/penciclovir. Acyclovir has become the therapeutic mainstay for the treatment and suppression of herpesvirus infections in immunocompromised patients [5].

Viral Resistance

Herpes simplex virus can develop resistance to acyclovir through mutations in the viral gene encoding thymidine kinase (TK), either through the generation of TK-deficient mutants or through the selection of mutants possessing a TK that is unable to phosphorylate acyclovir. Clinical isolates resistant to acyclovir are almost uniformly deficient in TK, although isolates with altered DNA polymerase have been recovered from HSV-infected patients. Drug resistance was considered rare and resistant isolates were thought to be less pathogenic until a series of acyclovir-resistant HSV isolates from patients with AIDS were characterized [22]. These resistant mutants were deficient in TK. Although sensitive to vidarabine and foscarnet *in vitro*, only foscarnet has been shown effective in the treatment of acyclovir resistant HSV [3]. Acyclovir-resistant HSV isolates have been identified as the cause of pneumonia, encephalitis, esophagitis, and mucocutaneous infections in immunocompromised patients. To date only a few isolates resistant to acyclovir have been cultured from the normal host [23, 24]. With progressive lesions while on intravenous acyclovir, foscarnet or cidofovir can be used for therapy, as reviewed [3, 11].

Toxicity

Acyclovir, valaciclovir and famciclovir therapies are associated with very few adverse effects. Renal dysfunction has been reported, especially in patients given large doses of acyclovir by rapid intravenous infusion, but appears to be uncommon and is usually reversible. The risk of nephrotoxicity can be minimized by administering acyclovir by slow infusion and by ensuring adequate hydration. Oral acyclovir therapy, even at doses of 800 mg five times daily, has not been associated with renal dysfunction. A few reports have linked intravenous administration of acyclovir with disturbances of the central nervous system, including agitation, hallucinations, disorientation, tremors, and myoclonus.

The Acyclovir in Pregnancy Registry has gathered data on prenatal exposure to acyclovir. No increase in the risk to the mother or fetus has been documented, but the total number of monitored pregnancies is too small to detect any low-frequency events. Since acyclovir crosses the placenta and is concentrated in amniotic fluid, there is concern about the potential for fetal nephrotoxicity, although none has been observed.

Prevention

Subunit Vaccines

Subunit vaccines evolved from attempts to remove viral DNA and eliminate the potential for cellular transformation, to enhance antigenic concentration and induce a stronger immunity, and, finally, to exclude any possibility of contamination with residual live virus [25]. Available subunit vaccines have been prepared using a variety of methods for antigen extraction from infected cell lysates by detergent and subsequent purification.

The immunogenicity of envelope glycoproteins, free of viral DNA, has been established in animal models [26-30]. These subunit vaccines, as well as others, have been studied in a variety of animal models, including mice, guinea pigs, and rabbits. Neutralizing antibodies can be detected in these systems in varying amounts, as can ELISA antibodies in some systems [30]. In these systems, the quantity of neutralizing antibody appears to correlate with the degree of protection upon challenge. Although there are many conflicting studies, generally the subunit vaccines elicited some protection, as evidenced by the amelioration of morbidity and reduction in mortality in the immunized animals. The predictability of these models for human studies is poor.

The results of studies in humans are disappointing. Envelope glycoproteins do not convey protection to uninfected sexual partners of individuals with genital HSV infection, as recently reported [31-33]. Subunit vaccines have failed in human experiments despite initial promising results. These data are summarized.

Studies have been completed with one of two gB and/or gD recombinant vaccines in humans. Initially, the gD-2 construct was administered to 24 human volunteers at the National Institutes of Health for reactogenicity and immunogenicity. These studies demonstrated an increase in the geometric mean antibody titer to gD-2; however, lymphocyte blastogenic responses were not consistent between populations. Either 30 μg or 100 μg of purified gD-2 was used as the immunogen with alum [34]. Extensive rodent experiments using the guinea pig genital herpes model have explored the utility of using viral glycoproteins gB and gD as vaccine components. If the dose is optimal, a mixture of gB and gD can protect against both primary and spontaneous recurrent disease after intravaginal viral inoculation [30]. However, in order to demonstrate this effect it was necessary to use complete Freund's adjuvant, a component not acceptable for human administration. More recently, investigators demonstrated that gD combined with a lipophilic muramyl tripeptide affords a high level of protection from HSV disease; [35, 36] however, this adjuvant was abandoned because of reactogenicity. In a series of experiments, investigators were able to demonstrate that the amount of antigen in the vaccine affects the host response. An important observation from these studies is that the quantity of neutralizing antibodies elicited by immunization and the total HSV antibody titer (as measured by ELISA) were higher after vaccination than after natural infection [33, 34].

These initial studies were expanded by further experiments using muramyl tripeptides with gB and gD in order to determine protective effects against recurrent infection. These studies show the development of immune responses similar to those of natural infection [34]. The use of these subunit vaccines for therapy of recurrent genital herpes appeared to decrease frequency of recurrence. Unfortunately, the failure of the gB and gD vaccine in a well performed clinical trial is disappointing [37] and has resulted in one vaccine company abandoning the approach.

More recently, an additional vaccine efficacy trial showed the gD with a proprietary SmithKline Beecham vaccine prevented both infection and disease in women seronegative for HSV. However, this vaccine had no effect in women seropositive for HSV-1 or any male population. These confounding results warrant further investigation [38].

Epstein-barr Virus

Introduction

Epstein-Barr virus is tropic for B-lymphocytes. Replication has been documented in the parotid gland, as well as other lymphatic tissues. Evidence of lytic disease, as evidenced by the formation of multinucleated giant cells, is not apparent with infection caused by EBV. The most significant clinical manifestations of EBV infection are those associated with classic mononucleosis. Epstein-Barr virus is the most common cause of the mononucleosis syndrome that occurs in humans. The predominant findings are malaise, myalgia, pharyngitis, cervical adenopathy, splenomegaly, and atypical lymphocytosis, as reviewed [39].

Epstein-Barr virus has been incriminated as a cause of lymphoproliferative disease in immunocompromised individuals [39, 40]. The development of lymphoproliferative malignancy in heart and bone marrow transplant recipients and children with AIDS has been documented. These lymphoproliferative disorders range from benign polyclonal B cell proliferations to malignant B cell lymphomas. The frequency of occurrence post transplant is a function of the degree and type of immunosuppression. Overall, approximately one to two per cent of bone marrow, liver, and renal transplant recipients will develop a lymphoproliferative disorder. The frequency is higher in individuals who have heart and long transplants where the reported frequency is approximately ten per cent. An unusual syndrome, known as the X-linked lymphoproliferative syndrome, has been identified in males and results in a fatal syndrome. The gene responsible for the syndrome has been identified. In addition, patients with Acquired Immunodeficiency Syndrome can develop a lymphoma of the central nervous system.

Malignancies associated with EBV infection include Burkitt's lymphoma for which 95 per cent of the tumor cells contain copies of the EBV genome. In addition, some forms of Hodgkin's disease and nasopharyngeal carcinoma are attributed to EBV infection.

Clinical Diagnosis (Table 3)

The clinical diagnosis of EBV infection resides on clinical findings compatible with a mononucleosis syndrome, particularly tonsil enlargement with diffuse generalized adenopathy, splenomegaly and malaise. Confirmation of the diagnosis is achieved by the utilization of appropriate laboratory tests.

Laboratory Diagnosis (Table 3)

The diagnosis is confirmed by demonstrating heterophile antibodies or type-specific antibodies to viral capsid antigen (VCA) but not nuclear antigen (NA) to EBV. Specific serologic tests include the evaluation of both VCA and NA studies for IgG and IgM as well as early antigen (EA) studies. Antibodies directed against viral capsid antigen (both IgG and IgM) as well as early antigen appear before those directed against EBV nuclear antigen. The heterophile antibody titer becomes positive after antibodies to EBV specific antigens appear (Table 3).

Of note, peripheral blood smears in patients with mononucleosis frequently, but not uniformly, reveal atypical lymphocytosis. Furthermore, individuals with a hemophagocytic syndrome will have detectable evidence on a peripheral smear.

Therapy

Antiviral treatment has not been proven of value for any EBV syndrome; however, drugs like acyclovir and ganciclovir have been tried in uncontrolled studies with

Table 3. Diagnosis of Epstein-Barr Virus Infections

Syndrome	Diagnosis	
	Clinical	Laboratory
Infectious Mononucleosis	Tonsillitis Adenopathy Splenomegaly Malaise	Seorology VCA and EBNA Or Heterophile and aypical lymphocytosis
Hemophagocytic Syndrome	Hemolysis Jaundice	Hemophagocytosis Serology: VCA and EBNA or Heterophile
Lymphoproliferative Disease	Seronegative transplant recipient from sero positive donor OR X-Linked family history	Biopsy PCR Histopathology Genetic studies
Oral Hairy Leukoplakia	White proliferation at tongue's lateral border	Histopathology

reported benefit. Nevertheless, all of the anti-herpes drugs have been administered to patients with lymphoproliferative diseases for which a polyclonal phenotype has been proven. The natural history of such disease indicates a progression from a polyclonal phenotype to one that is monoclonal. Once monoclonality has developed, therapy is of no value.

Short-term courses of both intravenous and oral acyclovir have been studied for the treatment of acute EBV infection; while therapy inhibits EBV replication transiently, no significant benefit can be demonstrated. Fundamentally, this is logical in that active viral replication has waned at the time of presentation with clinical symptomatology. In large part, the clinical symptoms are mediated immunopathologically.

Prevention

No vaccines are currently available for the prevention of EBV infections. Glycoprotein 350 is one of the most abundant late viral proteins present in lytically infected cell membranes. Most of the EBV neutralizing antibody response is directed against this glycoprotein. Currently, subunit vaccine studies of gp350 are in progress.

Human Herpesvirus 6 and 7

Introduction

Human herpesvirus 6 and 7 are associated with exanthem subitum, or roseola. This illness is characterized by 3-5 days of fever, followed by the appearance of a maculopapular "slapped cheek" rash. In pediatric ambulatory care settings, HHV-6 has been associated with high fevers (>40°C) and febrile convulsions. In addition, there has been an association between HHV-6 and rejection of transplanted livers, fulminant hepatitis and infections, multiple sclerosis of the central nervous system [41-43]. Importantly, HHV-6 infections have been linked to a variety of clinical syndromes in organ transplant recipients. Usually, virus becomes detectable in blood in approximately 2-4 weeks following organ transplantation. Clinical manifestations in the immunocompromised adult include high fever that may or may not be associated with rash. In additional, accumulating evidence suggests that HHV-6 may be an important cause of encephalitis in immunocompromised hosts, in general. These data reside on the detection of HHV-6 DNA in the cerebral spinal fluid by PCR [44].

Clinical Diagnosis (Table 4)

The diagnosis of roseola is made clinically. No laboratory studies exist to confirm these studies in a routine fashion.

Laboratory Diagnosis (Table 4)

While serologic tests are available for the diagnosis of HHV-6 infections, they are not routinely useful. The application of PCR to detection HHV-6 DNA has been applied to many prospective studies. A note of caution, however, is indicated. Since HHV-6 is latent in white blood cells, care must be utilized to select primers that detect replicating virus or utilize a reverse transcriptase procedure rather than alternative methods.

Table 4.   Diagnosis of HHV-6, HHV-7, and HHV-8 Infections

Syndrome	Diagnosis	
	Clinical	Laboratory
Roseola HHV-6 HHV-7	Slapped cheek rash and fever	Serology PCR on saliva/blood
Encephalitis HHV-6 HHV-7	Meningoencephalitis	PCR on CSF
Kaposi's Sarcoma HHV-8	Tumor in HIV infected person	Biopsy
Body Cavity Lymphoma HHV-8	Tumor in HIV infected person	Biopsy
Castleman's Syndrome HHV-8	Tumor in HIV infected person	Biopsy

Antiviral Therapy

No prospective controlled clinical trials of antiviral therapy for HHV-6 infections have been performed in transplant recipients. However, the proportion of HHV-6 positive specimens within three months of bone marrow transplantation has been reported to be significantly lower in those individuals who received acyclovir [41]. However, acyclovir is not the most active compound *in vitro* against HHV-6 infections. Indeed, the most active compounds are ganciclovir and the phosphonate series of drugs, particularly cidofovir [45].

Prevention

No vaccines exist for the prevention of HHV-6 infection at the present time. To the knowledge of these authors, no vaccines are under development.

Kaposi's Sarcoma Herpesvirus

Introduction

A new herpesvirus has been associated with Kaposi's Sarcoma and AIDS-related lymphomas of organ cavities [46]. The DNA of this virus is partially homologous to the DNA of Epstein-Barr virus and that of herpesvirus saimiri. This virus immortalizes B lymphocytes.

Clinical Diagnosis (Table 4)

Kaposi's sarcoma is diagnosed clinically. The clinical findings reflect the underlying histogenesis characterized by a proliferation of spindle-shaped cells and irregular slit-like vascular channels. These tumors first appear on the skin, particularly that of the extremities and face but can disseminate to lymphoid tissues and the viscera. Recently, there has been evidence of Kaposi's sarcoma herpes virus detected in the saliva of AIDS patients, indicating a source for transmission.

Laboratory Diagnosis

A laboratory diagnosis of Kaposi's sarcoma herpesvirus is confirmed by biopsy and histopathologic evaluation. The aforementioned spindle-shaped cells and vascular changes are characteristic of the tumor.

Therapy

Antiviral agents have not been routinely employed in the treatment of Kaposi's sarcoma. Of note, tumor regression has been documented in several patients receiving foscarnet, a viral DNA polymerase inhibitor in small but uncontrolled studies [47, 48].

Similarly, patients who receive both foscarnet as well as ganciclovir appear to have lower risk of developing Kaposi's sarcoma but these studies were neither controlled nor of adequate sample size.

Prevention

At the present time, no vaccines are under development for the prevention of Kaposi's sarcoma herpesvirus.

B-Virus

Introduction

B virus infections of humans are uncommon, because humans are not the natural reservoir of this infection [49]. Instead, the virus is found routinely in rhesus monkey colonies. Infection is transmitted to humans by the bite of an infected animal. Virus replicates locally in a fashion very similar to that of HSV infection. An important difference, however, is that there is a predisposition for rapid neuronal transport of virus to the central nervous system, with ensuing encephalitis in most cases.

B virus is resident in rhesus monkeys, particularly those obtained from Southeast Asia and India. In a manner similar to human herpesvirus infections, crowding and stress of monkeys lead to virus reactivation and excretion in saliva. Improper animal handling techniques can cause personnel to be exposed to this virus. Strict adherence to guidelines for the handling of rhesus monkeys is advised.

A major concern following exposure to B virus is the development of an almost uniformly fatal encephalitis in most individuals. The total number of cases reported in the world's literature is under 30, with a mortality of approximately 75 per cent. Survivors of B virus infection of the central nervous system have been left with a broad spectrum of neurologic impairment. Recurrent cutaneous disease has been noted, but generally only in patients who initially had a severe encephalitis [49].

Clinical Diagnosis

Because of the rapidity of neurologic progress of B virus infection of the central nervous system, clinical diagnosis is not usually made before demise in the absence of a history of a monkey bite. Most patients identify the presence of a monkey bite, alerting their medical care provider to the possibility of this disease.

Laboratory Diagnosis

Serologic evaluation of individuals of B virus antibodies can be obtained through the Centers for Disease Control and Prevention, Atlanta, Georgia, or the laboratory of Dr. Julia Hilliard at Georgia State University. These assays are either immunoblots or radioimmunoassays.

Alternatively, virus can be cultured from the saliva of either Rhesus monkeys or the skin wound itself. Two-known individuals have had cutaneous vesiclesfrom which B virus has been isolated.

Therapy

There are no proven therapies for B virus infections; however, the rapid introduction of an antiherpetic drug (primarily acyclovir) but, theoretically, also valaciclovir or famciclovir is imperative. While patients are being evaluated for the presence of B virus either in the saliva of the monkey that bit the animal-care provider or antibodies directed against B virus in the animal care provider, therapy should be started immediately. Therapy is generally continued until it is clear that there is no evidence of infection. One long-term survivor of B virus infection has continued to receive acyclovir, following introduction after the appearance of cutaneous vesicles. There is no distinction in clinical value between any of the three existing antiherpetic drugs.

Prevention

The most desirable mention of prevention is avoidance of contact with infected monkeys. A B virus-free community would be ideal; however, such colonies are only now being developed in the United States. Care and education of animal-care providers is essential if B virus infections are to be prevented.

References

1. Roizman B. Herpesviridae. In: Fields BN, Knipe DM, Howley PM, Chanock RM, Melnick JL, Monath TP, Roizman B, Straus SE, eds. Field's Virology. 3rd Edition ed. New York: Lippincott-Raven Publishers, 1996: 2221-2230.
2. Roizman B, Sears AE. Herpes simplex viruses and their replication. In: Fields BN, Knipe DM, Howley PM, Chanock RM, Melnick JL, Monath TP, Roizman B, Straus SE, eds. Fields Virology. Philadelphia: Lippincott-Raven Publishers, 1996: 2231-2295.
3. Balfour HH, Jr. Antiviral drugs. N Engl J Med 1999; 340: 1255-1268.
4. Whitley RJ. Herpes simplex virus. In: Fields BN, Knipe DM, Howley PM, Chanock RM, Melnick JL, Monath TP, Roizman B, Straus SE, eds. Fields Virology. Third ed. Vol. 2. Philadelphia: Lippincott-Raven publishers, 1996: 2297-2342.
5. Whitley RJ, Gnann J. Acyclovir: A decade later. N Engl J Med 1992; 327: 782-789.
6. Amir J, Harel L, Smetana Z, Varsano I. Treatment of herpes simplex gingivostomatitis with aciclovir in children: a randomized double blind placebo controlled study. BMJ 1997; 314: 1800-1803.
7. Spruance SL, Rea TL, Thoming C, Tucker R, Saltzman R, Boon R. Penciclovir cream for the treatment of herpes simplex labialis. A randomized, multicenter, double-blind, placebo-controlled trial. Topical Penciclovir Collaborative Study Group. JAMA 1997; 277: 1374-1379.
8. Spruance SL, Hamill ML, Hoge WS, Davis G, Mills J. Acyclovir prevents reactivation of herpes simplex labialis in skiers. JAMA 1988; 260: 1597-1599.
9. Fleming DT, McQuillan GM, Johnson RE, Nahmias AJ, Aral SO, Lee FK, St. Louis ME. Herpes simplex

virus type 2 in the United States, 1976-1994. N Engl J Med 1997; 337: 1105-1111.

10. Wald A, Corey L, Cone R, Hobson A, Davis G, Zeh J. Frequent genital herpes simplex virus 2 shedding in immunocompetent women: effect of acyclovir treatment. J Clin Investig 1997; 99: 1092-1097.

11. Abramowicz M. Drugs for non-HIV viral infections. Medical Letter on Drugs and Therapeutics 1999: 113-120.

12. Sacks SL, Aoki FY, Diaz-Mitoma F, Sellors J, Shafran SD. Patient-initiated, twice-daily oral famciclovir for early recurrent genital herpes. A randomized, double-blind multicenter trial. Canadian Famciclovir Study Group. JAMA 1996; 276: 44-49.

13. Straus SE, Rooney JF, Hallahan C. Acyclovir suppresses subclinical shedding of herpes simplex virus. Ann Intern Med 1996; 125: 776-777.

14. Douglas RM, Moore BW, Miles HB, Davies LM, Graham NM, Ryan P, Worswick DA, Albrecht JK. Prophylactic efficacy of intranasal alpha$_2$-interferon against rhinovirus infections in family setting. N Engl J Med 1986; 314: 65-70.

15. Straus SE, Croen KD, Sawyer MH, Freifeld AG, Felser JM, Dale JK, Smith HA, Hallahan C, Lehrman SN. Acyclovir suppression of frequently recurring genital herpes. Efficacy and diminishing need during successive years of treatment. JAMA 1988; 260: 2227-2230.

16. Herpetic Eye Disease Study Group. Acyclovir for the prevention of recurrent herpes simplex virus eye disease. N Engl J Med 1998; 339: 300-306.

17. Whitley RJ, Arvin A, Prober C, Burchett S, Corey L, Powell D, Plotkin S, Starr S, Alford C, Connor J, Jacobs RF, Nahmias AJ, Soong SJ, the National Institute of Allergy and Infectious Diseases Collaborative Antiviral Study Group. A controlled trial comparing vidarabine with acyclovir in neonatal herpes simplex virus infection. N Engl J Med 1991; 324: 444-449.

18. Kimberlin DW, Jacobs RF, Powell DA, Corey L, Gruber WC, Rathore M, Bradley J, Diaz P, Kumar M, Arvin AM, Gutierrez K, Shelton M, Weiner LB, Sleasman W, Sierra T, Soong S-J, Lin CY, Lakeman FD, Whitley RJ, the National Institute of Allergy and Infectious Diseases Collaborative Antiviral Study Group. The Safety and Efficacy of High-Dose (HD) Acyclovir (ACV) in Neonatal Herpes Simplex Virus (HSV) Infection. In: Society for Pediatric Research. San Francisco, California: , 1999.

19. Whitley RJ, Alford CA, Jr., Hirsch MS, Schooley RT, Luby JP, Aoki FY, Hanley D, Nahmias AJ, Soong S-J, the National Institute of Allergy and Infectious Diseases Collaborative Antiviral Study Group. Vidarabine *versus* acyclovir therapy in herpes simplex encephalitis. N Engl J Med 1986; 314: 144-149.

20. Meyers JD, Wade JC, Mitchell CD, Saral R, Lietman PS, Durack DT, Levin MJ, Segreti AC, Balfour HH, Jr. Multicenter collaborative trial of intravenous acyclovir for treatment of mucocutaneous herpes simplex virus infection in immunocompromised host. Am J Med 1982; 73: 229-235.

21. Saral R, Burns WH, Laskin OL, Santos GW, Leitman PS. Acyclovir prophylaxis of herpes simplex virus infections: A randomized, double-blind, controlled trial in bone-marrow-transplant recipients. N Engl J Med 1981; 305: 63-67.

22. Erlich KS, Mills J, Chatis P, Mertz GJ, Busch DS, Follansbee SE, Grant RM, Crumpacker CS. Acyclovir-resistant herpes simplex virus infections in patients with the acquired immunodeficiency syndrome. N Engl J Med 1989; 320: 293-296.

23. Kost RG, Hill EL, Tigges M, Straus SE. Brief report: recurrent acyclovir resistant genital herpes in an immunocompetent host. N Engl J Med 1993; 329: 1777-1781.

24. Kimberlin DW, Whitley RJ. Antiviral resistance — an emerging problem. Antiviral Res 1995; 26: 365-368.

25. Fenyves A, Strupp L. Heat-resistant infectivity of herpes simplex virus revealed by viral transfection.

Intervirology 1982; 17: 222-228.

26. Cappel R, DeCuyper F, Rikaert F. Efficacy of a nucleic acid free submit vaccine. Arch virol 1980; 65: 12-23.

27. Cappel R, Sprecher S, Rickaert F, DeCuyer F. Immune response to a DNA free herpes simplex vaccine in man. Arch Virol 1982; 73: 61-67.

28. Skinner GR, Williams DR, Moles AW, Sargent A. Prepubertal vaccination of mice against experimental infection of the genital tract with type 2 herpes simplex virus. Arch Virol 1980; 64: 329-338.

29. Hilfenhaus J, Moser H. Prospects for a subunit vaccine against herpes simplex virus infections. Behring Inst Mitt 1981; 69: 45.

30. Stanberry LR, Bernstein DI, Burke RL, Pachl C, Myers MG. Vaccination with recombinant herpes simplex virus glycoproteins: protection against initial and recurrent genital herpes. J Infect Dis 1987; 155: 914-920.

31. Mertz GJ, Peterman G, Ashley R, Jourden JL, Salter D, Morrison L, McLean A, Corey L. Herpes simplex virus type 2 glycoproteins-subunit vaccine: Tolerance and humoral and cellular responses in humans. J Infect Dis 1984; 150: 242-249.

32. Ashley R, Mertz GJ, Corey L. Detection of asymptomatic herpes simplex virus infections after vaccination. J Virol 1987; 61: 264-268.

33. Zarling JM, Moran PA, Brewer L, Ashley R, Corey L. Herpes simplex virus (HSV) specific proliferative and cytotoxic T-cell responses in humans immunized with an HSV type glycoprotein subunit vaccine. J Virol 1988; 2: 4481-4485.

34. Straus SE, Savarese B, Tigges M, Freifeld AG, Krause PR, Margolis DM, Meier JL, Paar DP, Adair SF, Dina D, et al. Induction and enhancement of immune responses to herpes simplex virus type 2 in humans by use of a recombinant glycoprotein D vaccine. J Infect Dis 1993; 167: 1045-1052.

35. Burke RL, Nest GV, Carlson J, Gervase B, Goldbeck C, Ng P, Sanchez-Pescador L, Stanberry L, Ott G. Development of herpes simplex virus subunit vaccine. In: Lerner RA, Ginsberg H, Chanock RM, Brown F, eds. Vaccines 89: Modern Approaches to New Vaccines Including Prevention of AIDS. Cold Springs Harbor, New York: Cold Springs Harbor Laboratory, 1989: 377-382.

36. Sanchez-Pescador L, Burke RL, Ott G, Nest GV. The effect of adjuvants on the efficacy of a recombinant herpes simplex virus glycoprotein vaccine. J Immun 1988; 141: 1720-1727.

37. Corey L, Langenberg AG, Ashley R, Sekulovich RE, Izu AE, Douglas JM, Jr., Handsfield HH, Warren T, Marr L, Tyring S, DiCarlo R, Adimora AA, Leone P, Dekker CL, Burke RL, Leong WP, Straus SE. Recombinant glycoprotein vaccine for the prevention of genital HSV-2 infection: two randomized controlled trials. Chiron HSV Vaccine Study Group. JAMA 1999; 28: 379-380.

38. Spruance SL, SmithKline Beecham (SB) Herpes Vaccine Efficacy Study Group. Gender-specific efficacy of a prophylactic SBAS4-adjuvanted gD_2 subunit vaccine against genital herpes disease (GHD): Results of two clinical efficacy trials. In: 40th Interscience Conference on Antimicrobial Agents and Chemotherapy. Toronto, Canada: , 2000 Sept 17-20.

39. Rickinson A, Kieff E. Epstein-Barr virus. In: Fields BN, Knipe DM, Howley PM, Chanock RM, Melnick JL, Monath TP, Roizman B, Straus SE, eds. Fields Virology. Third Edition ed. Philadelphia: Lippincott-Raven, 1996: 2397-2446.

40. Beaulieu B, Sullivan J. Epstein-Barr virus. In: Richman DD, Whitley RJ, Hayden FG, eds. Clinical Virology. New York: Churchill Livingstone, 1997: 485-527.

41. Gnann JW, Jr. Other Herpesviruses: Herpes simplex virus, varicella-zoster virus, human herpesvirus types 6, 7, and 8. In: Bowden RA, Ljungman P, Paya CV, eds. Transplant Infections. Philadelphia: Lippincott-Raven Publishers, 1998: 265-285.

42. Kimberlin DW, Gnann JW, Jr. Human herpesvirus-6 and -7 infections. In: Dolin R, Masur H, Saag MD, eds. AIDS Therapy. Philadelphia: Churchill Livingstone, 1999: 507-515.

43. Griffiths PD, Ait-Khaled M, Bearcroft CP, Clark DA, Quaglia A, Davies SE, Burroughs AK, Rolles K, Michael I, Knight SN, Noibi SM, Cope AV, Phillips AN, Emery VC. Human herpesviruses 6 and 7 as potential pathogens after liver transplant: prospective comparison with the effect of cytomegalovirus. J Med Virol 1999; 59: 496-501.

44. McCullers JA, Lakeman FJ, Whitley RJ. Human herpesvirus-6 is associated with focal encephalitis. Clin Infect Dis 1995; 21: 571-576.

45. Yoshida M, Yamada M, Tsukazaki T, S. C, Lakeman FD, Nii S, Whitley RJ. Comparison of antiviral compounds against human herpesvirus 6 and 7. Antiviral Res 1998; 40: 73-84.

46. Moore PS, Chang Y. Kaposi's sarcoma-associated herpesvirus. In: Richman DD, Whitley RJ, Hayden FG, eds. Clinical Virology. New York: Churchill Livingstone, 1997: 509-524.

47. Medveckzy NM. *In vitro* sensitivity of HHV-8. AIDS 1997; 11: 1327-1333.

48. Humphrey RW. Treatment of HHV-8 with foscarnet or ganciclovir. Blood 1996; 88: 297-304.

49. Whitley R, Chapman L. Cercopithecine herpes virus (B virus). In: Richman D, Whitley R, Hayden F, eds. Clinical Virology. New York: Churchill Livingstone, 1997: 411-420.

CHAPTER 7

CYTOMEGALOVIRUS

PAUL D. GRIFFITHS and RICHARD J. WHITLEY

"The development of CMV disease in an immunocompromised patient should be seen as a failure of medical management".

Table of Contents

Introduction

Cytomegalovirus (CMV) is a common infectious agent, which is well adapted to its host. It uses a variety of methods to down-regulate HLA class I and class II molecules, so that virus-infected cells can partially avoid the CD8 and CD4 restricted arms of the cell-mediated immune response. It also encodes genes which interfere with natural killer (NK) cells, antibody, complement and chemokines. Over an evolutionary time-scale, these multiple immune evasion genes have enabled the virus to persist and infect most individuals with normal immunity without usually producing any symptoms. CMV is thus only of medical relevance if this balance is altered because individuals have impaired cell-mediated immunity ie the fetus, recipients of solid organ transplants,

151

Practical Guidelines in Antiviral Therapy Ed. by Charles A.B. Boucher and George J. Galasso. 151 — 171
© 2002 *Elsevier Science. Printed in the Netherlands.*

recipients of bone marrow transplants, and HIV-positive patients. The pathogenesis of CMV disease in these patient groups includes factors common to them all, plus some distinct features in each, which will be discussed.

CMV was first isolated in 1956 when the "new" technology of cell culture became available. It was only possible to propagate CMV in fibroblast cell lines, and then with some difficulty, so cell-adapted strains such as Ad169 and Towne were used widely for their convenience. The fibroblast cell line, with its slow evolution of CMV cytopathic effect, provided a picture of an indolent virus which had an apparent parallel *in vivo* since CMV is slow to cause disease in patients also; typically appearing in the second month post-transplant; unlike HSV disease which appears in the first week. However, the last decade has seen the progressive application of modern molecular biology to define CMV as a rapidly replicating virus able to infect all nucleated cells in the body [1]. Laboratory-adapted strains have been important for defining the structure of the CMV genome and have given the nomenclature of each open reading frame numbered in the unique long (UL) and unique short (US) regions [2]. However, we now know that, in the process of adaptation to cell culture, at least 22 genes were lost [3], so cell culture experiments may not give an accurate picture of CMV pathogenesis. Furthermore, clinicopathological studies and the results of placebo-controlled clinical trials have demonstrated that the morbidity and mortality caused by CMV exceeds that which is recognized clinically as "CMV disease". In this chapter, we will use the term, *direct effects* to define end-organ involvement by CMV (synonymous with "CMV disease") and the term *indirect effects* to describe a variety of apparently distinct clinical syndromes [4] which are triggered by CMV (see Table 1). This chapter will emphasize how antiviral drugs can be deployed to reduce both the direct and indirect effects of CMV.

Table 1.   Clinical sequelae of CMV infection post-transplantation

Direct effects (= "CMV disease")	• hepatitis
	• enteritis
	• pneumonitis
	• bone marrow suppression
	• retinitis
	• encephalitis
Indirect effects	• allograft rejection
	• immunosuppressive state
	• atherosclerosis
	• malignancy

After: Rubin RH (1989)(4)

Clinical Diagnosis

There is an internationally agreed definition of CMV disease which applies to all patient groups [5]. It requires patients to have symptoms compatible with CMV end-organ involvement, signs of dysfunction of that organ, together with laboratory documentation of CMV infection of the affected organ (Table 2).

Table 2.   Definitions of CMV end-organ diseases

Disease	Symptoms or signs	*plus* Detection of virus
Pneumonitis	interstitial infiltration, hypoxia	BAL or biopsy
Gastrointestinal ulceration	fever, pain, blood	biopsy
Hepatitis	deranged liver function tests	biopsy
Retinitis	floaters, appearance	
CNS	lethargy, paresis	CSF-PCR

From: Ljungman P and Plotkin SA (1995)(5).

The relative importance of each disease in each patient group shows distinct differences (Table 3). In part, this reflects the predeliction of CMV for freshly dividing cells found under specific circumstances (in the brain of a neonate; in bone marrow following bone marrow transplant; in the lung following heart-lung transplant; in the liver following liver transplant). In part, it also reflects the ability of the cell-mediated immune system to limit CMV replication so that, in particular, its CNS tropism is controlled in all but the most immunodeficient (neonate; end-stage AIDS). In part, it also results from the ability of the dysfunctional immune system to mount inflammatory responses (pneumonitis post-bone marrow transplant; vitritis in AIDS patients given highly active anti-retroviral therapy (HAART)). However, not all of the differences shown in Table 3 can be explained by these factors; specifically, the high proportion of retinitis in AIDS patients (85% of CMV disease in this patient group) compared to all others (less than 5%) is both striking and perplexing.

Laboratory Diagnosis

Diagnosis of CMV Disease

As shown in Table 2, detection of CMV infection in clinically affected organs is an essential component of the diagnosis of CMV disease. A variety of diagnostic methods are available (Table 4). However, it should be emphasized that the main use of the laboratory is to identify those patients at risk of CMV disease and apply one of the treatment strategies described below to prevent disease from developing. Now that several controlled clinical trials have shown that CMV disease can be prevented effectively, we are convinced that we should set ourselves the tough assignment shown at the heading of this chapter. This is certainly true for most transplant patients; we believe the same potentially applied to AIDS patients in the pre-HAART era, and await evidence-based medicine to determine if the same applies now that HAART is available. Finally, we hope to reach the same conclusion for congenital CMV, once antiviral drugs safe enough to use in neonates and during pregnancy become available.

Table 3.   Relative incidence and anatomical locations of CMV disease in populations not receiving antiviral prophylaxis or HAART

Neonates	BMTx	Solid Tx	AIDS
BRAIN			brain
EAR	eye	eye	EYE
EYE	LUNGS	lungs	
GIT	GIT	GIT	
ORGAN	ORGAN		
	adrenal		

CAPS   = major problem
CAPS   = substantial problem
lc   = minor problem
GIT   = ulceration of gastrointestinal tract
ORGAN = disease in newly transplanted organ

Table 4.   Laboratory methods for diagnosing CMV infection

Method	Clinical presentation				
	Congenital	Pneumonitis	Hepatitis/GIT	Encephalitis	Retinitis
CCC	Urine		Biopsy		
DEAFF/shell vial		BAL			
PCR	Urine			CSF	(vitreus/ aqueous)
Histology			Biopsy		

CCC   = conventional cell culture
DEAFF = detection of early antigen fluorescent foci
PCR   = polymerase chain reaction
BAL   = bronchoalveolar lavage
CSF   = cerebrospinal fluid
GIT   = ulceration of gastrointestinal tract
(-)   = only required in atypical cases

Detection of Viremia

These optimistic statements above are possible because of the progressive recognition over more than a decade that: 1) CMV viremia is present in patients with CMV disease [6]; 2) viremia occurs before CMV disease develops [6-10]; 3) high CMV loads in blood correlate with disease [7, 9]; 4) a threshold value of viral load exists above which CMV disease becomes common [7, 8]; 5) sensitive and rapid methods can detect and quantify viremia in a timely fashion [8, 11]; 6) prospective surveillance for CMV viremia coupled with quantification of the first positive sample identifies those patients most at risk of CMV disease [12].

The early studies of viremia used cell culture to identify CMV [6]. This showed statistical correlation between viremia and CMV disease, but was too insensitive and slow to allow the management of individuals to be modified. Culture-confirmation methods (termed detection of early antigen fluorescent foci (DEAFF) in Europe and shell vial in the USA) are more rapid but less sensitive than conventional cell culture. Two newer methods, namely, antigenemia and polymerase chain reaction (PCR) have the characteristics required to allow rapid detection of viremia, coupled with sensitivity sufficient to detect all patients before CMV disease develops. Both have advantages and disadvantages, as summarized in Table 5. Various protocols have been shown to be robust when performed in several different laboratories, demonstrating that these assays can be performed on a routine basis [7, 9, 10] [12].

Table 5. Overview of the practical advantages and disadvantages of antigenemia and PCR assays for detecting CMV viremia

Method	Reagents	Rapidity	Precautions	Problems	Quantitative
Antigenemia	mAb pp65 (UL83)	Same day	Process cells within hours	Subjective BMTx have fewer cells	Semi-quantitative
PCR	One-round or nested Several primer sets evaluated	Next day	Prevent contamination Can be made too sensitive	Requires laboratory commitment of space and skilled staff	Can be fully quantitative

When To Treat

Several antiviral compounds inhibit CMV replication. Ganciclovir and acyclovir are nucleoside analogs which require anabolism *in vivo* to their active forms. They are monophosophorylated by the UL97 protein kinase and then converted to their triphosphates by cellular enzymes [13]. Each triphosphate is a potent inhibitor of CMV DNA polymerase (UL54). Like all nucleosides, acyclovir and, especially, ganciclovir, have low bioavailability, which can now be improved through use of their valine-ester produgs, termed valaciclovir and valganciclovir. Cidofovir is a phosphonate compound (structurally analogous to the monophosphate), which by-passes the UL97 step [14]. It is phosphorylated by cellular enzymes to cidofovir diphosphate (analogous to a nucleoside triphosphate) which acts as a competitive inhibitor of DNA polymerase. It is given intravenously. Foscarnet is a pyrophosphate analog which inhibits DNA polymerase directly and is administered intravenously. Fomivirsen is an antisense oligonucleotide, modified chemically to reduce enzymic cleavage, which is administered by intravitreal injection.

There is no single drug which is sufficiently potent and safe to be given to all patients at risk of CMV disease. When deciding whether to treat or prevent CMV disease, one therefore has to balance the proven efficacy of each candidate compound against its toxicity in the target population. Investigations to define the value of detecting CMV in the blood or at other body sites, such as urine or saliva, led to the development of distinct strategies for deploying anti-CMV drugs (Table 6).

Table 6.   Treatment strategies for CMV

Term used	When drug given	Risk of disease	Acceptable toxicity
True prophylaxis	before active infection	low	none
Suppression	after peripheral detection	medium	low
Pre-emptive therapy	after systemic detection	high	medium
Treatment	once disease apparent	established	high

Bone Marrow and Solid Organ Recipients

In Table 7, we present all of the double-blind, randomized, placebo-controlled trials which have been performed in transplant recipients according to the treatment strategies given in Table 6. Details of the dosages used and treatment durations are given in Table 8 for prophylaxis and Table 9 for treatment of established CMV disease. The overview provided in these tables shows that: 1) ganciclovir has activity against CMV infection and CMV disease in all populations studied; 2) foscarnet and cidofovir have not been subjected to the rigours of double-blind, randomized, placebo-controlled trials; 3) acyclovir and valaciclovir have activity against CMV infection *in vivo* as well as reduced disease after renal transplantation; 4) interferon-alpha also has some activity against CMV infection *in vivo*; 5) prophylactic immunoglobulin administration reduced CMV disease in one trial without reducing CMV infection in either, suggesting that, if it has a role to play in preventing CMV disease, it may not work by inhibition of CMV infection; 6) the mortality rate was high enough in the bone marrow transplant trials to provide the statistical power to determine whether these drugs could improve overall survival. When used for suppression, ganciclovir reduced mortality but had no effect in two trials of prophylaxis. The authors provide evidence that ganciclovir-induced

Table 7. Double-blind, placebo-controlled, randomized trials of CMV treatment strategies

Strategy	Drug	Bone marrow	Renal	Heart	Liver
Treatment	GCV	Reed [42]			
Suppressive/Pre-emptive	GCV	Goodrich [43]			
Prophylaxis	Interferon	Cheeseman [47]			
		Hirsch [48]			
		Lui [49]			
	ACV	Prentice [44]	Balfour [50]		
	VACV		Lowance [23]		
	Ig		Metselaar [51]		Snydman [53]
	GCV	Winston [45]		Merigan [20]	Gane [37]
		Goodrich [46]		Macdonald [52]	

GCV   =   ganciclovir
IFN   = interferon
ACV   = acyclovir
VACV = valaciclovir
Ig   = immunoglobulin

neutropaenia facilitated a fatal outcome to secondary bacterial infections which negated its beneficial effect on CMV disease. In contrast, acyclovir prophylaxis significantly reduced mortality because its modest efficacy was not offset by toxicity. In Table 9, the one randomized, double-blind, placebo-controlled trial of treatment of established CMV disease in transplant patients did not show a significant clinical benefit, attesting to the difficulty of resolving CMV disease in the immunocompromised host.

The results of these trials can be supplemented with information from: 1) a randomised, but not placebo-controlled, trial [15] of pre-emptive ganciclovir therapy after bone marrow transplant; 2) a placebo-controlled, but not randomised, trial [16] of acyclovir prophylaxis after bone marrow transplantation; 3) a successful trial of PCR to guide ganciclovir pre-emptive therapy in bone marrow transplant patients [17] but an unsuccessful trial of antigenemia [18] in the same patient population; 4) a head-to-head comparison of ganciclovir and acyclovir prophylaxis in liver transplant recipients, where the former was more successful [19].

Two of the double-blind, randomised, placebo-controlled trials have also shown inhibition of CMV indirect effects (Table 1). An early trial of 28-day intravenous ganciclovir in heart transplant recipients showed reduced CMV disease in the low risk CMV seropositive recipients, but not the high risk seronegative recipients [20]. Follow-up revealed significantly fewer fungal infections in the ganciclovir recipients [21]. Extended follow-up subsequently showed that ganciclovir administration reduced a syndrome of accelerated atherosclerosis [22]. A recent trial of valaciclovir prophylaxis for 90 days in renal allograft recipients showed reduced CMV disease in both the

Table 8. Double-blind, randomised, placebo-controlled trials of prophylaxis for CMV infection and disease after transplantation

Patient group	Study group	Dose	Planned duration of therapy (weeks)	No. of patients		Markers of efficacy in whole population				Reference
				Placebo	Drug	Reduced viremia	Reduced excretion	Reduced disease	Increased survival	
RT_x	IFN	3×10^6 U 2/w	6	20	21	Yes	Yes	No	No	(47)
RT_x	IFN	3×10^6 U 3/w 6w	14	22	20	No	Yes	Yes	No	(48)
RT_x	IFN	3×10^6 U 2/w 8w 3×10^6 U 3/w 6w	14	36	32	No	Yes	No	No	(49)
RT_x	ACV	800 - 3, 200 mg/d	12	51	53	Yes	Yes	Yes	No	(54)
RT_x	VACV	2 g qds	13	310	306	Yes	Yes	Yes	No	(23)
RT_x with rejection	Ig	100 mg/kg	15	16	11	No	No	No	Yes	(51)
LT_x	Ig	150 mg/kg	16	72	69	No	No	No	No	(53)
LT_x	GCV	1 g tds	14	154	150	NG	NG	Yes	No	(37)
HT_x	GCV	5 mg/kg bd 14 d 6mg/kg od 5/7 d until 28 d	4	73	76	No	Yes	Yes	No	(20)
HT_x	GCV	5 mg/kg od 3/7 d until 42 d plus 14d if rejection	6 (+ rejection)	28	28	NG	Yes	No	NG	(52)
BMT_x	GCV	2.5 mg/kg tds days - 7 to -1 then 6 mg/kg 5 d/w after engraftment	median 13.5	45	40	No	Yes	No	No	(45)
BMT_x	GCV	after engraftment 5mg/kg bd 5 d then od	median 10.9	31	33	No	Yes	Yes	No	(46)
BMT_x	ACV	500 mg/m² tds 1m then 800 mg qds 6 m or placebo. Third arm 200-400 mg 1m, then placebo	30	105	102*	Yes	Yes	Yes	Yes	(44)

BMT_x = bone marrow transplant   NG = not given   GCV = ganciclovir
RT_x = renal transplant   VACV = valaciclovir   ACV = aciclovir
HT_x = heart transplant   Ig = immunoglobulin   IFN = interferon-alpha

* Third arm

Table 9. Randomized, controlled trials of therapy for established CMV disease

Patient group	Organ affected	Drug 1	Drug 2	Planned duration of therapy (days)	No. of patients		Significant markers of efficacy reported					Reference
					Drug 1	Drug 2	Reduced viremia	Reduced excretion	Reduced disease	Reduced dissemination	Increased survival	
BMT$_x$	Upper GIT	GCV 2.5 mg/kg tds	Placebo	14	18	19	No	Yes	No	No	No	[42]
AIDS	Retina	GCV 5 mg/kg bd 14 *d* then od	Foscarnet 60 mg/kg tds 14*d* then 90 mg/kg od	14 induction then maintenance	127	107	ND	ND	No	No	Yes	[30]
AIDS	Lower GIT	GCV 5 mg/kg bd 14d then od	Placebo	14	32	30	No	Yes	No*	Yes	No	[32]
AIDS	Retina (relapsed or active retinitis despite maintenance)	GCV 5 mg/kg bd 14 *d* then 10 mg/kg od or foscarnet 90 mg/kg bd 14 *d* then 120 mg/kg od	GCV plus foscarnet: continue existing maintenance dose, add induction dose of second drug for 14 *d*. For maintenance: GCV 5 mg/kg od, foscarnet 90 mg/kg od	life	183	96	ND	ND	Yes	ND	No	[31]

BMT$_x$ = bone marrow transplant
GCV = ganciclovir
GIT = gastrointestinal tract
ND = not determined
* In intention-to-treat analysis. Yes for subsidiary analysis.

CMV seropositive and seronegative recipients [23]. In addition, the trial showed a significant reduction in biopsy-proven acute graft rejection among seronegative valaciclovir recipients. Taken together, these two controlled clinical trials demonstrate that the postulated indirect effects of CMV can be reduced by compounds with activity against CMV so that, by inference, CMV may well be the cause of these indirect effects. While much research remains to be done to prove this hypothesis formally, we suggest they support our contention that the morbidity caused by CMV exceeds that meeting the strict definition of CMV disease (Table 2) and that substantial clinical benefits could be obtained by the appropriate use of compounds active against CMV.

HIV-infected Patients

There are no double-blind, randomised, placebo-controlled trials in HIV-infected patients designed according to the virological criteria given in Table 6. Unfortunately, treatments for CMV in AIDS patients have evolved based upon clinical criteria uninformed by the impressive developments in the transplant community. Nevertheless, application of modern technology to natural history cohorts and controlled clinical trials shows that the underlying concepts behind the treatment strategies defined in Table 6 for allograft recipients can be applied directly to AIDS patients.

First, it is clear from the natural history studies that: 1) viremia, detected by whole blood PCR [8], plasma PCR [9] or antigenemia [10], precedes the onset of CMV disease in AIDS patients; 2) where the same laboratory method has been used in both transplant and AIDS patients, similar predictive values were obtained, despite the fact that CMV disease in AIDS patients is predominantly retinitis [8, 24]; 3) a similar positive predictive value of approximately 60% was obtained by 3 PCR techniques using different clinical samples (whole blood; plasma), different primer sets, and nested *versus* non-nested protocols, showing that, once assay parameters have been set, quite distinct PCR assays can give results of similar clinical significance [8-10]; 4) quantitative measures of CMV viremia show that increasing viral load represents an additional marker for CMV disease among those who are already viraemic [8].

Second, two controlled clinical trials of "clinical prophylaxis" (ie patients had no CMV disease before entering the study but baseline viral tests were not used to define which patients had active infection) show that: 1) patients who were PCR-positive at trial entry were at high risk of developing CMV disease [11, 25]; 2) patients with high viral loads at trial entry had a shortened incubation period to CMV disease [11, 25]; 3) oral ganciclovir was most efficacious in those initially PCR-negative, ie worked best for true prophylaxis [11]; 4) valaciclovir was most efficacious in those PCR-positive at trial entry, ie worked best for pre-emptive therapy [25]; 5) both drugs decreased CMV load once prophylaxis was begun [11, 26].

These results can be supplemented by data showing that: 1) high CMV loads were associated statistically with an increased death rate in AIDS patients [11, 27]; 2) the effect of high viral loads on death is greater for CMV than for HIV [28]; 3) patients who became PCR-negative with ganciclovir treatment had significantly improved survival [28]; 4) HAART reduces the risk of CMV disease by decreasing CMV viremia, presumably by allowing recovery of CMV-specific immunity [29].

Three double-blind, placebo-controlled trials of the treatment of established CMV disease were conducted in the pre-HAART era (Table 9). In patients with CMV retinitis, foscarnet was equivalent to ganciclovir in controlling retinitis but was associated with significantly improved survival [30]. This may reflect the anti-HIV activity of foscarnet and so, in retrospect, represents an early study of combination anti-retroviral therapy. In practice, ganciclovir is usually used for treating CMV retinitis because of its practical advantages and lower incidence of side-effects compared to foscarnet. Ganciclovir and foscarnet are synergistic *in vitro*. A randomised, controlled trial demonstrated results consistent with synergism *in vivo* [31] because the combination significantly delayed progression of retinitis (although most patients still progressed ultimately). No survival difference was apparent and the combination impaired quality of life because of the many hours required for daily infusion of both drugs. In AIDS patients with gastrointestinal ulceration, a placebo-controlled trial of ganciclovir did not improve clinical features in an intent-to-treat analysis (Table 9), although it did in a subsidiary analysis [32], again emphasizing that established CMV disease responds poorly to therapy, so that every effort should be made to prevent it developing.

Strains of CMV resistant to ganciclovir occur *in vitro* and *in vivo*. Most have single (or dual) mutations or small deletions in the UL97 region [33]. These strains are not cross-resistant to cidofovir or foscarnet. The replication of UL97 mutants is impaired compared to that of the wild-type but these mutants are nevertheless more fit than wild-type so long as the selective pressure of ganciclovir is maintained [1]. However, continued replication in the presence of the drug selects for UL54 mutants which may be cross-resistant to cidofovir [34]. One particular UL54 mutant is also cross-resistant to foscarnet. Note that the emergence of resistance is predictable, based upon knowledge of the dynamics of viral replication [35].

Treatment Alogorithms

The principles underlying these treatment algorithms are: to prevent CMV disease; to minimise toxicity; to avoid the selection of resistant strains. The algorithms focus strongly on the evidence-based medicine discussed above, updated where necessary in the light of new information. For example, the early trial of Merigan [20] could not administer iv ganciclovir on Saturdays or Sundays, producing a regimen now regarded as sub-optimal; we have therefore recommended daily administration of drug while retaining the dose and duration used in the clinical trial. Note that, for AIDS patients, we have assumed that the management of patients who fail HAART and develop CMV retinitis will follow the same principles defined in the pre-HAART era.

Allograft Recipients

Figure 1 shows the algorithm for transplant patients. Testing of donor and recipient for IgG antibodies against CMV defined patients with high, medium, low, and no risk of CMV disease. For patients in the first category, we recommend prophylaxis because there is a high probability of disease, CMV disease is most severe in this sub-group, and double-blind, randomized, placebo-controlled trials show that prophylaxis can be both efficacious and safe. For patients at medium or low risk, we recommend no prophylaxis but that patients are kept under clinical and virologic surveillance. Prophylaxis should be started if a patient requires any augmented immunosuppression for treatment of graft rejection/graft *versus* host disease. This strategy is termed, "delayed prophylaxis" because the drug is administered before there is evidence of systemic virus replication. If the patient becomes viremic, using a laboratory method demonstrated to correlate with the development of CMV disease, then the patient should be given a course of pre-emptive therapy.

Within this overview, some important differences between patient groups should be noted, as listed in the legend to Figure 1. Note that the sub-groups of patients at high, medium and low risk are different for recipients of solid organs *versus* bone marrow transplants. Note also that different drugs are indicated for different patient groups, as detailed in the legend. The dosing schedules for each course of prophylaxis or pre-emptive therapy are given in Table 10.

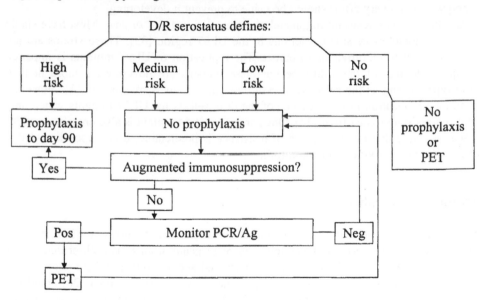

Figure 1.   Management algorithm for allograft recipients

Note: estimates of the number of patients in different risk groups is shown below for a theoretical population (n=100) where seropositivity = 60% for recipients and 55% for donors.

Risk category	BMTx*	Solid Tx **
High	D - R + n = 27	D + R - n = 22
Medium	D + R + n = 33	D + R + n = 33
Low	D + R - n = 22	D - R + n = 27
No	D - R - n = 18	D - R - n = 18

*   Prophylaxis = VACV (BMT$_x$),
** Prophylaxis = oral GCV (Liver T$_x$), VACV (Renal T$_x$), iv GCV (Heart T$_x$)

Table 10. Dosing Schemes

Strategy	Patient group	Drug	Dose	Duration	Recommendation category
Prophylaxis	Liver T$_x$	GCV-oral	1 g tds	14w	I
Prophylaxis	Bone marrow T$_x$	ACV	500 mg/m^2 tds 4w then 800 mg qds	26w	I
Prophylaxis	Renal T$_x$	VACV	2 g qds	90d	I
Prophylaxis	Heart T$_x$	GCV-iv	5 mg/kg bd	28d	I
Pre-emptive	Any T$_x$	GCV-iv	5 mg/kg bd	14d	II
Treatment	Any T$_x$ or AIDS*	GCV-iv	5 mg/kg bd	21d	I
Treatment	Any T$_x$ or AIDS*	Foscarnet	90 mg/kg bd	21d	I
Treatment	Pneumonitis	GCV-iv	5 mg/kg bd	21d	II
		Immunoglobulin	500 mg/kg (alternate days)	10 doses	
Treatment	Congenital	GCV-iv	6 mg/kg bd	6w	recommended only for those with CNS disease

* maintenance therapy may be required for CMV retinitis.
T$_x$ = transplant
ACV = acyclovir
VACV = valaciclovir
GCV = ganciclovir

HIV-infected Patients

Figure 2 shows how we believe the same principles should be applied to patients immunocompromised by ongoing HIV infection. Clearly, HAART is the most potent component of the total therapeutic prescription for these patients. Many patients have a good response to HAART, as shown by rapid decline of HIV RNA to undetectable levels, and an increase in CD4 count. However, some patients have inadequate responses for a variety of complex, inter-related reasons, discussed in Chapter 5. If, despite all medical attempts to provide effective control of HIV-induced damage, the CD4 count falls below 100, patients should be considered to be at risk for CMV disease. We suspect that serial monitoring for CMV viremia using antigenemia or PCR will identify those patients at risk of CMV disease, and natural history studies are currently underway to test this hypothesis. Assuming that these studies reaffirm the importance of CMV viremia in the post-HAART era, patients should be encouraged to enter controlled clinical trials of pre-emptive therapy to determine if such an antiviral intervention produces clinical benefits which outweigh the side-effects of drug administration. For example, pre-emptive therapy could involve a short, high-dose course of ganciclovir or such a course followed by long-term maintenance therapy with a lower dose of ganciclovir. One international double-blind, randomized, placebo-controlled trial has begun under the auspices of the AIDS Clinical Trials Group. Protocol 5030 will test the combined strategy of viremia detected by one method on one occasion (plasma PCR, Roche Molecular Systems) plus treatment with valganciclovir (high dose initially, reducing to maintenance levels).

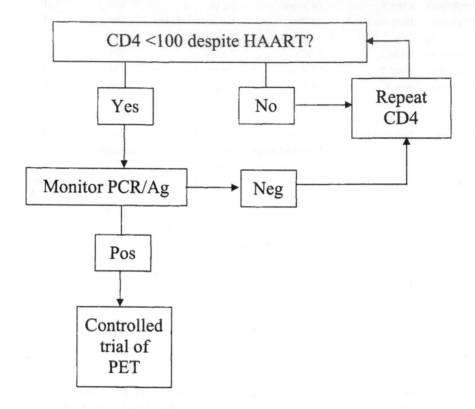

Figure 2.   Management algorithm for HIV-positive patients.
* Note ACTG 5030 is an international, placebo-controlled trial of valganciclovir pre-emptive therapy for patients plasma-PCR-positive by the Roche method.

AIDS Patients With CMV Retinitis

Figure 3 provides an algorithm for the suggested management of HIV-positive patients with a previous episode of CMV retinitis. Before HAART became available, most patients had progression of retinitis. Most patients with progression remained PCR-negative in blood, suggesting that virus persisting within the eye reactivated to cause disease [36]. A minority of patients became PCR-positive in blood, and this correlated with progression of retinitis [36], suggesting that, as with transplant patients, some cases of CMV disease may be caused by re-infection. Note that the CMV strains found in the eye may be multiple and distinct from those found in the blood at the same time, consistent with the occurrence of re-infection at some time. Of the patients who were PCR-positive, most had viruses in the blood which were genotypically resistant to ganciclovir [36] by virtue of changes in gene UL97. Such patients were significantly less likely to respond clinically to re-induction ganciclovir therapy than were viremic patients with wild-type CMV, illustrating the medical relevance of these molecular biological studies [36].

All of these observations have been used in the design of Figure 3. At the time of writing, it is possible to manage most patients with a past history of CMV retinitis without using maintenance ganciclovir. The algorithm, therefore, has been constructed to avoid this, at least for the first recurrence, by inviting clinicians to "consider" maintenance therapy. However, it seems likely that increasing numbers of patients who fail HAART will need maintenance options in the future, both to control CMV retinitis and to limit the effect of CMV on mortality [27, 28]. In the past, intraocular injections or slow-release devices were used to maintain vision in a pre-terminal AIDS patient. Indeed, the first antisense antiviral compound to be licensed was fomivirsen, which is administered by direct intra-vitreal injection. In our view, intraocular remedies should now be considered only as a component of holistic CMV therapy; it should be clear that CMV infection is systemic, with the retina being only one, albeit important, target organ. Furthermore, the performance of multiple procedures to replace intraocular devices now that patients live longer is impractical. We have also avoided the use of ganciclovir/foscarnet combination therapy at this time, although this therapeutic option may have to be deployed in the future control of HAART failures. Finally, the relative costs of different management regimens will require consideration.

Dosing Schemes

These are listed in Table 7.

Ganciclovir, foscarnet and acyclovir are eliminated by the kidneys. While there are no pharmacokinetic or pharmacodynamic drug interactions, the possibility of cumulative toxicity with other nephrotoxic drugs must be considered. Note that foscarnet and ganciclovir cannot be administered in the same intravenous fluid, so complicating their co-administration practically and by increasing fluid intake.

Side-effects

Ganciclovir is toxic to the bone marrow, inducing neutropenia frequently and thrombocytopenia occasionally. Initial treatment is with G-CSF followed by dose reduction or cessation of ganciclovir if neutropenia persists.

The nephrotoxicity of foscarnet can be reduced by pre-treatment with probenecid to decrease renal tubular secretion. Foscarnet also causes electrolyte abnormalities, particularly

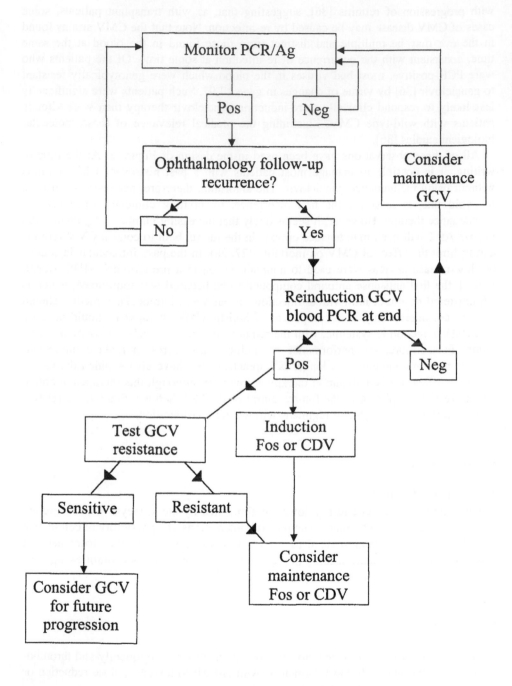

Figure 3. Management algorithm for AIDS patients with a past history of treated retinitis who are currently receiving HAART but not anti-CMV maintenance therapy.

changes in ionised magnesium concentration, and can cause a fixed drug eruption on genital skin due to local contamination with urine containing the excreted compound.

Cidofovir is nephrotoxic, and probenecid and fluid pre-hydration should always be used to decrease this. Administration is contra-indicated if the patient has proteinuria.

Special Considerations

Foscarnet has activity against HIV which might explain the improved survival seen in comparison with ganciclovir in AIDS patients [30].

Ganciclovir also inhibits HSV, so acyclovir prophylaxis can be stopped during ganciclovir administration [37].

For neonates with congenital CMV, a randomised, dose-comparative study showed 6 mg/kg iv bd to be as well tolerated as a lower dose [38]. A randomised comparison of 6 mg kg/kg bd *versus* no treatment has been conducted by the Collaborative Antiviral Study Group and reduced rate of hearing loss was reported on follow-up [39]. In our opinion, this protocol should be recommended for neonates meeting the inclusion criteria of the trial but that treatment of children without CNS symptoms or signs outside of a randomised, controlled clinical trial is not warranted because of the potential toxicity of this compound, including proven carcinogenicity in animals.

No clinical trials have studied the administration of anti-CMV therapy to pregnant women.

Vaccines

Neutralising antibodies against CMV are focused on glycoprotein B (gB), the product of UL55 and, less so, glycoprotein H (gH), the product of UL75. Cytotoxic T-cell activity is focused upon pp65 (ppUL83) and the major immediate early region (UL122/123).

Neutralising antibodies can be induced by gB presented as a soluble, truncated protein, or as part of a canarypox vector [40]. Phase I clinical trials have used these preparations alone or in a combined prime-boost mode.

Earlier work showed the live, attenuated Towne vaccine to be insufficiently protective against CMV infection and disease, although the severity of CMV disease in renal transplant recipients was reduced [41]. Towne lacked a series of genes found in wild strains [3]. These missing genes have now been engineered into Towne and phase I studies with the recombinant are planned.

References

1. Emery VC, Cope AV, Bowen EF, Gor D, Griffiths PD. The dynamics of human cytomegalovirus replication *in vivo*. Journal of Experimental Medicine 1999; 190: 177-182.

2. Chee MS, Bankier AT, Beck S, Bohni R, Brown CM, Cerny R, Horsnell T, Kouzarides T, Martignetti JA, et al. Analysis of the protein-coding content of the sequence of human cytomegalovirus strain

AD169. Current Topics in Microbiology & Immunology 1990; 154: 125-169.

3. Cha TA, Tom E, Kemble GW, Duke GM, Mocarski ES, Spaete RR. Human cytomegalovirus clinical isolates carry at least 19 genes not found in laboratory strains. Journal of Virology 1996; 70(1): 78-83.

4. Rubin RH. The indirect effects of cytomegalovirus infection on the outcome of organ transplantation. JAMA 1989; 261(24): 3607-3609.

5. Ljungman P, Plotkin SA. Workshop of CMV disease: definitions, clinical severity scores, and new syndromes. Scandinavian Journal of Infectious Diseases – Suppl. 1995; 99: 87-89.

6. Meyers JD, Ljungman P, Fisher LD. Cytomegalovirus excretion as a predictor of cytomegalovirus disease after marrow transplantation: importance of cytomegalovirus viremia. Journal of Infectious Diseases 1990; 162: 373-380.

7. Cope AV, Sabin C, Burroughs A, Rolles K, Griffiths PD, Emery VC. Interrelationships among quantity of human cytomegalovirus (HCMV) DNA in blood, donor-recipient serostatus, and administration of methylprednisolone as risk factors for HCMV disease following liver transplantation. Journal of Infectious Diseases 1997; 176(6): 1484-1490.

8. Bowen EF, Sabin CA, Wilson P, Griffiths PD, Davey C, Johnson MA, Emery VC. Cytomegalovirus (CMV) viraemia detected by polymerase chain reaction identifies a group of HIV-positive patients at high risk of CMV disease. AIDS 1997; 11: 889-893.

9. Shinkai M, Bozzette SA, Powderly W, Frame P, Spector SA. Utility of urine and leukocyte cultures and plasma DNA polymerase chain reaction for identification of AIDS patients at risk for developing human cytomegalovirus disease. Journal of Infectious Diseases 1997; 175(2): 302-308.

10. Dodt KK, Jacobsen PH, Hofmann B, Meyer C, Kolmos HJ, Skinhoj P, Norrild B, Mathiesen L. Development of cytomegalovirus (CMV) disease may be predicted in HIV-infected patients by CMV polymerase chain reaction and the antigenemia test. AIDS 1997; 11(3): F21-8.

11. Spector SA, Wong R, Hsia K, Pilcher M, Stempien MJ. Plasma cytomegalovirus (CMV) DNA load predicts CMV disease and survival in AIDS patients. Journal of Clinical Investigation 1998; 101: 497-502.

12. Emery VC, Sabin CA, Cope AV, Gor D, Hassan-Walker AF, Griffiths PD. Application of viral-load kinetics to identify patients who develop cytomegalovirus disease after transplantation. Lancet 2000; 355(9220): 2032-2036.

13. Littler E, Stuart AD, Chee MS. Human cytomegalovirus UL97 open reading frame encodes a protein that phosphorylates the antiviral nucleoside analogue ganciclovir. Nature 1992; 358: 160-162.

14. Safrin S, Cherrington J, Jaffe HS. Clinical uses of cidofovir. Reviews in Medical Virology 1997; 7(3): 145-156.

15. Schmidt GM, Horak DA, Niland JC, Duncan SR, Forman SJ, Zaia JA. A randomized, controlled trial of prophylactic ganciclovir for cytomegalovirus pulmonary infection in recipients of allogeneic bone marrow transplants; The City of Hope-Stanford-Syntex CMV Study Group. New England Journal of Medicine 1991; 324: 1005-1011.

16. Meyers JD, Reed EC, Shepp DH, Thornquist M, Dandliker PS, Vicary CA, Flournoy N, Kirk LE, Kersey JH, Thomas ED. Acyclovir for prevention of cytomegalovirus infection and disease after allogeneic marrow transplantation. New England Journal of Medicine 1988; 318(2): 70-75.

17. Einsele H, Ehninger G, Hebart H, Wittkowski KM, Schuler U, Jahn G, Mackes P, Herter M, Klingebiel T, Loffler J, et al. Polymerase chain reaction monitoring reduces the incidence of cytomegalovirus disease and the duration and side effects of antiviral therapy after bone marrow transplantation. Blood 1995; 86(7): 2815-2820.

18. Boeckh M, Gooley TA, Myerson D, Cunningham T, Schoch G, Bowden RA. Cytomegalovirus pp65

antigenemia-guided early treatment with ganciclovir *versus* ganciclovir at engraftment after allogeneic marrow transplantation: a randomized double-blind study. Blood 1996; 88(10): 4063-4071.

19. Winston DJ, Wirin D, Shaked A, Busuttil RW. Randomised comparison of ganciclovir and high-dose acyclovir for long-term cytomegalovirus prophylaxis in liver-transplant recipients. Lancet 1995; 346(8967): 69-74.

20. Merigan TC, Renlund DG, Keay S, Bristow MR, Starnes V, O'Connell JB, Resta S, Dunn D, Gamberg P, Ratkovec RM. A controlled trial of ganciclovir to prevent cytomegalovirus disease after heart transplantation. New England Journal of Medicine 1992; 326(18): 1182-1186.

21. Wagner JA, Ross H, Hunt S, Gamberg P, Valantine H, Merigan TC, Stinson EB. Prophylactic ganciclovir treatment reduces fungal as well as cytomegalovirus infections after heart transplantation. Transplantation 1995; 60(12): 1473-1477.

22. Valantine HA, Gao SZ, Menon SG, Renlund DG, Hunt SA, Oyer P, Stinson EB, Brown BW, Jr., Merigan TC, Schroeder JS. Impact of prophylactic immediate posttransplant ganciclovir on development of transplant atherosclerosis: a post hoc analysis of a randomized, placebo-controlled study. Circulation 1999; 100(1): 61-66.

23. Lowance D, Neumayer H-H, Legendre C, Squifflet J-P, Kovarik J, Brennan PJ, Norman D, Mendez R, Keating MR, Coggon GL, Crisp A, Lee IC, on behalf of the International Valaciclovir CMV Prophylaxis Transplantation Study Group. Valaciclovir reduces the incidence of cytomegalovirus disease and acute rejection in renal allograft recipients. New England Journal of Medicine 1999; 340: 1462-1470.

24. Kidd IM, Fox JC, Pillay D, Charman H, Griffiths PD, Emery VC. Provision of prognostic information in immunocompromised patients by routine application of the polymerase chain reaction for cytomegalovirus. Transplantation 1993; 56(4): 867-871.

25. Griffiths PD, Feinberg J, Fry J, Dix L, Gor D, Ansari A, Emery VC, on behalf of the ACTG 204/GlaxoWellcome 123-014 International CMV Prophylaxis Study Group. The effect of valaciclovir on cytomegalovirus viremia and viruria detected by polymerase chain reaction in patients with advanced human immunodeficiency virus disease. Journal of Infectious Diseases 1998; 177: 57-64.

26. Emery VC, Sabin C, Feinberg JE, Gryzwacz M, Knight S, Griffiths PD, on behalf of the ACTG 204/GlaxoWellcome 123-014 International CMV Prophylaxis Study Group. Quantitative effects of valaciclovir on the replication of cytomegalovirus in patients with advanced human immunodeficiency virus disease: baseline cytomegalovirus load dictates time to disease and survival. Journal of Infectious Diseases 1999; 180: 695-701.

27. Bowen EF, Wilson P, Cope A, Sabin C, Griffiths P, Davey C, Johnson M, Emery V. Cytomegalovirus retinitis in AIDS patients: influence of cytomegaloviral load on response to ganciclovir, time to recurrence and survival. AIDS 1996; 10: 1515-1520.

28. Spector SA, Hsia K, Crager M, Pilcher M, Cabral S, Stempien MJ. Cytomegalovirus (CMV) DNA load is an independent predictor of CMV disease and surival in advanced AIDS. Journal of Virology 1999; 73: 7027-7030.

29. Deayton JR, Mocroft A, Wilson P, Emery VC, Johnson MA, Griffiths PD. Loss of cytomegalovirus (CMV) viraemia following highly active antiretroviral therapy in the absence of specific anti-CMV therapy. AIDS 1999; 13: 1203-1206.

30. Mortality in patients with the acquired immunodeficiency syndrome treated with either foscarnet or ganciclovir for cytomegalovirus retinitis. Studies of Ocular Complications of AIDS Research Group, in collaboration with the AIDS Clinical Trials Group. New England Journal of Medicine 1992; 326: 213-220.

31. Combination foscarnet and ganciclovir therapy vs monotherapy for the treatment of relapsed cytomega-

lovirus retinitis in patients with AIDS. The Cytomegalovirus Retreatment Trial. The Studies of Ocular Complications of AIDS Research Group in Collaboration with the AIDS Clinical Trials Group. Archives of Ophthalmology 1996; 114(1): 23-33.

32. Dieterich DT, Kotler DP, Busch DF, Crumpacker C, Du Mond C, DearmandB., Buhles W. Ganciclovir treatment of cytomegalovirus colitis in AIDS: a randomized, double-blind, placebo-controlled multicenter study. Journal of Infectious Diseases 1993; 167: 278-282.

33. Chou S, Erice A, Jordan MC, Vercellotti GM, Michels KR, Talarico CL, Stanat SC, Biron KK. Analysis of the UL97 phosphotransferase coding sequence in clinical cytomegalovirus isolates and identification of mutations conferring ganciclovir resistance. Journal of Infectious Diseases 1995; 171(3): 576-583.

34. Chou S, Marousek G, Guentzel S, Follansbee SE, Poscher ME, Lalezari JP, Miner RC, Drew WL. Evolution of mutations conferring multidrug resistance during prophylaxis and therapy for cytomegalovirus disease. Journal of Infectious Diseases 1997; 176: 786-789.

35. Emery VC, Griffiths PD. Prediction of cytomegalovirus load and resistance patterns after antiviral chemotherapy. Proceedings of the National Academy of Science of the USA 2000; 97(14): 8039-8044.

36. Bowen EF, Emery VC, Wilson P, Johnson MA, Davey CC, Sabin CA, Farmer D, Griffiths PD. CMV PCR viraemia in patients receiving ganciclovir maintenance therapy for retinitis: correlation with disease in other organs, progression of retinitis and appearance of resistance. AIDS 1998; 12: 605-611.

37. Gane E, Saliba F, Valdecasas GJ, O'Grady J, Pescovitz MD, Lyman S, Robinson CA. Randomised trial of efficacy and safety of oral ganciclovir in the prevention of cytomegalovirus disease in liver-transplant recipients. The Oral Ganciclovir International Transplantation Study Group. Lancet 1997; 350(9093): 1729-1733.

38. Whitley RJ, Cloud G, Gruber W, Storch GA, Demmler GJ, Jacobs RF, Dankner W, Spector SA, Starr S, Pass RF, Stagno S, Britt WJ, Alford, C J, Soong S, Zhou XJ, Sherrill L, FitzGerald JM, Sommadossi JP. Ganciclovir treatment of symptomatic congenital cytomegalovirus infection: results of a phase II study. National Institute of Allergy and Infectious Diseases Collaborative Antiviral Study Group. Journal of Infectious Diseases 1997; 175(5): 1080-1086.

39. Kimberlin DW, Lin CY, Sanchez P, Demmler G, Dankner W, Shelton M, Edwards K, Jacobs RF, Robinson J, Wright J, Lakeman FD, Kiell JM, Soong SJ, Whitley RJ. Ganciclovir (GCV) treatment of asymptomatic congenital cytomegalovirus (CMV) infections; results of a phase III randomized trial. 40th ICAAC, Toronto, Canada, September 2000; 274. (Abstr.)

40. Pass RF, Duliege AM, Boppana S, Sekulovich R, Percell S, Britt W, Burke RL. A subunit cytomegalovirus vaccine based on recombinant envelope glycoprotein B and a new adjuvant. Journal of Infectious Disease 1999; 180(4): 970-975.

41. Plotkin SA, Smiley ML, Friedman HM, Starr SE, Fleisher GR, WlodaverC., Dafoe DC, Friedman AD, Grossman RA, Barker CF. Towne-vaccine-induced prevention of cytomegalovirus disease after renal transplants. Lancet 1984; 1: 528-530.

42. Reed EC, Wolford JL, Kopecky KJ, Lilleby KE, Dandliker PS, Todaro JL, McDonald GB, Meyers JD. Ganciclovir for the treatment of cytomegalovirus gastroenteritis in bone marrow transplant patients. A randomized, placebo- controlled trial. Annals of Internal Medicine 1990; 112: 505-510.

43. Goodrich JM, Mori M, Gleaves CA, Du-Mond C, Cays M, Ebeling DF, Buhles WC, DeArmond B, Meyers JD. Early treatment with ganciclovir to prevent cytomegalovirus disease after allogeneic bone marrow transplantation. New England Journal of Medicine 1991; 325: 1601-1607

44. Prentice HG, Gluckman E, Powles RL, Ljungman P, Milpied N, FernandezRanada JM, Mandelli F, Kho P, Kennedy L, Bell AR. Impact of long-term acyclovir on cytomegalovirus infection and survival

after allogeneic bone marrow transplantation. European Acyclovir for CMV Prophylaxis Study Group. Lancet 1994; 343: 749-753.

45. Winston DJ, Ho WG, Bartoni K, Du Mond C, Ebeling DF, Buhles WC. Ganciclovir prophylaxis of cytomegalovirus infection and disease in allogeneic bone marrow transplant recipients. Results of a placebo-controlled, double-blind trial. Annals of Internal Medicine 1993; 118: 179-184.

46. Goodrich JM, Bowden RA, Fisher L, Keller C, Schoch G, Meyers JD. Ganciclovir prophylaxis to prevent cytomegalovirus disease after allogeneic marrow transplant. Annals of Internal Medicine 1993; 118: 173-178.

47. Cheeseman SH, Rubin RH, Stewart JA, Tolkoff-Rubin NE, Cosimi AB, Cantell K, Gilbert J, Winkle S, Herrin JT, Black PH, Russell PS, Hirsch MS. Controlled clinical trial of prophylactic human-leukocyte interferon in renal transplantation. Effects on cytomegalovirus and herpes simplex virus infections. New England Journal of Medicine 1979; 300: 1345-1349.

48. Hirsch MS, Schooley RT, Cosimi AB, Russell PS, Delmonico FL, Tolkoff-Rubin NE, Herrin JT, Cantell K, Farrell ML, Rota TR, Rubin RH. Effects of interferon-alpha on cytomegalovirus reactivation syndromes in renal-transplant recipients. New England Journal of Medicine 1983; 308: 1489-1493.

49. Lui SF, Ali AA, Grundy JE, Fernando ON, Griffiths PD, Sweny P. Double-blind, placebo-controlled trial of human lymphoblastoid interferon prophylaxis of cytomegalovirus infection in renal transplant recipients. Nephrology, Dialysis, Transplantation 1992; 7: 1230-1237.

50. Balfour HHJ, Chace BA, Stapleton JT, Simmons RL, Fryd DS. A randomized, placebo-controlled trial of oral acyclovir for the prevention of cytomegalovirus disease in recipients of renal allografts. New England Journal of Medicine 1989; 320: 1381-1387.

51. Metselaar HJ, Rothbarth PH, Brouwer RM, Wenting GJ, Jeekel J, Weimar, W. Prevention of cytomegalovirus-related death by passive immunization. A double-blind placebo-controlled study in kidney transplant recipients treated for rejection. Transplantation 1989; 48(2): 264-266.

52. Macdonald PS, Keogh AM, Marshman D, Richens D, Harvison A, Kaan AM, Spratt PM. A double-blind placebo-controlled trial of low-dose ganciclovir to prevent cytomegalovirus disease after heart transplantation. Journal of Heart & Lung Transplantation 1995; 14(1 Pt 1): 32-38.

53. Snydman DR, Werner BG, Dougherty NN, Griffith J, Rubin RH, DienstagJL., Rohrer RH, Freeman R, Jenkins R, Lewis WD, et al. Cytomegalovirus immune globulin prophylaxis in liver transplantation. A randomized, double-blind, placebo-controlled trial. The Boston Center for Liver Transplantation CMVIG Study Group. Annals of Internal Medicine 1993; 119: 984-991.

54. Balfour HHJ, Chace BA, Stapleton JT, Simmons RL, Fryd DS. A randomized, placebo-controlled trial of oral acyclovir for the prevention of cytomegalovirus disease in recipients of renal allografts. New England Journal of Medicine 1989; 320 (21): 1381-1387.

CHAPTER 8

VARICELLA-ZOSTER VIRUS

MENNO D. DE JONG and ANN M. ARVIN

Table of Contents

Introduction

Varicella-zoster virus (VZV) is a human alpha herpes virus that causes varicella (chickenpox) during primary infection, following which the virus establishes latency in cells of the dorsal root ganglia. Reactivation of latent virus causes herpes zoster (shingles), a disease predominantly occurring in elderly and immunocompromised patients.

The highly temperature-sensitive viral particle is 180 to 200 nm in diameter, and consists of a lipid envelope, tegument, and an icosahedral nucleocapsid. The nucleocapsid

Practical Guidelines in Antiviral Therapy Ed. by Charles A.B. Boucher and George J. Galasso. 173 — 191
© 2002 *Elsevier Science. Printed in the Netherlands.*

contains a linear, double-stranded DNA genome of approximately 125.000 base pairs with at least 69 open reading frames [1].

Epidemiology

VZV is a highly contagious virus. It is transmissable by the respiratory route from patients with varicella, and by direct contact with vesicle fluids from patients with varicella or herpes zoster. The latter patients most likely are the source of annual epidemics of varicella, which occur in temperate climates during winter and spring. Approximately 95% of the population in temperate climates have acquired varicella before adulthood, usually during early childhood. In tropical areas, this percentage is substantially lower. Varicella provides life-long immunity against re-infection. However, rare cases of second varicella-episodes have been reported [2].

In otherwise healthy persons, herpes zoster is mainly a disease of the elderly. It is estimated that 75% of cases occur in individuals over 45 years of age [3]. The overall incidence ranges from 1.3 to 4.2 cases per 1000 persons per year, increasing to 10 cases per 1000 persons by the age of 75 [3-5]. Acquisition of varicella before birth or during the first year of life carries an increased risk of herpes zoster during childhood [6]. The risk of developing herpes zoster is increased in patients with impaired cellular immunity secondary to immunosuppressive treatment or disease. The highest risks are seen in human immunodeficiency virus-infected patients, recipients of transplants, most notably bone marrow transplants, and patients with leukemia or malignant lymphoma [7-9].

Pathogenesis and Clinical Features (Table 1)

Varicella

Inoculation of VZV occurs at respiratory tract mucous membranes, following which the virus presumably spreads to regional lymph nodes where it replicates and causes a primary cell-associated viremia [10]. During this viremia, VZV is transported to the liver and other cells of the reticuloendothelial system. A secondary viremia occurs during the last 4-5 days of the incubation period, which allows the virus to disseminate to cutaneous epithelial cells and produce the characteristic skin lesions [11-16]. The secondary viremia continues for some days after the appearance of the skin eruption [14, 17]. If viremia is not adequately controlled by the host immune response, disseminated infection may cause disease in lungs, liver, central nervous system and other organs.

The incubation period of varicella ranges from 10 to 21 days [10]. Prodromal symptoms of fever, malaise, headache, and abdominal pain may precede the onset of the skin rash by 24-48 hours. The typical exanthem of varicella usually begins on the scalp, face, or trunk, and consists of pruritic, erythematous macules that rapidly evolve to vesicles, containing clear fluid. After 1-2 days, the vesicles become cloudy in appearance, as crusting begins. Crusted lesions are ultimately sloughed, usually leaving intact, unscarred skin behind. The rash may also involve oropharyngeal, conjunctival, and vaginal mucous membranes.

Tabel 1. Clinical illnesses and complications caused by VZV infection

illness		most common complications	
		healthy children	high-risk patients[1]
primary infection	varicella	bacterial superinfection	protracted course
		meningoencephalitis	pneumonia
		cerebellar ataxia	hepatitis
			encephalitis
			thrombocytopenia/DIC[2]
reactivation	herpes zoster	postherpetic neuralgia	protracted course
	zoster ophtalmicus		multidermatomal zoster
	Ramsay-Hunt syndrome		disseminated disease[3]
	"zoster sine herpete"		acute retinal necrosis

1. high-risk patients include healthy adults, pregnant women, infants born within 2 days before to 4 days after onset of maternal varicella, and patients with compromised cellular immunity (see text); 2. DIC = disseminated intravascular coagulopathy; 3. see varicella

New lesions appear for 1-7 days. Although the total number of lesions usually ranges from 100 to 300, it may vary from fewer than 10 to more than 1500 lesions. Acquisition of varicella from househould contacts, or pre-existing skin damage, e.g. due to eczema or sunburn, predispose to more severe skin manifestations [18, 19].

In otherwise healthy children, the most frequent complication of varicella is secondary bacterial infection of the skin lesions, usually by *Streptococcus pyogenes* or *Staphylococcus aureus*. In addition, healthy children may develop signs of meningoencephalitis or cerebellar ataxia 2 to 6 days after the onset of the rash, which generally resolve completely within days to weeks. While subclinical hepatitis is common, the combination of vomiting and increased serum transaminase levels requires differentiation from Reye's syndrome [20]. Because of the risk of the latter syndrome, treatment with salicylates is contra-indicated in children with varicella. VZV pneumonia is extremely rare in healthy children, but represents an important complication in otherwise healthy adults with varicella [21, 22]. Although uncommon in otherwise healthy patients, hemorrhagic complications secondary to thrombocytopenia may occur. Rare complications of varicella include transverse myelitis, nephritis, arthritis, myocarditis, pericarditis, pancreatitis and orchitis.

While varicella usually is a relatively mild, self-limiting disease in healthy children, the risk of complications is increased in patients with lymphoproliferative malignancies, solid tumors, congenital cellular immunodeficiency, or AIDS, recipients of organ or bone marrow transplants, patients receiving high-dose steroids, otherwise healthy adults, pregnant women, and infants born within 2 days before to 4 days after the onset of maternal varicella. Without antiviral treatment, varicella in these patients can be associated with prolonged formation of new lesions, and a risk of potentially fatal disease with involvement of lungs, liver, central nervous system, and disseminated intravascular coagulopathy. VZV pneumonia represents the primary cause of death, and usually develops 3-7 days after the appearance of skin lesions [23]. Fulminant hepatitis and hemorrhagic complications are also associated with high mortality rates.

Herpes Zoster

During primary infection, VZV reaches cells of the dorsal root ganglia by hematogenous spread or travel from mucocutaneous sites of replication along the neuronal cell axon [10]. While the precise molecular mechanisms by which VZV establishes and maintains latency are unknown, it is clear from epidemiological observations that symptomatic reactivation of the virus is related to declining cell-mediated immunity. Upon reactivation, extensive replication occurs within the ganglion, following which the virus travels along the sensory nerve to cutaneous epithelial cells, where it produces the characteristic dermatomal skin vesicles. Herpes zoster most commonly is a localized disease, affecting one or two unilateral adjacent dermatomes. However, herpes zoster in immunocompromised patients is frequently accompanied by viremia, which, similar to varicella, may result in disseminated disease with widespread visceral involvement.

The onset of the skin rash of herpes zoster is preceeded or accompanied by neuritic pain, paresthesia, or pruritus. In some patients, cutaneous symptoms do not develop, and the symptoms remain restricted to neuropathic pain ("zoster sine herpete") [24]. The typical skin rash begins as clustered erythematous maculopapules, which rapidly evolve to vesicles, and then to pustules and crusts. New lesion formation ceases within 3-7 days. Healing of affected skin is usually complete within 2 weeks, but may take longer. In human immunodeficiency virus-infected persons, the skin eruption may persist as hyperkeratotic or verrucous lesions [25].

In approximately half of the cases, VZV reactivation occurs in thoracic ganglia [4, 5]. Cranial nerve involvement, particulary of the trigeminal nerve, is observed in 14-20% of patients [4, 5]. Involvement of the ophtalmic branch of the trigeminal ganglion (herpes zoster ophtalmicus) may cause conjunctivitis, keratitis, uveitis, or panopthalmitis [26]. Facial palsy is associated with herpes zoster of the seventh cranial nerve, but may also accompany involvement of other cranial nerves, sometimes without obvious skin manifestations [27, 28]. Herpes zoster oticus and facial palsy (Ramsay-Hunt syndrome) is caused by involvement of the eighth cranial nerve and the geniculate ganglion of the seventh nerve [28]. Lumbosacral herpes zoster may be associated with neurogenic urinary incontinence or ileus [27].

The most common complication of herpes zoster is postherpetic neuralgia, resulting in continuing pain which can be severe and last for several months. Overall, pain persists for more than 4 weeks after the resolution of herpes zoster in 10-15% of adult patients, 25-30% of whom still experience pain after 12 months [4, 5]. These percentages are substantially higher in elderly patients. Risk factors for the development of postherpetic neuralgia include increasing age, involvement of the ophtalmic trigeminal branch, the presence of prodromal symptoms, and the severity of pain as well as the number of skin lesions during herpes zoster [29, 30]. Most likely, postherpetic neuralgia is caused by neuronal cell damage inflicted during the acute phase of herpes zoster, rather than by continued viral replication. This may explain why the beneficial effects of antiviral treatment for this complication are disappointing.

In untreated immunocompromised patients, the skin rash of herpes zoster generally is more severe, often associated with hemorrhagic and necrotic lesions, and of longer duration. In addition, viremia may occur in up to 40% of patients, resulting in cutaneous and visceral dissemination. Hematogenous spread of the virus may result in the same complications as observed during varicella, including involvement of lungs, liver, central nervous system, and disseminated intravascular coagulopathy. In severely immunocompromized patients, acute retinal necrosis, potentially resulting in bilateral blindness, may occur with or without skin lesions. Particularly in bone marrow transplant recipients, who are at special risk for dissemination, the onset of the skin rash is frequently preceded by severe, unexplained epigastric pain, which may provide a clue for early diagnosis of disseminated herpes zoster [31].

Laboratory Diagnosis (Table 2)

In immunocompetent persons, the typical presentation of fullblown VZV infections usually allows for a clinical diagnosis without laboratory confirmation. However, in immunocompromised patients, rapid diagnostic techniques may be helpful for early diagnosis, thus guiding decisions about antiviral treatment. In addition, laboratory techniques are necessary for diagnosis of visceral involvement, e.g. pneumonia or encephalitis, and for clinical presentations of VZV infections without cutaneous involvement, e.g. isolated meningoencephalitis, zoster sine herpete, or retinal infection.

Table 2.   Laboratory diagnosis

diagnostic method	interpretation
viral culture	Isolation of virus from vesicles or other specimens using tissue culture methods is time-consuming and has limited sensitivity. Sensitivity and rapidity are improved by the shell vial culture method.
antigen detection	Immunofluorescent staining with mono- or polyclonal antibodies of vesicle scrapings or tissue specimens enables rapid diagnosis. Sensitivity dependent on stage of vesicle and quality of scraping.
nucleic acid amplification	PCR is highly sensitive and diagnostic method of choice in specimens such as CSF and vitreous fluid. No commercial assays available.
Serology	Important for determining immune status; limited role in diagnosis. IgM detection has limited sensitivity and specificity. FAMA assays[1] most sensitive. Several commercial ELISA's available, all with good specificity and sensitivities up to 90%.

1. FAMA = fluorescent antibody membrane antigen assay

Virologic Methods

The golden standard of diagnosis is the recovery of infectious virus from vesicles or other clinical specimens (e.g. cerebrospinal fluid, bronchial washing, peripheral blood mononuclear cells) using tissue culture methods. However, the sensitivity of viral culture is limited, especially in matrices such as cerebrospinal fluid, and dependent on the stage of the vesicle, and the handling-time of the specimen. Furthermore, it may take 1-2 weeks before VZV is isolated from clinical specimens, which precludes the use of viral culture for clinical decision-making. The shell vial culture method may improve both sensitivity and rapidity of VZV isolation [32].

A rapid diagnosis of cutaneous VZV infections can be made by immunofluorescent or immunoperoxidase staining with mono- or polyclonal antibodies of epithelial cells from a vesicle. Since the sensitivity of this procedure is dependent on the stage of the vesicle and the presence of sufficient numbers of epithelial cells on the slide, care must be given to rigorous scraping of cells from the base of a newly formed vesicle. In solubilized preparations of cells and vesicle fluid, VZV antigens can be detected by enzyme immunoassay methods. Immunologic staining can also be used on tissue specimens for diagnosis of visceral infection.

The detection of VZV DNA in clinical specimens by *in situ* hybridization or PCR provides highly sensitive methods for diagnosis [14, 33-37]. VZV-specific PCR is the diagnostic method of choice in biological matrices such as cerebrospinal- or vitreous fluid. The detection of VZV DNA in blood may enable diagnosis of disseminated VZV infections during the stage of prodromal symptoms, such as abdominal pain, thereby allowing for early treatment [38]. The role of quantitative PCR for the purpose of therapeutic monitoring is under study [36].

Serologic Methods

Although valuable for determining the immune status of exposed individuals, the role of serologic testing for diagnosis of acute varicella or herpes zoster is limited. IgM, IgG, and IgA antibodies become detectable within 3 days after the onset of varicella in most patients, but are often not present at the onset of the skin rash. Detection of IgM antibodies has limited sensitivity and specificity; in the presence of high titers of VZV-specific IgG, false-positive reactions are common. Since IgM antibodies may also be produced during VZV reactivation, their presence in serum does not differentiate primary from recurrent infection. While varicella may be clinically indistinguishable from disseminated herpes zoster in immunocompromized patients, the presence of VZV-specific IgG in pre-illness sera points to the latter. If such sera are unavailable, primary infection may be differentiated from disseminated recurrent disease by measuring the avidity of antibodies [39]. However, avidity-testing of VZV-specific IgG is currently restricted to research settings; commercial assays are not available.

Antiviral Agents

Acyclovir

Acyclovir is the drug of choice for the treatment of VZV infections. Clinical efficacy has been demonstrated in immunocompromized as well as immunocompetent patients with varicella or herpes zoster (see *treatment algorithms*). Since the antiviral activity of acyclovir against VZV is less than it is against herpes simplex viruses, higher doses are required for treatment of VZV infections [40]. Because the oral bioavailability of the drug is low (approximately 20%), oral administration requires high and frequent dosing [41]. Acyclovir levels achieved in cerebrospinal fluid are approximately 50% of those in plasma. Since acyclovir is excreted through the kidneys, doses should be adjusted in case of renal function impairments.

The safety profile of acyclovir is excellent, even at high doses [41]. Although side effects are uncommon, acyclovir treatment may be associated with allergic cutaneous reactions, nausea, vomiting, diarrhea, abdominal pain, or headache. Very rarely, reversible neurologic reactions may occur, manifested by dizziness, confusion, agitation, hallucinations, tremors, or convulsions [42]. Neurotoxicity is strongly associated with underlying renal function impairment, resulting in high plasma acyclovir levels. Rare adverse reactions include hematologic abnormalities and hepatitis. Acute renal insufficiency may occur in dehydrated patients and patients with pre-existing impairments of renal function, especially in case of rapid infusion of acyclovir. This extremely rare complication is probably caused by precipation of acyclovir-crystals in the renal tubuli, and can be prevented by adequate hydration and slow infusion (appr. 60 minutes), and adjusting the dose if the serum creatinine level is elevated. Caution is warranted during high-dose oral treatment in the elderly, since plasma levels may be considerably high despite apparently normal renal function, as measured by serum creatinine and urea levels [43]. Acute renal failure and coma during oral treatment in this setting has been described [44].

Co-administration of probenecid increases the bio-availability of acyclovir by prolonging the elimination rate [45]. High plasma acyclovir concentrations during oral treatment have been observed in patients also receiving diuretics, which may suggest that diuretics and acyclovir compete for active renal secretion, resulting in reduced clearance of the latter [43].

Antiviral resistance to acyclovir is rare, but has been reported in severely immunocompromized patients, most notably AIDS patients, who received prolonged treatment with acyclovir for recurrent or chronic episodes of herpes zoster [46-49]. Drug resistance to acyclovir is caused by deficiency of-, or amino acid changes in the viral thymidine kinase [48-50].

Valaciclovir

Valaciclovir is the L-valine ester of acyclovir, which is rapidly converted to acyclovir after oral administration [51]. Compared to acyclovir, the oral bioavailability of valaciclovir is markedly improved, such that an oral dose of 1000 mg yields plasma levels of acyclovir which are similar to those observed after intravenous acyclovir administration. As expected, the clinical efficacy of valaciclovir in healthy adults with herpes zoster is at least equal to oral acyclovir (see *treatment algorithms*) [52]. The same may be expected in healthy persons with varicella, but formal studies have not been performed. At present, valaciclovir is not licensed for pediatric use. Since the efficacy of valaciclovir has not been studied in immunocompromized patients at high risk of complications, intravenous treatment with acyclovir remains the mainstay of therapy in this patient group. Side effects and drug interactions of valaciclovir are identical to acyclovir [51].

Famciclovir

Famciclovir is an oral prodrug of penciclovir [53]. The latter is a nucleoside analogue with an anti-VZV activity equivalent to acyclovir [54]. Similar to valaciclovir, famciclovir is well-absorbed after oral administration, and rapidly converted to the active metabolite [53]. The clinical efficacy of famciclovir in otherwise healthy patients with herpes zoster is at least equal to oral acyclovir treatment (see *treatment algorithms*) [55]. Clinical studies comparing famciclovir and valaciclovir treatment have not been performed. Famciclovir has not been studied in patients with varicella or VZV-infected patients at high risk of complications. Famciclovir is well tolerated [56]. Reported side effects include headache, nausea, diarrhea, abdominal pain, dizziness, and insomnia. Allergic cutaneous reactions, hallucinations, and confusion have very rarely been reported. There are no known drug interactions with famciclovir.

Others

In initial studies of antiviral treatment for VZV-infections, vidarabine and interferon-alpha were shown to exert antiviral activities [57-60], but the improved tolerance and efficacy of acyclovir has eliminated their use for anti-VZV therapy [61, 62]. Ganciclovir has equal *in vitro* activity against VZV as acyclovir, but clinical studies have not been performed because of its greater toxicity. Treatment with intravenous foscarnet is indicated in case of acyclovir resistance [63]. Brivudin and sorivudine have shown to be effective in healthy adults with varicella, as well as in HIV-infected patients with herpes zoster [64-68]. However, bromovinyl uracil, a metabolite of these agents, inhibits the metabolism of 5-fluorouracil (5-FU), which has resulted in lethal 5-FU toxicities in patients receiving concommittant treatment with 5-FU and sorivudine [69]. Due to this drug interaction, further clinical development of the latter drug has been halted.

Treatment Algorithms

The treatment algorithms for varicella and herpes zoster in different patient groups are summarized in Tables 3 and 4. Dosing schedules are shown in Table 5.

Table 3. Antiviral treatment of varicella

otherwise healthy		high-risk	complications
children	adults (incl. pregnant women)	incl. hematologic malignancies, transplant recipients, AIDS, high dose steroids, neonatal varicella	incl. pneumonia, encephalitis, hepatitis, thrombocytopenia
no treatment[a]	oral acyclovir[b, c]	intravenous acyclovir[d]	intravenous acyclovir

a. oral acyclovir is recommended for children with chronic cutaneous or pulmonary disease, and children requiring chronic treatment with corticosteroids or salicylates
b. valaciclovir is probably at least as effective, but is not licensed for treatment of varicella. The same may be true for famciclovir.
c. treatment should be started within 24 hours after onset of the rash
d. treatment should ideally be started within 24-72 hours, but delayed treatment may also confer clinical benefit

Table 4. Antiviral treatment of herpes zoster

otherwise healthy [a]	low-risk [a]	high-risk [b]	dissemination
	incl. low-dose steroids, and HIV-infection	incl. hematologic malign., and transplant recipients	incl. cutaneous dissemin., and visceral disease
oral acyclovir *or* valaciclovir *or* famciclovir	oral acyclovir *or* valaciclovir *or* famciclovir	intravenous acyclovir	intravenous acyclovir

a. treatment should be started within 48-72 hours after onset of the rash
b. treatment should ideally be started 48-72 hours after onset of the rash, but delayed treatment may also confer clinical benefit

Varicella

Based on proven clinical safety and efficacy in large, placebo-controlled studies, oral acyclovir is licensed for the treatment of varicella in healthy children and adults [19, 22, 70, 71]. When started within 24 hours after onset of the skin rash, oral acyclovir treatment reduces the duration of fever and new lesion formation, as well as the total number of lesions in these patient groups. However, in view of the mild,

Table 5. Dosing schedules of anti-VZV agents

antiviral agent	dosage — children	dosage — adults	duration	remarks
acyclovir	intravenous: 500 mg/m² q8hrs or 10 mg/kg q8hrs oral: 20 mg/kg 4 times daily	intravenous: 500 mg/m² q8hrs or 10 mg/kg q8hrs oral: 800 mg, 5 times daily	varicella: 7 days, or until no new lesion formation for 48 hours. herpes zoster: idem	1. for pediatric use, an oral solution (40 mg/ml) is available 2. infusion time should be appr. 60 minutes 3. adequate hydration is important 4. adjust dosing in case of renal function impairment, hemodialysis or CAPD
valaciclovir	-	1000 mg, 3 times daily	herpes zoster: 7 days, or until no new lesion formation for 48 hours.	1. adjust dosing in case of renal function impairment, hemodialysis or CAPD.
famciclovir	-	500 mg, 3 times daily	herpes zoster: 7 days, or until no new lesion formation for 48 hours.	1. adjust dosing in case of renal function impairment, hemodialysis or CAPD.

self-limiting course and low risk of complications in otherwise healthy children with varicella, there is no need for antiviral treatment in these patients. Supportive and hygienic measures usually suffice. The American Academy of Pediatrics recommends that acyclovir therapy should only be considered for children with chronic pre-existing cutaneous or pulmonary disease, and children receiving chronic salicylate treatment or courses of systemic or aerosolized corticosteroids [72]. Since the illness is usually more severe in adolescents, and even more so in adults, the clinical impact of acyclovir treatment in these patients is greater. More importantly, early treatment in this age group carries the potential of reducing the risk of varicella pneumonia. For these reasons, oral treatment with acyclovir should be considered in adolescents and adults with varicella, when it is possible to start treatment within 24 hours after onset of the illness. Adolescents or adults who develop a varicella pneumonia require intravenous treatment with acyclovir [73]. Valaciclovir and famciclovir probably are at least as effective as oral acyclovir, but have not been studied in this patient group, and are not licensed for the treatment of varicella.

Intravenous treatment with acyclovir is strongly indicated in patients at high risk of developing complications, most notably patients with lymphoproliferative malignancies, solid tumors, congenital cellular immunodeficiency, or AIDS, recipients of organ or bone marrow transplants, patients receiving high-dose steroids, and infants born within 2 days before to 4 days after the onset of maternal varicella. Early intravenous treatment has been shown to prevent progressive varicella and visceral dissemination, and to decrease the mortality rate, especially by reducing the risk of varicella pneumonia [23, 74, 75]. Since visceral dissemination of VZV occurs within the first 24-72 hours after the onset of the rash, treatment should be started within this time interval. However, when started later in the course of the disease, intravenous acyclovir may still reduce viral replication and associated tissue destruction.

Herpes Zoster

In immunocompetent persons, treatment of herpes zoster with oral acyclovir at a dosage of 800 mg five times daily has been shown to reduce the duration of new lesion formation and acute zoster-associated pain when started within 48-72 hours after onset of the rash [76-79]. The beneficial effects of oral acyclovir on postherpetic neuralgia are subject to controversy. However, reanalysis and meta-analyses suggest that acyclovir reduces the duration of this major cause of zoster-related morbidity [79-81]. The addition of corticosteroids or prolongation of antiviral treatment does not provide additional benefits in preventing or alleviating postherpetic neuralgia [82, 83].

In a study comparing valaciclovir and acyclovir for the treatment of herpes zoster, there were no differences in the effects on rash-healing parameters, but the duration of zoster-associated pain was significantly shorter in valaciclovir-treated patients [52]. However, the incidence of pain at several timepoints after the acute phase of herpes zoster was similar in both treatment groups.

Compared to placebo, treatment with famciclovir at dosages of 500 or 750 mg q8h accelerates lesion healing, especially when initiated within 48 hours after onset of the rash [84]. While the 500 mg dose also showed a statistically significant effect on resolution of acute pain, this was not observed for the higher dose. In the subgroup of patients who were 50 years of age or older, both dosages also seemed to reduce the duration of postherpetic neuralgia. When compared to acyclovir, the effects of famciclovir on the cutaneous manifestations and zoster-associated pain were similar [55]. However, in the subgroup of patients who were treated within 48 hours after rash onset, the duration of zoster-associated pain was significantly reduced in famciclovir-treated patients, also after adjusting for risk factors of postherpetic neuralgia.

Overall, the present data suggest that the clinical efficacies of oral acyclovir, valaciclovir and famciclovir in immunocompetent patients with herpes zoster are largely similar. Therefore, the choice between them may depend on convenience of administration and costs.

In patients with herpes zoster ophtalmicus, oral acyclovir has proven effects on ocular complications, such as anterior uveitis or stromal keratitis, even when treatment is delayed beyond 72 hours after onset of symptoms [85, 86]. Although valaciclovir and famciclovir likely are as effective, data on the treatment of herpes zoster ophtalmicus with these compounds are scarce.

Severely immunocompromised patients with localized herpes zoster, including transplant recipients, especially of bone marrow transplants, and patients with hematologic malignancies, should be treated with intravenous acyclovir. In these patients, intravenous acyclovir has been shown to terminate local progression in the affected dermatome and to prevent cutaneous and visceral dissemination [61, 62, 87]. Although optimal benefit of treatment will be obtained when treatment is started within 72 hours after the onset of the rash, delayed treatment still is likely to provide clinical benefit. Similar to immunocompetent persons, the beneficial effects of antiviral treatment on the development of postherpetic neuralgia are equivocal. Valaciclovir and famciclovir have not been evaluated in severely immunocompromised patients, and should not be used as initial treatment in these patients.

In patients with minimal degrees of immunosuppression, as well as in HIV-infected patients with dermatomal herpes zoster, oral treatment with acyclovir usually will suffice. Valaciclovir most likely is equally effective in the latter patient groups, but has not been formally evaluated. The same is true for famciclovir. All immunocompromised patients with signs of cutaneous or visceral dissemination should receive intravenous treatment with acyclovir.

Evaluation of Treatment Efficacy

In patients with varicella, the efficacy of antiviral treatment is assessed by the cessation of new lesion formation. Immunocompromised patients may develop new lesions shortly after withdrawal of therapy, which may require the reinstitution of treatment. Especially in immunocompromised patients, the development of visceral disease and other complications should be monitored by careful clinical examinations and routine blood chemistry and hematology. Suspected involvement of lungs or central nervous system warrants radiologic examinations and virologic tests of bronchial washings and cerebrospinal fluid respectively. The potential role of quantitative PCR in evaluating treatment efficacy is under study [35, 36]. In case of suspected bacterial superinfection, gram-stain and culture of vesicle fluid should be performed. The spectrum of empiric antibiotic treatment should cover *S. aureus* and *S. pyogenes*.

The efficacy of antiviral treatment for herpes zoster is monitored by new lesion formation and resolution of pain. In practice, patients are unable to differentiate the acute pain of herpes zoster from postherpetic neuralgia. For this reason, it seems more appropriate to monitor the duration of pain as a whole, defined as zoster-associated pain. Similar to varicella, severely immunocompromised patients should be closely clinically monitored for evidence of cutaneous or visceral dissemination and other complications.

Prevention

Infection Control

Since VZV is a highly contagious virus which causes potentially life-threatening disease in high-risk patients, appropriate measures for infection control should be taken immediately when a VZV-infected patient is hospitalized. Prevention of VZV transmission to susceptible persons is complicated by the fact that patients with varicella are contagious for 24-48 hours before the onset of clinically evident disease.

Infection control measures include strict isolation of patients with varicella or disseminated herpes zoster. Drainage and secretions precautions are sufficient for patients with dermatomal herpes zoster. Isolation precautions should continue until the last skin lesion is completely crusted. VZV susceptibility of exposed patients and health personnel is assessed by serology in case of a negative or unknown history of chickenpox. Susceptible patients who are exposed to a VZV-infected patient and are at risk for complications of varicella should receive hyperimmunoglobulin as soon as possible to prevent transmission of infection (see *prophylaxis*). Since the usual incubation time of varicella is 9-21 days, all susceptible, exposed patients should be placed in strict isolation from 9 days after the first to 21 days after the last possible exposure. Some experts recommend that susceptible immunocompromised patients should be placed in strict isolation immediately, because the incubation period in these patients may be shorter. Exposed VZV seronegative health personnel should be reassigned to a low-risk department or placed on administrative leave from 9 days after the first to 21 days after the last exposure. Vaccination of seronegative health care workers in high-risk clinical departments is highly recommended.

Prophylaxis

Varicella-zoster immune globulin (VZIG) is prepared from high titer immune human serum, and is recommended as prophylaxis for VZV-susceptible individuals who have been exposed to a patient with varicella or herpes zoster, and who are at risk for complications of varicella [88]. These include immunocompromised persons, pregnant women, and newborns exposed to maternal varicella. VZIG is administered intramuscularly at a dose as recommended by the manufacturer, and is only effective when administered within 96 hours, and preferably within 48 hours after exposure. It is not effective when given after the onset of varicella. A second dose of VZIG should be given if renewed VZV exposure occurs more than two weeks following the initial administration. Especially in immunocompromized patients, breakthrough infection may occur despite VZIG administration [89, 90]. The incubation period in these patients may be prolonged up to 28 days [90].

The use of antiviral prophylaxis for preventing varicella is not recommended, because the safety and efficacy of antiviral agents for this purpose have not been properly established. The use of oral acyclovir for preventing herpes zoster or frequently relapsing disease has been evaluated in immunocompromized patients, most notably bone marrow transplant recipients and HIV-infected patients [91, 92]. Although the incidence of herpes zoster is decreased in bone marrow transplant recipients during acyclovir prophylaxis, the overall annual incidence in this patient group has been shown not to change due to the occurrence of VZV reactivations after discontinuation of the drug [91]. Long-term prophylaxis with acyclovir may prevent frequently relapsing or chronic herpes zoster in HIV-infected persons [92], but is also associated with the emergence of acyclovir-resistant VZV strains [46-49]. In view of the latter observation, chronic low-dose administration of acyclovir or other antiviral agents should be avoided.

Vaccination

An effective live attenuated varicella vaccine, made from the Oka strain of VZV, has been licensed for clinical use in several countries [93]. While universal administration to children 12-15 months of age is advised in the United States, recommendations of vaccination are restricted to susceptible adolescents and adults in other countries. The vaccine is highly protective against household exposure to varicella in healthy children [93]. Serocoversion rates after a single dose of vaccine are more than 95% in children under 12 years of age. In adolescents and adults, similar levels of protection are only obtained when two doses are given at an interval of at least 4 weeks. While persistence of immunity has been documented for up to six years in healthy children, antibody titers decrease to undetectable levels in a large proportion of adult vaccinees during this time. In children with leukemia, most of whom required two doses to elicit sufficient immunity, vaccination during remission reduced the attack rate following household exposure to 13% [94]. However, the Oka vaccine is not yet licensed for use in this patient group. Since symptomatic VZV reactivation is related to declining cellular immunity, vaccination may also prevent the development of herpes zoster by boosting the VZV-specific immunity [95]. Clinical studies evaluating this potential use of VZV vaccination are ongoing.

Since the vaccine contains infectious virus, careful attention must be given prior to administration to the presence of underlying diseases and concomittant immunosuppressive treatment. While mild breakthrough infections after vaccination uncommonly occur in healthy children and adults [96], vaccine-related rashes, sometimes progressing to varicella-like illnesses, were observed in approximately 50% of leukemic children in remission [94]. During vaccine-related rashes, the vaccine strain can be transmitted to susceptible contacts [97]. Reactivation of the vaccine virus has also been reported, but appears to be less common than reactivation of wild-type virus [98]. Since the Oka strain of VZV is susceptible to acyclovir, varicella-like illnesses or herpes zoster caused by vaccine virus can be treated with this drug.

References

1. Davison AJ, Scott JE. The complete DNA sequence of varicella-zoster virus. J gen Virol 1986; 67: 1759-816.

2. Gershon AA, Steinberg SP, Gelb L. Clinical reinfection with varicella-zoster virus. J Infect Dis 1984; 149: 137-42.

3. McGregor RM. Herpes zoster, chickenpox, and cancer in general practice. BMJ 1957; 1: 84-7.

4. Hope-Simpson RE. The nature of herpes zoster: a long-term study and a new hypothesis. Proc R Soc Med 1965; 58: 9-20.

5. Ragozzino MW, Melton LJ, Kurland LT, Chu CP, Perry HO. Population-based study of herpes zoster and its sequelae. Medicine 1982; 61: 310-6.

6. Brunell PA. Varicella in pregnancy, the fetus, and the newborn: problems in management. J Infect Dis 1992; 166 (Suppl 1): S42-S47

7. Dolin R, Reichman RC, Mazur MH, Whitley RJ. Herpes zoster-varicella infection in immunosuppressed patients. Ann Intern Med 1978; 89: 375-88.

8. Schuchter LM, Wingard JR, Piantadosi S, Burns WH, Santos GW, Saral R. Herpes zoster infection after autologous bone marrow transplantation. Blood 1989; 74: 1424-7.

9. Rogues A-M, Dupont M, Ladner J, Ragnaud J, Pellegrin J, Dabis F. Herpes zoster and human immunodeficiency virus infection: a cohort study of 101 coinfected patients. J Infect Dis 1993; 168: 245

10. Arvin AM. Varicella-zoster virus. In: Fields Virology. Fields BN, Knipe DM, Howley PM, eds. 1996; Philadelphia: Lippincot-Raven Publishers

11. Asano Y, Itakura N, Hiroishi Y, et al. Viremia is present in incubation period in nonimmunocompromised children with varicella. J Pediatr 1985; 106: 69-71.

12. Feldman S, Epp E. Detection of viremia during incubation of varicella. J Pediatr 1979; 94: 746-8.

13. Gershon AA, Steinberg S, Silber R. Varicella-zoster viremia. J Pediatr 1978; 92: 1033-6.

14. Koropchak CM, Graham G, Palmer J, et al. Investigation of varicella-zoster virus infection by polymerase chain reaction in the immunocompetent host with acute varicella. J Infect Dis 1991; 163: 1016-22.

15. Ozaki T, Ichikawa T, Matsui Y, et al. Lymphocyte-associated viremia in varicella. J Med Virol 1986; 19: 249-53.

16. Vonsover A, Leventon-Kriss S, Langer A, Smetana Z, Zaizov R, Potaznick D, Cohen IJ, Gotlieb-Stematsky T. Detection of varicella-zoster virus in lymphocytes by DNA hybridization. J Med Virol 1987; 21: 57-66.

17. Sawyer MH, Wu YN, Chamberlin CJ, et al. Detection of varicella-zoster virus DNA in the oropharynx and blood of patients with varicella. J Infect Dis 1992; 166: 885-8.

18. Boyd AS, Neldner KH, Zemtsov A, Shihada B. Photolocalized varicella. J Am Acad Derm 1992; 26: 772-4.

19. Dunkle LM, Arvin AM, Whitley RJ, et al. A controlled trial of acyclovir for chickenpox in normal children. N Engl J Med 1991; 325: 1539-44.

20. Hurwitz I, Goodman RA. A cluster of cases of Reye syndrome associated with chickenpox. Pediatrics 1982; 70: 901-10.

21. Gogos CA, Bassaris HP, Vagenakis AG. Varicella pneumonia in adults. A review of pulmonary manifestations, risk factors, and treatment. Respiration 1992; 59: 339-43.

22. Wallace MR, Bowler WA, Murray NB, Brodine SK, Oldfield EC. Treatment of adult varicella with oral acyclovir: a randomized, placebo-controlled trial. Ann Intern Med 1992; 117: 358-63.

23. Feldman S, Lott L. Varicella in children with cancer: impact of antiviral therapy and prophylaxis. Pediatrics 1987; 80: 465-72.

24. Gilden DH, Dueland AN, Devlin ME, Mahalingam R, Cohrs R. Varicella-zoster virus reactivation without rash. J Infect Dis 1992; 166 (Suppl 1): S30-S34

25. Alessi E, Cusini M, Zerboni R, et al. Unusual varicella zoster virus infection in patients with the acquired immunodeficiency syndrome. Arch Dermatol 1988; 124: 1011-3.

26. Womack LW, Leisegang TJ. Complications of herpes zoster ophtalmicus. Arch Ophthalmol 1983; 101: 42-9.

27. Reichman RC. neurologic complications of varicella-zoster infections. Ann Intern Med 1978; 375: 89-96.

28. Feldman SR, Ford MJ, Briggaman RA. Herpes zoster and facial palsy. Cutis 1988; 42: 523-4.

29. Choo PW, Galil K, Donahue JG, Walker AM, Spiegelman D, Platt R. Risk factors for postherpetic neuralgia. Arch Intern Med 1997; 157: 1217-24.

30. Whitley RJ, Weiss HL, Soong SJ, Gnann JW. Herpes zoster: risk categories for persistent pain. J Infect Dis 1999; 179: 9-15.

31. David DS, Tegtmeier BR, O'Donnell MR, Paz IB, McCarty TM. Visceral varicella-zoster after bone marrow transplantation: report of a case series and review of the literature. Am J Gastroenterol 1998; 93: 810-3.

32. Schirm J, Meulenberg JJ, Pastoor GW, van Voorst V, Schroder FP. Rapid detection of varicella-zoster virus in clinical specimens using monoclonal antibodies on shell vials and smears. J Med Virol 1989; 28: 1-6.

33. Puchhammer-Stockl E, Popow-Kraupp T, Heinz FX, Mandl CW, Kunz C. Detection of varicella-zoster virus DNA by polymerase chain reaction in the cerebrospinal fluid of patients suffering from neurological complications associated with chicken pox or herpes zoster. J Clin Microbiol 1991; 29: 1513-6.

34. Sawyer MM, Wu YN, Chamberlin CJ, et al. Detection of varicella-zoster virus DNA in the oropharynx and blood of patients with varicella. J Infect Dis 1992; 166: 885-8.

35. De Jong MD, Weel JFL, Schuurman T, Wertheim-van Dillen PME, Boom R. Quantitation of varicella zoster virus DNA in whole blood, plasma and serum by PCR and electrochemiluminescence. J Clin Microbiol 2000; 38: 2568-73.

36. Hawrami K, Breuer J. Development of a fluorogenic polymerase chain reaction assay (TaqMan) for the detection and quantitation of varicella zoster virus. J Virol Meth 1999; 79: 33-40.

37. Mainka C, Fuss B, Geiger H, Hofelmayr H, Wolff MH. Characterization of viremia at different stages of varicella-zoster virus infection. J Med Virol 1998; 56(1): 91-8.

38. De Jong MD, Weel JFL, Van Oers MHJ, Boom R, Wertheim-van Dillen PME. Molecular diagnosis of visceral herpes zoster. Lancet, in press.

39. Kangro HO, Manzoor S, Harper DR. Antibody avidity following varicella-zoster virus infections. J Med Virol 1991; 33: 100-5.

40. Biron KK, Elion GB. *In vitro* susceptibility of varicella-zoster virus to acyclovir. Antimicrob Agents Chemother 1980; 18: 443-7.

41. Wagstaff AJ, Faulds D, Goa KL. Aciclovir. A reappraisal of its antiviral activity, pharmacokinetic properties and therapeutic efficacy. Drugs 1994; 47: 153-205.

42. Adair JC, Gold M, Bond RE. Acyclovir neurotoxicity: clinical experience and review of the literature. South Med J 1994; 87: 1227-31.

43. Wood MJ, McKendrick MW, Freris MW, Jeal SC, Jones DA, Gilbert AM. Trough plasma acyclovir concentrations and safety of oral acyclovir, 800 mg five times daily for 7 days in elderly patients with herpes zoster. J Antimicrob Chemother 1994; 33: 1245-9.

44. Eck P, Silver SM, Clark EC. Acute renal failure and coma after a high dose of oral acyclovir. N Engl J Med 1991; 325: 1178.

45. Laskin OL, de Miranda P, King DH, Page DA, Longstreth JA, Rocco L, Lietman PS. Effects of probenecid on the pharmacokinetics and elimination of acyclovir in humans. Antimicrob Agents Chemother 1982; 21: 804-7.

46. Linnemann CCJ, Biron KK, Hoppenjans WG, Solinger AM. Emergence of acyclovir-resistant varicella zoster virus in an AIDS patient on prolonged acyclovir therapy. AIDS 1990; 4: 577-9.

47. Jacobson MA, Berger TG, Fikrig S, et al. Acyclovir-resistant varicella zoster virus infection after chronic oral acyclovir therapy in patients with the acquired immunodeficiency syndrome (AIDS). Ann Intern Med 1990; 112: 187-91.

48. Talarico CL, Phelps WC, Biron KK. Analysis of the thymidine kinase genes from acyclovir-resistant mutants of varicella-zoster virus isolated from patients with AIDS. J Virol 1993; 67: 1024-33.

49. Sawyer MH, Inchauspe G, Biron KK, Waters DJ, Straus SE, Ostrove JM. Molecular analysis of the pyrimidine deoxyribonucleoside kinase gene of wild-type and acyclovir-resistant strains of varicella-zoster virus. J gen Virol 1988; 69: 2585-93.

50. Boivin G, Edelman CK, Pedneault L, Talarico CL, Biron KK, Balfour HH, Jr. Phenotypic and genotypic characterization of acyclovir-resistant varicella-zoster viruses isolated from persons with AIDS. J Infect Dis 1994; 170: 68-75.

51. Perry CM, Faulds D. Valaciclovir. A review of its antiviral activity, pharmacokinetic properties and therapeutic efficacy in herpesvirus infections. Drugs 1996; 52: 754-72.

52. Beutner KR, Friedman DJ, Forszpaniak C, Andersen PL, Wood MJ. Valaciclovir compared with acyclovir for improved therapy for herpes zoster in immunocompetent adults. Antimicrob Agents Chemother 1995; 39: 1546-53.

53. Pue MA, Benet LZ. Pharmacokinetics of famciclovir in man. Antiviral Chem Chemother 1993; 4 (suppl. 1): 47-55.

54. Boyd MR, Bacon TH, Sutton D, Cole M. Antiherpesvirus activity of 9-(4-hydroxy-3-hydroxy-methylbut-1-yl)guanine (BRL 39123) in cell culture. Antimicrob Agents Chemother 1987; 31: 1238-42.

55. Degreef H FHZCSG. Famciclovir, a new oral antiherpes drug: results of the first controlled clinical study demonstrating its efficacy and safety on the treatment of uncomplicated herpes zoster in immunocompetent patients. Int J Antimicrob Agents 1994; 4: 241-6.

56. Saltzman R, Jurewicz R, Boon R. Safety of famciclovir in patients with herpes zoster and genital herpes. Antimicrob Agents Chemother 1994; 38: 2454-7.

57. Arvin AM, Kushner JH, Feldman S, Baehner D, Hammand D, Merigan TC. Human leukocyte interferon for the treatment of varicella in children with cancer. N Engl J Med 1982; 306: 761-5.

58. Whitley RJ, Soong SJ, Dolin R, Betts R, Linnemann CC, Alford C. Early vidarabine therapy to control the complications of herpes zoster in immunosuppressed patients. N Engl J Med 1982; 307: 971-5.

59. Whitley RJ, Hilty M, Haynes R, et al. Vidarabine therapy of varicella in immunosuppressed patients. J Pediatr 1982; 101: 125-31.

60. Merigan TC, Rand KH, Pollard RB, Abdallah PS, Jordan GW, Freid RP. Human leukocyte interferon for the treatment of herpes zoster in patients with cancer. N Engl J Med 1978; 298: 981-7.

61. Shepp DH, Dandliker PS, Meyers JD. Treatment of varicella-zoster virus infection in severely immunocompromised patients. A randomized comparison of acyclovir and vidarabine. N Engl J Med 1986; 314: 208-12.

62. Whitley RJ, Gnann JWJ, Hinthorn D, et al. Disseminated herpes zoster in the immunocompromised host: a comparative trial of acyclovir and vidarabine. J Infect Dis 1992; 165: 450-5.

63. Breton G, Fillet AM, Katlama C, Bricaire F, Caumes E. Acyclovir-resistant herpes zoster in human immunodeficiency virus-infected patients: results of foscarnet therapy. Clin Infect Dis 1998; 27: 1525-7.

64. Wallace MR, Chamberlin CJ, Sawyer MH, et al. Treatment of adult varicella with sorivudine: a randomized, placebo-controlled trial. J Infect Dis 1996; 174: 249-55.

65. Wutzler P, De Clercq E, Wutke K, Farber I. Oral brivudin vs. intravenous acyclovir in the treatment of herpes zoster in immunocompromised patients: a randomized, double-blind trial. J Med Virol 1995; 46: 252-7.

66. Heidl M, Scholz H, Dorffel W, Hermann J. Antiviral therapy of varicella-zoster virus infection in immunocompromised children — a prospective randomized study of aciclovir *versus* brivudin. Infection 1991; 19: 401-5.

67. Bodsworth NJ, Boag F, Burdge D, et al. Evaluation of sorivudine (BV-AraU) *versus* acyclovir in the treatment of acute localized herpes zoster in human immunodeficiency virus-infected adults. J Infect Dis 1997; 176: 103-11.

68. Gnann JW, Crumpacker CS, Lalezari JP, et al. Sorivudine *versus* acyclovir for treatment of dermatomal herpes zoster in human immunodeficiency virus-infected patients: results from a randomized, controlled clinical trial. Antimicrob Agents Chemother 1998; 42: 1139-45.

69. Okuda H, Nishiyama T, Ogura K, et al. Lethal drug interactions of sorivudine, a new antiviral drug, with oral 5-fluorouracil prodrugs. Drug Metab Dispos 1997; 25: 270-3.

70. Balfour HHJ, Kelly JM, Suarez CS, et al. Acyclovir treatment of varicella in otherwise healthy children [see comments]. J Pediatr 1990; 116: 633-9.

71. Balfour HHJ, Rotbart HA, Feldman S, et al. Acyclovir treatment of varicella in otherwise healthy adolescents. J Pediatr 1992; 120: 627-33.

72. American Academy of Pediatrics Committee on Infectious Diseases. The use of oral acyclovir in otherwise healthy children with varicella. Pediatrics 1993; 91: 674-6.

73. Haake DA, Zakowski PC, Haake DL, Bryson YJ. Early treatment with acyclovir for varicella pneumonia in otherwise healthy adults: retrospective controlled study and review. Rev Infect Dis 1990; 12: 788-98.

74. Nyerges G, Meszner Z, Gyarmati E, Kerpel-Fronius S. Acyclovir prevents dissemination of varicella in immunocompromised children. J Infect Dis 1988; 157: 309-13.

75. Prober CG, Kirk LE, Keeney RE. Acyclovir therapy of chickenpox in immunosuppressed children: a collaborative study. J Pediatr 1982; 101: 622-5.

76. Huff JC, Bean B, Balfour HH, et al. Therapy of herpes zoster with oral acyclovir. Am J Med 1988; 85 (2A): 79-83.

77. Wood MJ, Ogan PJ, McKendrick MW, Care CD, McGill JI, Webb EM. Efficacy of oral acyclovir in the treatment of acute herpes zoster. Am J Med 1988; 85 (2A): 79-83.

78. Morton P, Thomson AN. Oral acyclovir on the treatment of herpes zoster in general practice. N Z Med J 1989; 102: 93-5.

79. Huff JC, Drucker JL, Clemmer A, et al. Effect of oral acyclovir on pain resolution in herpes zoster: a reanalysis. J Med Virol 1993; suppl. 1: 93-6.

80. Wood MJ, Kay R, Dworkin RH, Soong SJ, Whitley RJ. Oral acyclovir therapy accelerates pain resolution in patients with herpes zoster: a meta-analysis of placebo-controlled trials. Clin Infect Dis

1996; 22: 341-7.

81. Jackson JL, Gibbons R, Meyer G, Inouye L. The effect of treating herpes zoster with oral acyclovir in preventing postherpetic neuralgia: a meta-analysis. Arch Intern Med 1997; 157: 909-12.

82. Wood MJ, Johnson RW, McKendrick MW, Taylor J, Mandal BK, Crooks J. A randomized trial of acyclovir for 7 days or 21 days with and without prednisolone for treatment of acute herpes zoster. N Engl J Med 1994; 330: 896-900.

83. Esmann V, Geil JP, Kroon S, et al. Prednisolone does not prevent post-herpetic neuralgia. Lancet 1987; ii: 126-9.

84. Tyring S, Barbarash RA, Nahlik JE, et al. Famciclovir for the treatment of acute herpes zoster: effects on acute disease and postherpetic neuralgia. Ann Intern Med 1995; 123: 89-96.

85. Harding JC, Porter SM. Oral acyclovir in herpes zoster ophtalmicus. Curr Eye Res 1991; 10: 177-82.

86. Cobo LM, Foulks GN, Liesegang TJ, et al. Oral acyclovir in the treatment of acute herpes zoster ophtalmicus. Ophthalmol 1986; 93: 763-70.

87. Balfour HH, Bean B, Laskin OL, et al. Acyclovir halts progression of herpes zoster in immunocompromised patients. N Engl J Med 1983; 308: 1448-53.

88. Centers for Disease Control. Varicella-zoster immune globulin for the prevention of chickenpox: recommendations of the immunization practices advisory committee. Ann Intern Med 1984; 100: 859-65.

89. Miller E, Cradock-Watson JE, Ridehalgh MK. Outcome in newborn babies given anti-varicella-zoster immunoglobulin after perinatal maternal infection with varicella-zoster virus. Lancet 1989; ii: 371-3.

90. Zaia JA, Levin MJ, Preblud SR, et al. Evaluation of varicella-zoster immune globulin: protection of immunosuppressed children after household exposure to varicella. J Infect Dis 1983; 147: 737-43.

91. Ljungman P, Wilczek H, Gahrton G, et al. Long-term acyclovir prophylaxis in bone marrow transplant recipients and lymphocyte proliferation responses to herpes virus antigens *in vitro*. Bone Marrow Transplant 1986; 1: 185-92.

92. Ioannidis JP, Collier AC, Cooper DA, et al. Clinical efficacy of high-dose acyclovir in patients with human immunodeficiency virus infection: a meta-analysis of randomized individual patient data. J Infect Dis 1998; 178: 349-59.

93. White CJ. Varicella-zoster virus vaccine. Clin Infect Dis 1997; 24: 753-61.

94. Gershon AA, Steinberg SP, Gelb L, et al. Live attenuated varicella vaccine: efficacy for children with leukemia in remission. JAMA 1984; 252: 355-62.

95. Levin MJ, Hayward AR. The varicella vaccine. Prevention of herpes zoster. Inf Dis Clin N Am 1996; 10: 657-75.

96. Watson BM, Piercy SA, Plotkin SA, Starr SE. Modified chickenpox in children immunized with the Oka/Merck varicella vaccine. Pediatrics 1993; 9: 17-22.

97. Tsolia M, Gershon AA, Steinberg SP, Gelb L. Live attenuated varicella vaccine: evidence that the virus is attenuated and the importance of skin lesions in transmission of varicella-zoster virus. J Pediatr 1990; 116: 184-9.

98. Hardy I, Gershon AA, Steinberg SP, LaRussa P. The incidence of zoster after immunization with live attenuated varicella vaccine. A study in children with leukemia. N Engl J Med 1991; 325: 1545-50.

CHAPTER 9

VIRAL HEPATITIS

KENNETH R. HIRSCH and TERESA L. WRIGHT

Table of Contents

Viral hepatitis is the leading cause of chronic liver diseases worldwide. At the present time, numerous different hepatitis-causing viruses have been identified, with assignations ranging from hepatitis A through hepatitis G. Some of these viruses, such as HAV and HEV, cause acute, self-limited infections which never result in a chronically infected state. Others of these viruses such as hepatitis G are not clearly pathologic in human hosts. Finally, hepatitis C and hepatitis B (+/- Hepatitis D) can cause chronic, persistent infection and a wide spectrum of disease. Interestingly, not all persons infected with these latter viruses will invariably develop chronic infection. Also, even in those individuals who do develop persistent infection, the manifestations of their infections

193

Practical Guidelines in Antiviral Therapy Ed. by Charles A.B. Boucher and George J. Galasso. 193 — 221
© 2002 *Elsevier Science. Printed in the Netherlands.*

can be protean, ranging from prolonged asymptomatic infection to severe, debilitating hepatitis and progression to end stage liver disease and/or hepatocellular carcinoma.

There are numerous similarities between infection with hepatitis B and hepatitis C. First and foremost is the ability of each of these viruses to effect an escape from the host immune system. This appears to be a more consistently effective strategy for HCV, however both viruses persist in the host not because of sequestration in immune-privileged sites but because of the absence of an effective host immune response or the development of host immune tolerance to the infecting virus and its expressed antigens. Another similarity is that both viruses are transmitted through exposure to infected bodily fluids, although the relative efficiency of transmission differs between them. Infection with either virus can lead to the development of a number of extrahepatic disease manifestations, most commonly in the form of autoimmunity. Finally, both of these viruses demonstrate significant genetic heterogeneity both within populations and even in individual patients. This diversity appears to have more practical significance in the case of hepatitis C, however many believe it also plays some role in the pathogenesis of disease due to hepatitis B [1]. The lower rate of mutation with HBV *versus* HCV is also due in part to the presence of multiple overlapping open reading frames in the genome of HBV rather than the single ORF found in HCV (see below). Such diversity has implications both for development of an effective immune response or vaccine as well as for the sustained efficacy of pharmacologic therapies for these infections.

Although there are clear similarities between HBV and HCV, these are in fact very different viruses which have unique structures, life cycles, epidemiology, and treatments. In the remainder of this chapter, we shall individually address the specific features of each virus and discuss the available therapeutic interventions for control and/or eradication of these chronic infections.

Introduction and History of Hepatitis B

The first modern recognition of a form of hepatitis that was transmissible through blood or blood products was reported in 1883 by Lurman in Germany [2]. He reported on a large group of persons who received smallpox vaccine that had been prepared from human sera. Fifteen percent of that group developed jaundice over the next several weeks to months while none of their coworkers who did not undergo immunization developed jaundice over the same period. A vaccine derived from human serum was again implicated in the transmission of hepatitis during World War II. In this case, there was a high incidence of jaundice development among a specific group of soldiers who received yellow fever vaccination that was made from human serum [3, 4].

The alphabet of viral hepatitis was started in 1947 with the work of MacCallum and Bauer [5]. They introduced the assignation of hepatitis A for "infectious hepatitis", with fecal-oral transmission and short incubation. They contrasted this with what they termed hepatitis B or "homologous serum" hepatitis that they proposed was transmitted parenterally and had an incubation time measured in months. In the late 1960s, a unique antigen was identified in the serum of an Australian aborigine patient with acute leukemia, and subsequently this antigen was found to occur most commonly in patients who received multiple blood transfusions [6, 7]. This antigen was called the Australia antigen. Further studies established a relationship between the Australia antigen and the development of hepatitis B, and this association eventually led to the development of the first specific diagnostic tests for HBV infection [8]. Ultimately, it was recognized that the Australia antigen was the HBsAg protein. Confirmation of the hypothesis that hepatitis B was a viral infection and that it was associated with the Australia antigen was achieved through the recognition by electron microscopy of specific virions which reacted with serum directed against the Australia antigen [9]. These virions were termed "Dane particles, " and they were subsequently shown to be in fact the etiologic agents responsible for hepatitis B infection.

The worldwide number of persons who have been affected by hepatitis B is staggering. Over 2 billion people who are alive today have been infected with hepatitis B at some time, and over 350 million of them are chronically infected [10]. This comprises approximately 5% of the world's population, making HBV infection the number one worldwide cause of chronic hepatitis, cirrhosis, and hepatocellular carcinoma [10]. Annually, approximately 500,000 to 1,000,000 people die from complications of hepatitis B infection with only approximately 5,000 of those annual deaths occurring in the United States.

The likelihood of developing acute *versus* chronic HBV infection is dependent largely on the patient's age at the time of initial infection as well as the immune competency of the host. Geographic locales where hepatitis B infection is highly endemic (defined as an HBsAg prevalence greater than 8%) include most of Asia, sub-Saharan Africa, the Pacific Islands, and Alaska [11, 12]. In these highly endemic areas, the lifetime risk of HBV infection is greater than 60%, and most infections occur either perinatally or in infancy/early childhood. Infection early in life is typically asymptomatic, but it carries the highest risk for the development of chronic infection and the eventual sequelae of chronic hepatitis, cirrhosis, and/or hepatocellular carcinoma [4]. In geographic areas with low endemic rates of HBV, such as the United States, the pattern of disease and chronicity is opposite. Most Western patients are infected during their adult years, and they typically fall into a high risk group such as intravenous drug users, homosexual men, or patients with hemophilia. Most infections with HBV in the United States are associated with acute, symptomatic hepatitis and result in the development of persistent infection in fewer than 5% of cases. In the U.S., the prevalence of chronic HBV infection is only 0.35% and only 5% of the general population has evidence of prior HBV infection [13].

Virology of Hepatitis B

Hepatitis B is a member of the family *Hepadnavirdae*, which includes other hepatitis-causing viruses including the duck hepatitis virus (DHBV), the ground squirrel hepatitis virus (GSHV), the woodchuck hepatitis virus (WHV), and the heron hepatitis virus (HHV). HBV, along with all the members of this family, is a partially double-stranded, enveloped DNA virus. It is the smallest known DNA virus, with a genome comprised of only 3200 base pairs. The structure of HBV's genomic DNA is unusual. It has an almost complete circular minus DNA strand which encodes both the structural and enzymatic proteins of the virus. The plus DNA strand typically forms an incomplete circle which varies in length from virion to virion. The incomplete plus strand has a defined 5' end but a variable 3' end [14].

The HBV genome is comprised of four open reading frames which encode the nucleocapsid proteins, the envelope proteins, the polymerase, and the so-called X protein. The structural proteins of the HBV virion include the core antigen (HBcAg) and the e antigen (HBeAg), as well as the various envelope glycoproteins, HBsAg, pre-S1, and pre-S2. The infectious virions are composed of the viral DNA associated with the viral polymerase and the core proteins surrounded by an envelope made of the three surface glycoproteins embedded in cellular lipids. In the course of infection, in addition to producing complete virions, the liver produces large excesses of viral proteins in tubular and spherical forms. These particles are very important both because they are easily detectable markers of infection as well as the fact that they are highly immunogenic. The capacity of many hosts to generate a neutralizing antibody response to these particles provides an effective mechanism either to prevent or clear infection. The success of vaccination for hepatitis B is due to the presence of neutralizing epitopes in the HBsAg molecule that can induce protective and amnestic immune responses, even in the absence of actual HBV infection. The larger envelope proteins are believed to be important in mediating viral attachment and entry into hepatocytes.

The hepatitis B core protein (HBc) is critical in maintenance of the HBV life cycle. It is the presence of HBc protein in newly assembled nucleocapsid particles which facilitates envelopment of the new particles by the surface proteins thus completing the reproduction of intact virus particles [15]. In addition to its clear role in envelopment of nascent viral particles, some also hypothesize that HBcAg plays a role in delivery of the mature viral genome to the host cell nucleus, leading to a stable state of infection, replication and persistence. Furthermore, the expression of HBcAg-derived peptides on the surface of hepatocytes leads to the development of a cytotoxic T cell response in many hosts, and this response can lead to killing of infected cells. The HBeAg is formed by cleavage of the same translational product which produces HBcAg. However, unlike HBcAg, the HBe protein product is not essential to the virus life cycle. The function of the HBeAg appears to be the induction of immune tolerance by the host. HBeAg is found in all cellular compartments in infected hepatocytes and it can also be excreted from the cells into the bloodstream. High levels of HBe antigenemia are seen in patients with minimally symptomatic but highly viremic infections. In such patients, loss of HBe antigenemia and acquisition of anti-HBe antibodies (termed HBe seroconversion) is typically associated with a flare of hepatitis (manifest by elevated transaminases as a marker of necroinflammation) as well as an eventual diminution of viremia. These observations have led to the hypothesis that continued presence of HBeAg in the serum of infected patients somehow prevents effective immune attack of infected hepatocytes [16]. Once HBeAg is suppressed or eliminated, the host defenses can react against the infected cells, killing them in order to clear productive infection. It is known that HBeAg can cross the placenta, and it is postulated that exposure to high levels of HBeAg early in infection leads to the development of a prolonged period of neonatal T cell tolerance to nucleocapsid peptides. This tolerance results in little immune recognition of the infection, leading to insignificant hepatic inflammation or viral clearance until the time of seroconversion, which usually takes decades.

The hepatitis B polymerase is a remarkably polyfunctional enzyme. It possesses the capacity to catalyze RNA dependent DNA synthesis (reverse transcription), DNA dependent DNA synthesis, self-priming for reverse transcription, and RNase-H activity. The processing of viral nucleic acids is a complex, multi-step process. Following new viral infection of a hepatocyte, the viral genome is transformed from partially double stranded DNA into supercoiled covalently closed circular DNA (cccDNA). Host cell enzymes accomplish this step. The cccDNA is the template for the transcription of the pregenomic viral mRNA, again by cellular enzymes. The pregenomic mRNA is then transported to the cytoplasm, where the HBV polymerase acts upon it. Specifically, the reverse transcriptase function of the polymerase uses the mRNA as a template to form a full-length negative-sense DNA strand. Next, the polymerase uses its DNA-dependent DNA polymerase activity to synthesize the positive-sense strand from the negative-sense template. The new genomic DNA can then be packaged into nucleocapsid cores, assembled with envelope proteins and excreted from the infected cell.

The final HBV protein product is the X protein. Unlike the aforementioned structural and enzymatic proteins, the X protein is not found in all members of the hepadnavirus family and it does not appear to play any role in genetic replication nor viral assembly. It appears that HBx is a transcriptional activator which can mediate numerous effects on both viral and host genes [17], and it may play a significant role in development of hepatocellular carcinoma in non-cirrhotic patients with HBV, although this remains very controversial.

Pathogenesis of Hepatitis B Associated Liver Disease

HBV is not a cytopathic virus for the most part, and most of the diseases which are recognized as being caused by HBV infection are really due to the host immune response to the viral infection rather than any direct toxic effects of the virus itself [18]. In fact, a vigorous immune response on the part of the infected host is the only way to clear infection with HBV, but it is the same vigorous immune activation which leads to the most severe acute liver injury en route to resolution of infection. The vital role of immune competence in the development of either acute or chronic infection is demonstrated by the following statistics: 95% of neonatal infections are associated with the development of asymptomatic chronic HBV infections. This occurs in the context of an almost completely naïve immune system. This pattern is in stark contrast to infection in adults with mature, competent immune systems. In those cases, most patients have acute symptomatic hepatitis with subsequent viral clearance and development of protective immunity while only 3-5% go on to develop chronic HBV infection.

Given the fact that hepatitis B associated disease is really due to a dynamic interaction between the virus and the host immune system, one needs to consider the different phases of disease progression or resolution in terms which take both host immunity and virus into consideration [19]. The first phase of HBV/host interaction occurs in all hosts immediately upon infection, and it is a period of incubation for the virus and immune tolerance on the part of the infected host. The duration of this first phase is variable. In the immune competent adult it will typically last from 2-4 weeks, while in the immune naïve neonate this period of immune escape and viral proliferation can persist for decades.

In the second phase, the host mounts an immune response to the HBV infection. During this period, there is activation of both humoral and cellular immunity, with increased inflammatory mediator production and immune-mediated hepatocyte killing. Given that the immune system is targeting and destroying infected hepatocytes during this time, it is unsurprising that this is also the phase in which acute symptomatic hepatitis is recognized. Throughout this portion of the cycle, patients will have elevated transaminases and they may have jaundice. Serial measurements of HBV DNA during this period will demonstrate falling levels, although HBeAg may still be detectable in serum. The duration and outcome of this phase is dependent on the pre-infection status of the host's immune system. In immune competent adults, the vast majority will mount a fully effective immune response to HBV infection, resulting in death of all infected hepatocytes and resolution of infection within 3-4 weeks. In contrast, when those patients with neonatal infection do eventually mount an immune response to HBV, it is a suboptimal response which is frequently incapable of leading to clearance. Such cases can result in chronic hepatitis, with constant but not total turnover of infected cells, and this state can persist for decades, ultimately resulting in cirrhosis and its attendant complications.

The third phase of the host/HBV interaction occurs once the host has mounted an effective immune response to infection viral replication is no longer readily detected. This stage is serologically characterized by the absence of HBeAg and HBV DNA. At this point, most patients also become positive of HBeAb and they are said to have undergone e antigen seroconversion. In patients with chronic HBV infection, the rate of spontaneous seroconversion is approximately 5% per year [20]. During this phase, some patients may still be positive for HBsAg, and this is thought to occur due to integration of HBV DNA into the host genome and/or ongoing low level replication. The likelihood of HBV integration is in large part dependent on the duration of infection, and it is not typically seen unless the patient has been infected for 2 or more years [21]. The integrative step does not occur in all patients, and the mechanism by which it occurs as well as its ultimate consequence is still the topic of substantial debate.

The fourth and final phase is the development of protective immunity. During this period, patients are negative for HBeAg, HBV DNA, and HBsAg, and they develop antibodies to the HBs antigen and HBc antigen. If a patient reaches this phase, they are unlikely to ever be reinfected by HBV nor are they likely to have reactivation disease even if they had integrated HBV genomic DNA, so long as substantial immune compromise does not develop in the future [22].

Natural History & Treatment of HBV Infection

Human liver diseases caused by hepatitis B are essentially caused by one of two mechanisms. The first mechanism is immune system activation leading to hepatocyte killing. This is the mechanism responsible for acute hepatitis due to HBV, and as previously noted, it usually results in clearance of infection. However, if the immune-mediated attack is present but ineffective/less than complete, then a state of chronic hepatitis develops. This chronic hepatitis persists until (a) the virus ceases to produce antigens that the host immune system recognizes, (b) the virus is cleared, or (c) the host immune system stops recognizing the presence of infection (i.e. increased immunosuppression). If chronic hepatitis persists long enough, progressive hepatic fibrosis will develop and can eventually lead to the development of cirrhosis and hepatocellular carcinoma. The rate of these developments is dependent on a variety of factors including the repertoire of the host immune system, the age of the patient, the serologic state of the infection, and likely other environmental and genetic factors [23].

The second mechanism by which HBV can cause liver disease is through integration of portions of its DNA into the host genome. This process can lead to the development of hepatoma in the absence of cirrhosis. Hypotheses to explain this phenomenon include the possible disruption of host oncogenes, introduction of exogenous promoters which dysregulate host cell cycle enzymes, and many others [24, 25]. The true mechanism remains to be determined definitively.

The primary goal of treatment for patients with hepatitis B infection is to improve liver histology if possible with associated eradication of virus from the host hepatocytes. Presently, there are two main strategies used in attempts to accomplish this goal. The first strategy involves the use of immune stimulants, the best known of which is interferon. The idea behind this strategy is that the host immune response is present but deficient in some respect, and through exogenous, generalized upregulation of the host immune system, that effective viral clearance can be achieved. An important caveat to the use of agents that rely on this mechanism is that it presupposes the presence of some endogenous immune response. If a given patient is either immune tolerant to the virus (as occurs in neonatal infection) or if they are no longer producing HBV antigens (as can happen after stable integration of hepatitis B DNA), then there will be no immune response for stimulants to augment, and this approach to treatment will be unsuccessful.

The second widely used approach to the treatment of hepatitis B infection involves the use of nucleoside analogues which suppress the replication of the virus. A variety of agents with these characteristics have been identified, and one of them, lamivudine, is in regular clinical use. As will be discussed in greater detail below, problematic issues in the use of these agents include potentially prolonged duration of therapy as well as the likelihood of viral development of resistance.

Interferon-α

Interferons were first discovered in 1957, when researchers observed that virus infected cells released some substance which could react with other non-infected cells and render those cells resistant to infection by a variety of viruses [26]. Interferons are actually a large family of proteins which can be divided into three species: α, β, and γ, each of which differ in regard to the cell types which produce them, their cellular effects, and the stimuli which induce their endogenous production. Interferons α and β are both derived from genes on chromosome 9, and both of these have been used to treat hepatitis B infections. However, the vast majority of work has focused on the use of IFN-α. There are two main methods for the commercial production of IFN-α. One method is through viral stimulation of immortalized cell lines. The other method, most commonly in use currently, is through the use of recombinant technology in which the relevant interferon gene is transfected into a culture of *Escherichia coli* with resultant high-level expression of the protein product.

In the treatment of hepatitis B, interferon appears to have two important mechanisms of action. The first mechanism is directly antiviral. IFN-α induces an increase in intracellular production of 2', 5'-oligoadenylate synthetase, which activates cellular ribonucleases that cleave viral mRNA and thus prevents effective viral replication and production [27, 28]. The second major mechanism of IFN-α for the treatment of HBV infection is immunomodulatory. There are probably numerous immunomodulatory effects of IFN treatment, but one major mechanism is the upregulation of major histocompatibility complex (MHC) class I antigens on hepatocytes. The complex of HBV antigens and MHC class I antigens allows immune recognition of infected hepatocytes and thus it facilitates lysis of infected cells by CD8+ cytotoxic lymphocytes [29].

The two most common regimens for administration of IFN-α in HBV infected persons are 5 million international units given daily or 10 million international units given three times per week. Interferon is administered as an intramuscular or deep subcutaneous injection. Use of this medication is associated with numerous adverse effects in most patients. Almost all patients report the development of flu-like symptoms with initial use of the drug. These symptoms include fever, chills, myalgia, and fatigue. The flu-like symptoms are usually most severe when therapy is initiated, and they decrease in most patients as use continues. Furthermore, these symptoms can be minimized by the use of antipyretics, such as acetaminophen, as well as by timing of administration at bedtime, so that the most severe side effects will hopefully occur while the patient is sleeping. A potentially serious adverse effect of interferon therapy is the development of myelosuppression. This is typically a dose-dependent phenomenon, and it is one of the more common indications for dose reduction while on therapy. Development of myelosuppression can be completely asymptomatic. Therefore it is vital that patients undergo routine laboratory monitoring while on therapy. Other side effects of interferon therapy include alterations in mood, exacerbation of underlying autoimmune disease (overt or occult), alopecia, arthralgia, fatigue, and rarely, hypersensitivity reactions. It is important to note that severe depression with suicidality has occurred in a few patients treated with interferon. It is therefore important to screen patients carefully for pre-existing psychiatric disease and ensure that any depression is being optimally managed prior to the initiation of interferon therapy.

Treatment of hepatitis B with interferon has been demonstrated to result in clearance of infection and resolution of disease in a small subset of infected patients. It has been convincingly demonstrated that patients who do not demonstrate a significant endogenous immune response to infection at the time of treatment will not benefit from administration of interferon α-2 [30, 31]. Patients' whose infection are in phase 1, as described above, are immune tolerant to HBV, and therefore generalized immune activation during this period would not be unlikely to result in amplification of a specific anti-HBV response of sufficient magnitude to clear infection. During phase 3 & 4 infection, patients do not have significant amounts of actively replicating virus, so that treatment would not be expected to have substantial efficacy. Therefore, response to interferon treatment is only seen during phase 2 of the host-virus interaction, when there is pre-existing activation of a specific anti-HBV immune response on the part of the host in the context of ongoing viral replication.

In those patients who respond to interferon therapy, administration of the drug leads to rapid inhibition of viral replication and a decrease in detectable serum HBV DNA levels. Approximately 1-2 months into therapy, responders may manifest a "flare" of hepatitis, with significant increases in their transaminase levels. This phenomenon is due to immune recognition of infected hepatocytes and resultant enhancement of CD8+ lymphocyte mediated killing of these cells. These serum enzyme elevations are typically asymptomatic, so long as the patient has reasonably intact hepatic reserve (i.e. does not have advanced cirrhosis). Finally, in successfully treated patients, the loss of serum HBeAg and the eventual development of anti-HBe antibodies follow the hepatitis flare. In adult patients who are chronically infected for only a few years, HBeAg seroconversion is usually followed by HBsAg seroconversion as well. In those patients who had been infected for prolonged periods of time (generally greater than 3-5 years), detectable HBsAg persists, likely due to HBV integration into the host genome and/or ongoing low level replication. This HBsAg positivity does diminish over time in some patients, probably due normal elimination of the hepatocytes bearing the integrated DNA [32].

There have been numerous studies examining the efficacy of interferon treatment for the eradication or suppression of HBV infection. In general, the loss of HBeAg with treatment of adult-acquired chronic hepatitis B infection is between 30-40% [33-36]. A meta-analysis of randomized trials utilizing a variety of interferon regimens showed that HBeAg loss occurred in 33% of chronic hepatitis B patients who were treated as compared with a rate of 12% in untreated patients [37]. The same meta-analysis demonstrated that clearance of HBsAg occurred in 8% of treated patients but only 2% of controls. Long term follow-up of interferon-treated patients who underwent HBeAg seroconversion demonstrated that the remission of chronic hepatitis induced by this treatment is durable over many years, with only 5-10% of responders having reactivation over the subsequent 10 years [32, 38]. In the few cases where reactivation did occur, it was typically transient and was followed by subsequent spontaneous seroconversion.

The many studies examining the effectiveness of interferon therapy for hepatitis B have led to the identification of clinical characteristics which predict positive response to treatment. These include: (a) high pretreatment ALT levels (>100 IU/ml), (b) detectable levels of HBeAg in serum, (c) low serum levels of HBV DNA (<200 pg/ml), (d) short duration of infection and acquisition of infection in adulthood, and (e) evidence of active hepatitis on liver biopsy [39]. It is important to note that the majority of patients infected with HBV worldwide are not described by these characteristics. Interferon is generally ineffective in the treatment of patients who are immunosuppressed, and Asian patients, who typically have normal serum transaminase levels, also tend not to respond to interferon therapy [40]. The ineffectiveness of interferon treatment for the majority of patients has fueled the search for alternative treatment strategies, and that search has borne fruit with the application of nucleoside analogs to the treatment of HBV infection.

Nucleoside Analogs

As described earlier in this chapter, the replication of the hepatitis B viral genome is accomplished by the HBV polymerase, which possesses both reverse transcriptase activity as well as DNA-dependent DNA polymerase activity. Recognition of this enzyme and the lack of comparable host cellular enzymes led to the targeting of the HBV polymerase for pharmacologic intervention. The identification of an obligate reverse transcription step in the HBV life cycle suggested that the reverse transcriptase inhibitors which were being developed for use against HIV may have comparable efficacy *versus* hepatitis B [41]. Despite demonstrated efficacy of many of these agents *in vitro*, most of these agents have hepatic metabolism which limits their practical utility as anti-HBV agents [42]. The HIV reverse transcriptase inhibitor with good *in vivo* activity against HBV is β-L-2', 3'-dideoxy-3'-thiacytidine, better known as lamivudine or 3TC.

Another potential source of candidate anti-hepatitis B pharmaceuticals was identified in the group of acyclic deoxyguanosine analogs which were originally developed to treat herpesvirus infections [43, 44]. These drugs include acyclovir, ganciclovir, and penciclovir (whose oral form is famciclovir), and they were known to have activity against the DNA-dependent DNA polymerases of the herpesviruses [45]. These three compounds are quite structurally similar. However they possess differing mechanisms of action for inhibition of the HBV polymerase. Furthermore, these agents demonstrate markedly different activities for the inhibition of hepatitis B replication [46, 47]. Of this group of compounds, famciclovir has shown promise in the treatment of chronic HBV infection.

Lamivudine

Lamivudine belongs to the family of nucleoside inhibitors which possess of the "unnatural" L-enantiomeric structure. The orally administered compound is an inactive prodrug that gains functionality once it is converted into its triphosphorylated form. It has been shown in multiple *in vitro* studies that the activated drug is a potent inhibitor of the HBV reverse transcriptase functionality [48, 49]. Lamivudine 5'-triphosphate is a competitive inhibitor of dCTP incorporation into viral DNA, and its incorporation results in chain termination of the elongating nucleic acid strand [50]. Fortunately, it has also been shown that lamivudine 5'-triphosphate is a poor substrate for both nuclear and mitochondrial DNA polymerases, thus at least partially explaining its low toxicity profile. Early clinical trials showed that 4-12 week courses of orally administered 3TC were well tolerated, and treatment resulted in a rapid and pronounced inhibition of HBV replication [51, 52]. However, these studies also showed that the response was transient, and almost all patients had recurrence of detectable serum HBV DNA after cessation of treatment. Fewer than 10% of treated patients underwent HBeAg seroconversion.

Studies of the kinetics of hepatitis B viral clearance during treatment with lamivudine predicted that prolonged treatment of 1-5 years duration would be required in order to reliably clear infection [53]. However, it is known from *in vivo* experience with HIV as well as HBV that prolonged use of 3TC can lead to development of viral mutations conferring resistance to this agent [54]. The hepatitis B virus has a high rate of viral turnover and its polymerase is error prone, (particularly the reverse transcriptase functionality. Therefore acquisition of resistance mutations would be predicted [53]. The most common mutation leading to lamivudine resistance is a specific point mutation in the conserved YMDD motif of the HBV polymerase in which a methionine residue is changed to a valine or isoleucine [55]. The identical mutation has also been identified in the YMDD motif of the HIV reverse transcriptase enzyme, and it confers 3TC resistance to that virus as well. The emergence of the YMDD mutants in the context of lamivudine therapy results in diminished therapeutic effect [56]. However the HBV DNA and transaminase levels are typically lower in the presence of the mutant virus when compared with wild type infection, suggesting reduced replication of the YMDD variant [57].

A number of trials examining extended duration lamivudine therapy have been undertaken. Two placebo controlled trials of one year of continuous lamivudine administration to patients with chronic hepatitis B demonstrated substantial benefit [58, 59]. These studies demonstrated that treatment with lamivudine, when compared with untreated controls, resulted in total suppression of HBV DNA, normalization of ALT values, improved necroinflammatory scores and decreased rates of hepatic fibrosis. The histologic improvements occurred even in the absence of HBe seroconversion, a marked contrast from the case with interferon therapy. Fortuitously, these studies also demonstrated an HBeAg loss of approximately 32%, which was very similar to the rate observed with interferon treatment. Finally, these trials demonstrated similar effects of lamivudine treatment in both U.S. and Asian populations, unlike the situation with interferon in which the beneficial effects seemed mostly confined to non-Asian patients [40]. The beneficial results demonstrated in these studies came at the price of the expected induction of resistant mutant virus. The rate of development of the YMDD mutation was between 14-32% of patients treated for one year in these two studies. Even in the absence of the YMDD mutation, those patients who did not undergo HBeAg seroconversion had recrudescence of viremia once lamivudine was discontinued. It is important to note, that all patients treated with 3TC had suppression of serum HBV DNA below the level of detection by hybridization assays prior to either the development of resistance or the withdrawal of drug. This suggests that continued therapy beyond one year would continue to result in viral suppression and which may in turn increase the number of patients who eventually undergo full seroconversion. However, extension of the duration of therapy would also be expected to lead to the increased development of resistance. One small study which looked at prolonging duration of treatment to 18 months confirmed these hypotheses [60]. They found that after 18 months of treatment, 9 of 24 patients (38%) underwent HBeAg seroconversion, and this conversion was durable after withdrawal of therapy. Approximately 13% of patients in this study developed lamivudine resistance due to the YMDD mutation. Larger studies looking at such prolonged treatment regimens are currently in progress.

Famciclovir

As previously mentioned, research on anti-herpesvirus agents led to the recognition of a purine nucleoside analogue called penciclovir. This agent is a highly selective antiviral compound with clear activity *versus* herpesviruses [61]. Subsequent work *in vitro* and *in vivo* demonstrated that penciclovir and its oral formulation, famciclovir, had potent anti-hepadnavirus activity in the duck hepatitis B model (DHBV) [62, 63]. Penciclovir is a prodrug which must be phosphorylated intracellularly in order to assume its active form. In herpes viruses, the virus encodes the kinase responsible for this phosphorylation. Hepadnaviruses encode no comparable kinase, yet the prodrug nevertheless becomes triphosphorylated, likely through the activity of a host cellular kinase. Study of the interaction between penciclovir triphosphate and the HBV polymerase revealed a mechanism of viral inhibition distinct from that observed with lamivudine. Whereas lamivudine competes for integration into the reverse transcribed DNA strand with resultant chain termination, penciclovir is not a candidate for incorporation into the viral nucleic acid at that stage of replication. Instead, penciclovir acts by inhibiting the priming step of the reverse transcription process. This step is normally accomplished by the polymerase enzyme itself, so this compound essentially competes against the enzyme to block its function [64]. PCV also inhibits the activity of the DNA-dependent DNA polymerase activity of the HBV polymerase, much in the same way it does in the inhibition of herpesviruses [47]. However, the true contribution of this activity to famciclovir's anti-HBV properties is uncertain.

Clinical experience with famciclovir has demonstrated that this medication can effectively reduce serum HBV DNA levels in patients with chronic hepatitis B as well as those who are status post liver transplantation [65-67], however overall clinical efficacy of this agent is probably less than that of lamivudine. The benefit of famciclovir treatment was demonstrated in one large, multicenter placebo-controlled trial examining a 16 week course of famciclovir [68]. In this study, famciclovir was found to have a dose-dependent antiviral effect, with decreased serum ALT levels, decreased serum HBV DNA levels, and a small but significant increase in HBeAg seroconversion. However, as is the case with 3TC, ongoing treatment is associated with the emergence of mutant virus resistant to penciclovir inhibition, while withdrawal of drug after a short course of treatment is associated with rapid replicative recurrence. The mutations of the HBV polymerase which result in resistance to penciclovir do not occur in the YMDD motif. Given the fact that PCV inhibits the polymerase via a distinct mechanism from 3TC, it is unsurprising that the emergence of resistant mutants would develop in differing areas of the polymerase as well. There are a number of mutations associated with resistance to famciclovir. Most of them are clustered in the B domain region of the HBV polymerase (as opposed to the C domain which contains the YMDD motif) [69], but there are other resistance mutations scattered throughout the polymerase/reverse transcriptase domain of the viral genome [70-72]. There are some famciclovir associated variants which demonstrate mutations in the C domain, conferring cross resistance to both famciclovir and lamivudine.

It appears to be unlikely that either famciclovir or lamivudine monotherapy will be successful in eradication of HBV infection in the majority of chronically infected patients. The paradigm of combination therapy for enhancement of drug efficacy and prevention of resistance has been used for decades in cancer chemotherapy, and it has been validated in the treatment of HIV over the last 5-10 years. In HIV, it has been clearly demonstrated that combination therapy with multiple reverse-transcriptase inhibitors and protease inhibitors leads to a marked increase in CD4+ cell counts and a substantial diminution of HIV RNA levels when compared with monotherapy involving only one of these agents [73, 74]. Furthermore, in the HIV model, it has been shown that combination therapy can prevent the development of viral resistance to the constituent drugs, and in some cases complementary resistance patterns have been observed in which the mutation conferring viral resistance to one medication enhances viral susceptibility to another drug in the combination [75]. A recent *in vitro* study demonstrated synergistic activity of lamivudine and famciclovir in the DHBV model [75], and clinical trials of combination therapies are currently underway.

Adefovir

Adefovir dipivoxil is the oral prodrug of an acyclic nucleotide monophosphate analog, (9-(2-phosphonylmethoxyethyl)-adenine (PMEA). The active drug is a selective inhibitor of numerous species of viral nucleic acid polymerases and reverse transcriptases. It has been shown to have broad-spectrum antiviral activity against retroviruses, hepadnaviruses, and herpesviruses [76]. Orally administered adefovir dipivoxil exhibits an inhibitory effect on both the HIV and HBV reverse transcriptases. Importantly, it appears that adefovir is capable of inhibiting the enzymatic activity of both wild type and YMDD mutant variants of both of these viruses [77].

Studies of this medication for treatment of HIV infection include induction of renal insufficiency as well as frequent development of hypophospatemia. However, doses being examined for use in HBV infection are significantly lower than those used in the HIV studies. Phase II clinical trials of adefovir for use against hepatitis B demonstrated a dose dependent antiviral effect associated with an increased rate of HBe seroconversion when compared with placebo controls [78]. In one study of 15 HBV patients, 12 weeks of treatment with 30 mg of adefovir daily was associated with a 4.1 log reduction in serum HBV DNA [79]. *In vitro* studies have demonstrated synergistic inhibitory activity of adefovir and lamivudine or famciclovir against duck HBV, and it has further been shown that adefovir retains activity against various HBV strains which have acquired both lamivudine or famciclovir resistance [80].

Clearly, further large-scale clinical trials are necessary before the safety and efficacy of adefovir are clearly established in the treatment of hepatitis B infected humans.

However, this does appear to be a promising therapeutic with novel, non-overlapping resistance characteristics when compared with agents already in use against this infection. The safe and effective dose of adefovir appears to be 10 mg po q day.

Introduction and History of Hepatitis C

As was already described, the appreciation of a transmissible agent or agents responsible for hepatitis was first recognized in the mid-19th century. The routine application of blood and blood product transfusions in the mid-20th century led to the recognition of the syndrome of transfusion-associated hepatitis. With the identification of the etiologic agents responsible for hepatitis A and hepatitis B infections in the 1960s and 1970s, as well as specific diagnostic tests to detect their presence, it became clear that neither one of these viruses was responsible for the vast majority of cases of transfusion-associated hepatitis. This led to the eventual designation of this pathologic entity as non-A, non-B hepatitis (NANBH) [81]. There have been numerous prospective studies of transfusion-associated hepatitis [82, 83], and these were important in initially defining the natural history of this illness. It became clear from analysis of these studies that NANBH was responsible for most cases of transfusion-associated hepatitis and that this infection was the most common complication of transfusion therapy. Importantly, these studies also demonstrated that acquisition of NANBH was frequently associated with the development of chronic hepatitis.

Initially, NANB hepatitis was defined as a clinical entity, and it was characterized more as an exclusionary diagnosis (i.e. clinical criteria of hepatitis without serologic evidence of HAV, HBV, or other known causes of acute hepatitis) rather than a clear individual pathologic entity. Shortly after recognition of this entity, numerous putative indirect diagnostic tests were proposed [84]. However none of them were sufficiently reproducible nor reliable to be introduced as actual markers of NANB hepatitis. An animal model for NANB hepatitis was identified through the inoculation of chimpanzees with serum of patients who had NANBH [84, 85]. This model allowed researchers to define more clearly the natural history of acute NANBH as well as its propensity for chronicity in some and resolution in others. Obviously, a transmissible agent caused this illness, and it was widely presumed that the agent was a virus. However, proving this hypothesis was beyond the reach of classic virologic methodology available at the time. Various studies were able to demonstrate infectivity/inactivation characteristics of the agent [86, 87]. However virus-like particles were not observed in electron microscopic studies looking at both liver tissue and blood from affected subjects. Serial filtration studies were able to determine that the agent was between 30-60 nm in diameter and this finding supported the characterization of the agent as a virus and suggested possible structures based upon presumed homology with known viruses of comparable size [88]. The virus which was eventually named hepatitis C was finally identified through the application of molecular biologic techniques [89]. In this experiment, the researchers collected liters of pooled serum from a chimpanzee with NANB hepatitis and extracted total RNA from serum. The RNA was then reverse transcribed into cDNA and the resultant nucleic acids were transfected into an expression vector. Enormous numbers of colonies of the expression vector were screened with antisera from a patient with chronic NANB hepatitis, and this led to the identification of a single clone expressing viral specific immunoreactive proteins. This clone was amplified and sequenced, and it was shown to be a previously undescribed viral genome. This monumental achievement represented the first time that a virus was identified primarily by molecular means, before visualization by electron microscopy or expression in culture.

Epidemiology and Natural History of Hepatitis C

In the United States, HCV infection is the most common blood borne infection. It is estimated that 3.9 million persons in the U.S., or 1.8% of the total population, has been infected with hepatitis C at some point in time [90]. Of this group, approximately 2.7 million persons remain chronically infected with HCV. During the 1980s, prior to the recognition of hepatitis C as the cause of NANB hepatitis, the incidence of new infections was approximately 230,000 per year [91]. This has been demonstrated by retrospective analysis of serum samples collected during that period from patients with NANBH [92]. In the period from 1989-1997, the incidence of acute infection has plummeted. Presently, it is estimated that there are approximately 38,000 new cases of HCV infection in the U.S. per year [93]. One explanation for the marked decline in incident infection is changes in the practice of blood banking during that period, initially with indirect screening of donors (i.e. exclusion of donors with high risk behaviors, exclusion of samples with elevated transaminase values), and eventually with direct screening of donated blood for specific HCV antibodies [94]. Despite the virtual elimination of HCV risk from blood transfusion, other risk factors for acquisition of HCV infection persist, such as intravenous drug use, application of tattoos with unsterile needles, occupational exposure, and incarceration.

Currently, there are between 8,000-10,000 deaths annually in the United States which are due to HCV-associated liver disease. However, the majority of currently infected persons are between the ages of 30 and 49 years old. As this population ages, a fraction of them will be expected to develop severe complications from their infection. Because of the size of this group, even if only the expected 20% of them develop severe hepatic disease, the total number of persons dying from this disease or requiring liver transplantation is likely to rise substantially over the next 10-20 years.

The natural history of infection with hepatitis C is highly variable. It has been observed that only between 15-20% of persons who are infected with HCV will spontaneously clear the virus after acute infection. In the remaining large majority, a state of chronic infection develops. This chronic infection is characterized by the presence of continuous viral replication despite the typical presence of a vigorous humoral and cellular immune response directed against many specific viral antigens [95]. There is substantial controversy over the pathologic and pathophysiologic correlates of this chronically infected state. Some patients have persistent viremia without any histologic or symptomatic sequelae, some have chronically elevated transaminases without appreciable progression of fibrosis over time, and still others have progressive fibrosis with eventual development of cirrhosis and/or hepatocellular carcinoma. Even among patients who develop progressive fibrosis, there appears to be substantial heterogeneity in rate of fibrosis progression and development of disease [96]. In the study by Poynard, three distinct groups of patients were identified: rapid, intermediate, and slow fibrosers. In patients described as rapid fibrosers, the median time from infection to development of cirrhosis was less than 20 years while those in the slow fibroser group will not develop cirrhosis for at least 50 years. A major deficiency of these data is the fact that in most patients, time of infection could not be accurately identified, and therefore statements about duration of disease are only estimates. No validated model for estimation of time of infection has been proposed, therefore this limitation continues to make interpretation of most natural history data problematic. In Poynard's study, a number of risk factors that predicted fibrosis progression were identified. These included older age, male sex, and alcohol consumption. There have been a number of other studies which have identified variables which may have prognostic value for fibrosis progression in HCV infection, and these have included sex, host immune status, duration of infection, route of transmission, volume of infecting dose, and viral genotype [97-99]. However, substantial controversy persists about the applicability of these putative prognostic variables in the general population of infected patients.

One ongoing study circumvents the aforementioned difficulty regarding the timing of infection. This study from Ireland involves the occurrence of HCV infection in a group of young women who received HCV-tainted anti-D immune globulin to prevent Rh isoimmunization in childbirth from 1977-1978 [100]. In this group whose duration of infection was known to be approximately 17 years, mild fibrosis was apparent on liver biopsy in 51% of them while cirrhosis was present in 2%, and inflammation was present in 98% of the biopsies. This study also showed that 81% of the infected women reported symptoms attributable to HCV including fatigue, myalgias, and arthralgias.

The clinical significance of progressive fibrosis appears to rest on the fact that progressive fibrosis can eventually lead to cirrhosis and patients with HCV-related cirrhosis demonstrate a substantial excess mortality over the general population [101]. A study by Niederau showed that the overall liver-related morbidity and mortality in a large cohort of HCV infected patients was a reasonably low 7.3%. However mortality was increased fourfold in all patients and 20-fold increased in cirrhotic patients under the age of 50.

Virology of Hepatitis C

Hepatitis C is a member of the Flaviviridae family, which includes the flaviviruses and pestiviruses. The genomic nucleic acid is comprised by a positive, single stranded RNA molecule of approximately 9,500 nucleotides [89]. There are at least 6 distinct genotypes of HCV which have been identified, and there are at least an order of magnitude greater number of subtypes.

The genomic RNA possesses 3' and 5' untranslated regions (UTR) which show little variability between different strains or genotypes. The 5' UTR appears to play an important role in interfacing the viral genomic RNA with host ribosomes, thus facilitating translation of viral peptides [102]. The function of the 3' UTR remains unclear. The translated region of the HCV genome consists of a single open reading frame (ORF) which encodes a large polypeptide of approximately 3,00 amino acids. The N-terminal portion of this translational product contains the HCV structural proteins: the core protein and the two envelope proteins, E1 and E2. The C-terminal portion of the polypeptide possesses the viral enzymes, including the proteases (NS2/3 and NS3), the helicase (NS3), and the RNA-dependent RNA polymerase (NS5B) [103, 104]. Cleavage of the structural proteins is accomplished by host cell peptidases, however the enzymatic portions of the polypeptide are post-translationally processed by the viral protease, and this step is actually an attractive potential site for pharmacologic intervention into the viral life cycle. However, at present, no such pharmaceutical agent exists.

The virus enters hepatocytes via an interaction between the viral envelope proteins and a presumed receptor on the cell surface, [105] which is believed to be CD81, although this has not been conclusively established. Once within the cell, the virus sheds its outer envelope, uncoating the nucleocapsid within. This exposure of the genomic RNA permits cellular ribosomal attachment to the 5' UTR leading to the initiation of viral polyprotein translation [106]. As it is formed, the 5' end of the viral polyprotein is directed into the cellular endoplasmic reticulum, and it is within this structure that host signal peptidases cleave the HCV structural proteins from the larger translational product [107]. Next, the nonstructural viral proteins are cleaved by a combination of cellular and viral enzymes, and the resultant products form the replication initiation complex [108]. The NS5B enzyme in the replication complex provides RNA-dependent RNA polymerase activity, and this results in the generation of negative-stranded RNA. The nascent negative-stranded RNA subsequently serves as the template for the NS5B catalyzed production of new positive RNA strands which can then be incorporated into nucleocapsids and eventually complete new virions.

As is the case with hepatitis B, HCV is not directly cytopathic to hepatocytes. Continuing the analogy to HBV, it appears that hepatocyte damage or destruction in patients with hepatitis C infection is due to host immune-mediated responses [109]. It is clear that in most immunocompetent patients with chronic hepatitis C infection, there is a polycolonal antigen-specific T cell response with vigorous CD4+ and CD8+ activity against a large variety of viral epitopes [110]. Cytotoxic T-cell mediated killing of infected hepatocytes is clearly a mechanism by which chronic hepatitis develops, with ongoing hepatic inflammation and eventual fibrosis. However, despite the development of a polyclonal T cell response, the efficacy of the attack is low, and spontaneous clearance of infection almost never occurs once chronic hepatitis develops [95, 111]. The humoral immune system is no less activated by the presence of HCV infection, but unfortunately it is also typically no more efficacious in preventing or eradicating infection than its cellular counterpart. [112-114]

Treatment of Hepatitis C Infection

Before beginning a discussion of how to treat chronic HCV infection, we must first address the question of if and when to treat a given patient. As discussed in some detail above, the natural history of this infection is quite variable, and there is a large subset of individuals who will never develop severe morbidity nor premature mortality due to their infection. Presently, clinical practitioners lack many tools with which to predict clinical outcomes accurately for any given patient with HCV, but what does appear clear is that advanced fibrosis/cirrhosis is a precondition for the development of substantial morbidity/mortality in most patients. Therefore, in order to predict the likelihood of benefit of treatment in a particular individual, one needs to first establish the degree of histologic damage that has already occurred and also make predictions about the probability of further progression. If the therapeutic interventions available for the treatment of hepatitis C were both completely effective and very well tolerated, these determinations would be unnecessary, because practitioners would be able to treat all patients with infection, rationally expecting to cure the majority of cases. In reality, presently available therapeutics have only limited efficacy and marked side effects associated with their use, and we must therefore select patients for treatment based upon their demonstration of predilection for histologic progression as well as their ability to tolerate the medicines. According to the 1997 NIH Consensus Conference, only those patients between the ages of 18-60 who have abnormal alanine aminotransferase levels, HCV RNA in serum, and evidence of chronic hepatitis on liver biopsy should be considered for therapy [115]. These recommendations are undergoing reconsideration. However they do underscore the importance of ascertaining liver histology prior to deciding on the implementation of specific therapy. Patients without evidence of fibrosis or significant inflammatory activity are at extremely low risk for the development of cirrhosis or serious hepatic complications, and they can reasonably defer therapy. Conversely, patients with advanced cirrhosis are poor candidates for current interferon-based treatment regimens because of the increased treatment associated morbidity seen in these patients and the possible precipitation of decompensation or frank hepatic failure.

Interferon α

Presently, the cornerstone of all treatment regimens for chronic hepatitis C involves the administration of interferon α. Interestingly, the use of interferon for the treatment of HCV-related disease predates the discovery of HCV itself, and it had been advocated as intervention in the management of NANB hepatitis [116]. Subsequent virologic assays of serum from interferon treated NANBH patients demonstrated that therapy usually led to rapid decreases in serum HCV RNA[117], which in turn led to long term clearance of virus in a small subset of patients [118]. Controlled trials of interferon alpha treatment for chronic hepatitis C demonstrated that 6 months of treatment with 3 million units three times per week led to decreases in serum ALT in the majority of patients and normalized liver function tests in 40-50% of those treated [119-121]. Disappointingly, once treatment was discontinued, at least 50% of patients who had responded with normalization of their transaminases had recurrent elevation of these serum enzymes. Therefore, the actual sustained response to a 6 month course of interferon monotherapy was estimated to be approximately 15%.

Recognition of these dismal response rates led investigators to examine a wide variety of methodologies for enhancing the response to interferon. Explored strategies included longer courses of therapy[122-124], higher doses of interferon[121, 125], and utilization of different formulations of interferon [126-128]. These studies found that increasing the duration of treatment and/or the dose of interferon did result in improved response rates, but they still saw durable remissions in less than one quarter of the treated patients. Also, patients tolerated the prolonged regimens or higher dosing schedules poorly. Furthermore, there did not appear to be a significant difference in efficacy or tolerability between different forms of interferon.

Ribavirin

Ribavirin is a purine nucleoside analog which has been used over the last 20-30 years in the treatment of a variety of viral infections. It has a broad spectrum of activity against numerous RNA and DNA viruses, but prior to its use for the treatment of HCV infection, the main clinical application of this drug was in the treatment of respiratory syncytial virus in children. Ribavirin is available in an oral formulation, and this is generally well tolerated. Minor side effects associated with its use include irritability, fatigue, upper respiratory symptoms, and pruritus. The major adverse effects of ribavirin therapy include a dose dependent hemolytic anemia, which is not severe in the majority of patients, and the possibility of teratogenicity, which has been observed in animal models.

A pilot study in 1991 suggested that oral ribavirin may have efficacy in the treatment of HCV infection [129], and subsequent clinical trials demonstrated that short courses of treatment were associated with improvement in serum transaminase values when administered to patients with chronic HCV. These findings were confirmed in placebo-controlled clinical trials. However administration of ribavirin as monotherapy did not result in any decrement in HCV RNA levels nor were investigators able to demonstrate any improvement in hepatic fibrosis after 12 months of treatment [130]. Furthermore, once therapy was discontinued serum transaminase levels quickly returned to the pretreatment values in all patients who had responded.

Treatment with ribavirin was clearly associated with decreased direct and indirect measures of hepatic necroinflammation without any appreciable modulation of viral replication or infectivity. This finding led to the hypothesis that ribavirin's potential benefit in the therapy of hepatitis C was as an immunomodulatory agent rather than as a specific antiviral. Although the attenuated immune response was clearly insufficient for resolution of infection, it led to the development of interest in utilizing ribavirin as a component of multi-drug therapy in the treatment of HCV.

Combination Therapy with Interferon and Ribavirin

In 1998, three reports were published on the results of blinded, placebo-controlled trials of hepatitis C treatment with combination therapy utilizing interferon and ribavirin [131-133]. These large, well-designed studies clearly demonstrated that treatment with a combination of interferon α (3 million IU three time per week) and ribavirin (1000-1200 mg daily) resulted in substantially increased rates of sustained viral clearance when compared against interferon therapy alone for the same duration of therapy. Sustained virologic response (SVR) was defined as the absence of detectable HCV RNA in the serum six months after the completion of therapy. This goal was reached in approximately 33% of those treated with interferon/ribavirin for 24 weeks and approximately 41% of those treated with combination therapy for 48 weeks, as compared with 6% and 16% respectively in the interferon monotherapy groups. When the results of these trials were stratified by the genotype of infecting virus (genotype 1 or non-1), even more striking outcomes were observed. 65% of patients with non-1 genotype infections had sustained response to therapy with both 24 and 48 week treatment durations, whereas those with genotype 1 infection had a 17% sustained response rate at 24 weeks of therapy with improvement to 30% sustained response after 48 weeks of therapy. These studies also demonstrated significant improvements in histologic inflammatory scores which correlated with virologic response to treatment.

Analysis of the data from these studies led to the recognition of five independent factors that predicted sustained virologic response to combination therapy. These factors included (1) infection with genotypes 2 or 3, (2) pre-treatment serum HCV RNA level of less than 3.5 million copies/mL, (3) age less than 40 years, (4) minimal evidence of fibrosis on liver biopsy, and (5) female sex [134]. Furthermore, it was shown that all patients who ultimately had sustained response to treatment had undetectable serum HCV RNA levels before 24 weeks into therapy. This led to the practice guideline that recommends rechecking HCV RNA at six months into therapy (for genotype 1 patients who require 12 months of treatment), and terminating further therapy at that time if HCV RNA is still detectable, because the probability of sustained virologic response is less than 2%. These guidelines further recommend that if a patient is negative for HCV RNA at 24 weeks into therapy, the decision to continue or terminate treatment should be based upon evaluation of the five independent risk factors. If a patient has four or more of the items pre-treatment, then they may terminate treatment at 24 weeks without decreasing likelihood of sustained response. On the other hand, if a patient had fewer than four of the characteristics, then the guidelines recommend continuing therapy to 48 weeks in order to maximize probability of achieving sustained virologic response. These recommendations are based upon reanalysis of the original combination therapy data and they have not yet been validated prospectively in clinical trials.

Pegylated Interferon

Although the advent of combination interferon/ribavirin therapy has led to significant improvement in our ability to clear serum HCV RNA and improve both biochemical and histologic evidence of chronic hepatitis, there are still a substantial proportion of patients with chronic infection who are not adequately treated with current strategies. A very active avenue of research in the last few years has been examining methodologies for enhancing the effectiveness of interferon-based treatments. The most promising of these explorations has been the development of pegylated interferon(PEG-IFN). This compound is formed through the attachment of polyethylene glycol, a large organic moiety, to an interferon molecule, thus changing the pharmacokinetic and pharmacodynamic properties of the drug.

PEG-IFN was thought to have advantages over conventional interferon α because of its different pharmacologic characteristics. Specifically, PEG-IFN has a more sustained blood level compared with standard IFN α regimens without the peaks observed with standard interferon, and it is thought that some of the typical interferon-related side effects are mediated by high peak levels. Therefore, PEG-IFN would be expected to be better tolerated than standard IFN α. Further enhancing tolerability and patient compliance, PEG-IFN only needs to be injected once weekly rather than thrice weekly. Finally, the trough levels of PEG-IFN are significantly higher than those observed for conventional IFN α, and it is thought that these sustained and higher trough levels may contribute to the increased efficacy of PEG-IFN by providing more constant antiviral pressure, thus minimizing opportunities for mutational escape.

Presently, there are two formulations of PEG-IFN in commercial development for use in HCV infected patients. These formulations differ in terms of size of the PEG moiety, molecular structure of the PEG moiety (straight *versus* branched), the means of attachment of the moiety to the interferon molecule, as well as the exact amino acid position in interferon to which the PEG molecule is attached. Specifically, the two formulations are a 12 kDalton PEG-IFNα2b with a linear PEG moiety (Schering-Plough) and a 40 kDalton PEG-IFNα2a with a branched PEG moiety (Roche). At the time of this writing, the 12kD PEG-IFNα2b has been approved for use as a monotherapeutic agent in Europe, and it the U.S.

One study comparing monotherapy with the 12 kD PEG-IFNα2b (1.0 µg/kg qweek) against standard IFN (3 million I.U. tiw) for 48 weeks demonstrated a statistically significant improvement in sustained virologic response for the PEG-IFN treated group. As had been typical in all previous interferon-based trials, the magnitude of the response rate was largest in those patients with genotype 2 or 3 infection who had a low viral load (<2 million copies/mL). However, a statistically significant improvement in SVR was seen in all genotype and viral load groups examined (Clinical Symposium, European Association for the Study of Liver Disease, 2000). An investigation comparing monotherapy with the 40kD PEG-IFNα2a (180 µg qweek) with standard IFN (6 then 3 million I.U. t.i.w.) for 48 weeks also showed an improved SVR rate for those treated with the PEG-IFN formulation.[136]

At present, there has been no head-to-head comparison trial looking at the two different PEG-IFN formulations. Based upon the work that has already been completed, it is reasonable to assert that both formulations more effective than conventional IFN monotherapy but less effective than interferon plus ribavirin combination therapy. However, until a true comparison is undertaken, it would be inappropriate to assume that either formulation has specific advantages over the other.

The efficacy of PEG-IFN monotherapy led naturally to the investigation of whether addition of ribavirin would augment its antiviral efficacy. One study compared various dosing regimens of the 12kD PEG-IFN with the same doses of PEG-IFN plus ribavirin. This study found a dose-response relationship for the PEG-IFN (up to 1.4 μg/kg in this case), and it further noted that for each dose of PEG-IFN, the SVR was increased significantly by the addition of ribavirin.[137] Another investigation compared treatment with 1.5 μg/kg of 12kD PEG-IFN plus ribavirin with standard combination therapy of interferon plus ribavirin. This study found a small but statistically significant improvement in SVR in the PEG-IFN ribavirin group. [138] A thought provoking sub-analysis of this study demonstrated the largest improvement in SVR was realized in patients with genotype 1 infection, a group that has typically been most recalcitrant to previously available therapies. Based upon the results of these recent trials, it seems clear that in the near future, the backbone of treatment for chronic hepatitis C is going to consist of some formulation of PEG-IFN plus one or more additional drugs. In the near term, it is highly probable that ribavirin will be the additional drug in clinical practice, however other adjunctive agents are being explored, including other IMPDH inhibitors (mycophenylate, VX 497) as well as other antiviral compounds such as amantidine.

Future Directions In The Treatment of HCV

There are a number of other putative strategies for combating hepatitis C infection which are still in the preclinical or phase I clinical arenas of development. These include construction of agents which directly target the HCV protease or HCV helicase. Specific targeting of viral protein processing enzymes has been an extraordinarily effective method for controlling HIV-related disease. Researchers hope that agents with efficacy similar to that of HIV protease inhibitors can be identified for HCV. Unfortunately, at the present time, no such compounds have been identified. Another avenue of attack which appears promising is the use of ribozymes to disrupt viral nucleic acid replication and translation. Ribozymes are RNA molecules that catalyze sequence-specific cleavage of RNA through the combination of a conserved catalytic site flanked by engineered antisense sequences that mediate site-specific binding to target RNA molecules. These constructs have been shown to cleave HCV RNA in hepatocyte cultures[135], however the ability to deliver effectively and consistently these agents to the intracellular milieu of infected cells has not been established. Phase I trials of this approach are underway.

Another approach to treatment of patients with HCV infection that is under investigation is the administration of antifibrotic agents. The presumption with such a course of treatment is to prevent the disruptive pathology rather than (or in addition to) directly combating the virus. Candidate compounds with antifibrotic activity include IL-10, possibly some other cytokines, as well as possibly some medications such as ursodeoxycholic acid. It should be emphasized that this is a putative, unproven method for treating HCV infected patients. There is also enthusiasm for the development of an anti-HCV vaccine that may be used either prophylactically or therapeutically.

Unfortunately, this enthusiasm is tempered by numerous technical obstacles including the absence of an animal model for HCV infection nor a good cell culture system as well as the high mutational rate of the virus' envelope proteins. These obstacles make the actual realization of such a vaccine unlikely any time in the foreseeable future.

References

1. Alexopoulou A, Karayiannis P, Hadziyannis, SJ, et al. Emergence and selection of HBV variants in an anti-HBe positive patient persistently infected with quasi-species. 1997; 26: 748-753.
2. Lurman A. Eine icterus Epidemic. Wochenschr 1855; 22: 20-23.
3. Neefe J, Gellis, SS, Stokes J. Homologous serum hepatitis and infectious (epidemic) hepatitis: studies in volunteers bearing on immunological and other characteristics of etiologic agents. Am J of Med 1946; 1: 3-22.
4. Seef L, Koff RS. Evolving concepts of the clinical and serologic consequences of hepatitis B infection. Semin Liver Dis 1986; 6: 11-22.
5. MacCallum FO, Bauer DJ. Homologous serum hepatitis. Lancet 1947; 691-692.
6. Blumberg BS, Alter HJ. A "new" antigen in leukemic serum. JAMA 1967; 191: 541-546.
7. Prince AM. An antigen detected in the blood of patients during the incubation of serum hepatitis. Proc Natl Acad Sci USA 1968; 60: 814-821.
8. Blumberg BS. Australia antigen and the biology of hepatitis B. Science 1977; 197: 17-25.
9. Dane DS, Cameron CH, Briggs M. Virus-like particles in serum of patnts with Australia antigen associated hepatitis. Lancet 1970; i: 695-698.
10. Maynard JE, Kane MA, Alter MJ, Hadler SC. Control of hepatitis B by immunization: global perspectives. New York, NY: Grune and Stratton Inc, 1988.
11. Hadler SC, Margolis HS. Epidemiology of hepatitis B virus infection. New York, NY: Marcel Dekker, Inc, 1993.
12. Sung JL. Hepatitis B eradication strategy for Asia. Vaccine 1990; 8 (suppl): 96-99.
13. Margolis H, Alter MJ, Hadler SC. Hepatitis B: evolving epidemiology and implications for control. Semin Liver Dis 1991; 11: 84-92.
14. Landers T, Greenberg HB, Robinson WS. Structure of hepatitis B Dane particle DNA and nature of the endogenous DNA polymerase reaction. J Virol 1977; 23: 368-376.
15. Hatton T, Zhou S, Standring DN. RNA and DNA binding activities in hepatitis B virus capsid protein: a model for their roles in viral replication. J Virol 1992; 66: 5232-5241.
16. Milich D, Jones JE, Hughes JL, et al. Is a function of the secreted hepatitis B e antigen to induce immunologic tolerance in utero? Proc Natl Acad Sci USA 1990; 87: 6599-6603.
17. Rossner M. Review: hepatitis B virus X-gene product: a promiscuous transcriptional activator. J Med Virol 1992; 36: 101-117.
18. Chisari F, Ferrari C. Hepatitis B virus immunopathology. Semin Immunopathol 1995; 17: 261-281.
19. Lee W. Hepatitis B Virus Infection. N Engl J Med 1997; 337: 1733-1743.
20. Wong J, Koff RS, Tine F, Pauker SG. Cost-effectiveness of interferon-alpha 2b treatment of hepatitis B e antigen-positive chronic hepatitis B. Ann Intern Med 1995; 122: 664-675.
21. Caselmann W, Eisenberg J, Hofschneider PH, et al. Beta and gamma interferon in chronic active hepatitis B: a pilot trial of short term combination therapy. Gastroenterology 1989; 96: 449-455.
22. Davis G, Hoofnagle JH, Waggoner J. Spontaneous reactivation of hepatitis B virus infection.

Gastroenterology 1986; 86: 230-235.

23. Villeneuve J-P, Desrochers M, Infante-Rivard C, et al. A long-term followup-up study of asymptomatic hepatitis B surface antigen-positive carriers in Montreal. Gastroenterology 1994; 106: 1000-1005.

24. Dejean A. Specific hepatitis B virus integration in hepatocellular carcinoma DNA through a viral 11-base pair direct repeat. Proc Natl Acad Sci USA 1996; 81: 5350-5358.

25. Chisari F, Klopchin K, Moriyama T, et al. Molecular pathogenesis of hepatocellular carcinoma in hepatitis B virus transgenic mice. Cell 1989; 59: 1145-1156.

26. Issacs A, Lindemann J. Virus interference. I. The interferon. Proc R Soc London (Biol) 1957; 147: 258-267.

27. Fujisawa K, Yamkazi K, Kawaze H, et al. Interferon therapy for chronic viral hepatitis and the use of peripheral lymphocytic 2'5'-oligoadenylate synthetase. In: Zuckerman A, ed. Viral Hepatitis and Liver Disease. New York: Alan R Liss, 1987: 834-839.

28. Greenberg H, Pollard RB, Lutwick LI, Gregory PB, Robinson WS, Merigan TC. Effect of human leukocyte interferon on hepatitis B virus infection in patients with chronic active hepatitis. N Engl J Med 1976; 295: 517-522.

29. Chisari F. Cytotoxic T cells and viral hepatitis. J Clin Invest 1997: 1472-1477.

30. Lok A, Chung H-T, Liu VWS, Ma OCK. Long-term follow-up of chronic hepatitis B patients treated with interferon alfa. Gastroenterology 1993; 105: 1833-1838.

31. Carreno V, Castillo I, Molina J, Porres JC, Bartolome J. Long-term follow-up of hepatitis B chronic carriers who responded to interferon therapy. J Hepatol 1992; 15: 102-106.

32. Korenman J, Baker B, Waggoner J, et al. Long term remissions of chronic hepatitis B after alpha interferon. Ann Intern Med 1991; 114: 629-634.

33. Alexander G, Brahm J, Fagan E, et al. Loss of HBsAg with interferon therapy for chronic HBV. Lancet 1987; ii: 66-69.

34. Anderson M, Harrison TJ, Alexander GJM, et al. Randomised controlled trial of lymphoblastoid interferon for chronic active hepatitis B. B J Hepatol 1986; 3(suppl): S225-S227.

35. Hoofnagle J, Peters M, Mullen KD, et al. Randomized controlled trial of a four month course of recombinant alpha interferon in patients with chronic type B hepatitis. Hepatology 1985; 5: 1033-1039.

36. Hoofnagle J, Peters M, Mullen KD, et al. Randomized controlled trial of recombinant human alpha-interferon in patients with chronic hepatitis B. Gastroenterology 1988; 95: 1318-1325.

37. Wong D, Cheung AM, O'Rourke K, Naylor CD, Detsky AS, Heathcote J. Effect of alpha-interferon treatment in patients with hepatitis B e antigen-positiive chronic hepatitis B: a meta-analysis. Ann Intern Med 1993; 119: 312-323.

38. Niederau C, Heintges T, Lange S, et al. Long-term follow-up of HBeAg-positive patients treated with interferon alfa for chronic hepatitis B. N Engl J Med 1996; 334: 1422-1427.

39. Hoofnagle J, DiBisceglie AM. The treatment of chronic viral hepatitis. N Engl J Med 1997; 336: 347-356.

40. Perrillo R. Factors influencing response to interferon in chronic hepatitis B: implications for Asian and western populations. Hepatology 1990; 12: 1433-1435.

41. Summers J, Mason WS. Replication of the genome of a hepatitis B-like virus by reverse transcription of an RNA intermediate. Cell 1982; 29: 403-415.

42. Shaw T, Locarnini S. Hepatic purine and pyrimidine metabolism: Implications for chemotherapy in viral hepatitis. Liver 1995; 15: 169-184.

43. Shaw T, Locarnini S. Hepatic purine and pyrimidine metabolism. Implications for chemotherapy in viral hepatitis. Liver 1995; 15: 169-184.

44. Sommadossi J-P. Treatment of hepatitis B by nucleoside analogs: still a reality. Curr Opin Infect Dis 1994; 7: 678-682.

45. Martin J, Brown CE, Matthews-Davis N, Reardon JE. Effects of antiviral nucleoside analogs on human DNA polymerases and mitochondrial DNA synthesis. Antimicrob Agents Chemother 1994; 38: 2743-2749.

46. Korba B, Boyd MR. Penciclovir is a selective inhibitor of hepatitis B virus replication in cultured human hepatoblastoma cells. Antimicrob Agents Chemother 1996; 40: 1282-1284.

47. Shaw T, Mok SS, Locarnini SA. Inhibition of hepatitis B virus DNA polymerase by enantiomers of penciclovir triphosphate and metabolic basis for selective inhibition of HBV replication by penciclovir. Hepatology 1996; 24: 996-1002.

48. Zoulim F, Dannaoui E, Borel C, Hantz O, LIn T-S, Liu S-H, et al. 2', 3'-dideoxy-b-L-5-fluorocytidine inhibits duck hepatitis B virus reverse transcription and suppresses viral DNA synthesis in hepatocytes, both *in vitro* and *in vivo*. Antimicorb Agents Chemother 1996; 40: 448-453.

49. Doong S, Tsai CH, Schinazi RF, Liotta DC, Cheng YC. Inhibition of the replication of hepatitis B virus *in vitro* by 2', 3'-dideoxy-3'thiacytidine and related analogues. Proc Natl Acad Sci USA 1991; 88: 8495-8499.

50. Severini A, Liu XY, Wilson JS, Tyrrell LJ. Mechanism of inhibition of duck hepatitis B virus polymerase by 2', 3'-dideoxy-3'-thiacytidine. Antimicrob Agents Chemother 1995; 39: 1430-1435.

51. Dienstag J, Perillo R, Schiff E, Bartholomew M, Vicary C, Rubin M. A preliminary trial of lamivudine for chronic hepatitis B infection N Engl J Med 1995; 333: 1657-1661.

52. Lai C, Ching CK, Tung ANM, Li E, Young J, et al. Lamivudine is effective in suppressing hepatitis B virus DNA in Chinese hepatitis B surface antigen carriers: a placebo-controlled trial. Hepatology 1997; 25: 241-244.

53. Nowak M, Bonhoeffer S, Hill A, Boehme R, et al. Viral dynamics in hepatitis B virus infection. Proc Natl Acad Sci USA 1996; 93: 4398-4402.

54. Zoulim F, Trepo C. Drug therapy for chronic hepatitis B: antiviral efficacy and the influence of hepatitis B virus polymerase mutations on the outcome of therapy. J Hepatol 1998; 29: 151-168.

55. Ling R, Mutimer D, Ahmed M, et al. Selection of mutations in the hepatitis B virus polymerase during therapy of transplant recipients with lamivudine. Hepatology 1996; 24: 711-713.

56. Chayama K, Suzuki Y, Kobayashi M, et al. Emergence and takeover of YMDD motif mutant hepatitis B virus during long-term lamivudine therapy and re-takeover by wild type after cessation of therapy. Hepatology 1998; 27: 1711-1716.

57. Allen M, Deslauriers M, Andrews CW, et al. Identification and characterization of mutations in hepatitis B virus resistant to lamivudine. Hepatology 1998; 27: 1670-1677.

58. Dienstag J, Schiff ER, Wright TL, Perrillo RP, et al. Lamivudine as initial treatment for chronic hepatitis B in the United States. N Engl J Med 1999; 341: 1256-1263.

59. Lai C-L, Chien R-N, Leung NWY, Chang T-T, Guan R, et al. A one year trial of lamivudine for chronic hepatitis B. N Engl J Med 1998; 339: 61-68.

60. Dienstag J, Schiff ER, Mitchell M, Casey DE, Gitlin N, et al. Extended lamivudine retreatment for chronic hepatitis B: Maintenance of viral suppression after discontinuation of therapy. Hepatology 1999; 30: 1082-1087.

61. Boyd M, Bacon T, Sutton D, Cole M. Antiherpesvirus activity of 9-(4-hydroxy-3-hydroxy-methylbut-1-yl)guanine (BRL 39123) in cell culture. Antimicrob Agents Chemother 1987; 31: 1238-1242.

62. Shaw T, Amor P, Civitico G, Boyd M, Locarnini S. *In vitro* antiviral activity of penciclovir, a novel purine nucleoside against duck hepatitis B virus. Antimicrob Agents Chemother 1994; 38: 719-723.

63. Tsiquaye K, Sutton D, Maung M, Boyd M. Antiviral activities and pharmacokinietics of penciclovir and famciclovir in Pekin ducks chronically infected with duck hepatitis B virus. Antiviral Chem Chemother 1996; 7: 153-159.

64. Zoulim F, Dannaoui E, Trepo C. Inhibitory effect of penciclovir on the priming of hepadnavirus reverse transcription, 35th Interscience conference on antimicorbial agents and chemotherapy, Washington, D.C., 1995. American Society Microbiology.

65. Lai C, Yuen MF, Cheng CC, Wong WM, et al. An open comparative study of lamivudine and famciclovir in the treatment of chronic hepatitis B infection (Abstract). Hepatology 1998; 28(suppl): 318A.

66. Main J, Brown JL, Howells C, Glassini R, et al. A double blind, placebo-controlled study to assess the effect of famciclovir on virus replication in patients with chronic hepatitis B: results of a dose finding study (Abstract). J Viral Hepat 1996; 3: 211-215.

67. Rayes N, Seehofer D, Bechstein WO, Muller AR, et al. Long-term results of famciclovir for recurrent or de novo hepatitis B virus infection after liver transplantation. Clin Transplantation 1999; 13: 447-452.

68. Trepo C, Jezek P, Atkinson G, Boon R. Efficacy of famciclovir in chronic hepatitis B: results of a dose finding study. Hepatology 1996; 24: 188A.

69. Tillmann H, Trautwein C, Bock T, Boker KH, Jackel E, et al. Mutational pattern of hepatitis B virus on sequential therapy with famciclovir and lamivudine in patients with hepatitis B virus reinfection occurring under HBIg immunoglobulin after liver transplantation. Hepatology 1999; 30: 244-256.

70. Xiong X, Yang H, Westland CE, Zou R, Gibbs CS. *In vitro* evaluation of hepatitis B virus polymerase mutations associated with famciclovir resistance. Hepatology 2000; 31.

71. Aye T, Bartholomeusz A, Shaw T, Bowden S, et al. Hepatitis B virus polymerase mutations during antiviral therapy in a patient following liver transplantation. J Hepatol 1997; 26: 1148-1153.

72. Bartholomeusz A, Locarnini S. Mutations in the hepatitis B virus polymerase gene that are associated with resistance to famciclovir and lamivudine3. Internatl Antiviral News 1997; 5: 123-124.

73. Corey L, Holmes KK. Therapy for the human immunodeficiency virus infection - what have we learned? N Engl J Med 1996; 335: 1142-1144.

74. Richman D. Consensus symposium on combined antiviral therapy. Antiviral Res 1995; 29: 5-29.

75. Larden B, Kemp SD, Harrigan PR. Potential mechanism for sustained antiretroviral efficacy of AZT-3TC combination therapy. Science 1995; 269: 696-699.

76. De Clercq E. Antiviral activity spectrum and target of action of different classes of nucleoside analogues. Nucleosides Nucleotides 1994: 1271-1295.

77. Xiong X, Flores C, Yang H, Toole JJ, et al. Mutations in hepatitis B DNA polymerase associated with resistance to lamivudine do not confer resistance to adefovir *in vitro*. Hepatology 1998; 28: 1669-1673.

78. Heathcote E, Jeffers L, Wright T, Sherman M, et al. Loss of serum HBV DNA and HBeAg and seroconversion following short-term (12 week) adefovir dipivoxil therapy in chronic hepatitis B: two placebo controlled phase II studies (Abstr). Hepatology 1998; 38: 317A.

79. Jeffers L, Heathcote E, Wright T, et al. A phase II dose-ranging, placebo-controlled trial of adefovir dipivoxil for the treatment of chronic hepatitis B virus infection [Abstract]. Antiviral Res 1998; 37: A197.

80. Shaw T, Colledge D, Locarnini SA. Synergistic inhibition of *in vitro* hepadnaviral replication by PMEA and penciclovir or lamivudine [Abstract]. Antiviral Res 1997; 34: A33.

81. Feinstone SK AZ, Purcell RH, Alter HJ, Holland PV. Transfusion-associated hepatitis not due to viral hepatitis type A or B. N Engl J Med 1975; 292: 767-770.

82. Alter H. Chronic consequences of non-A, non-B hepatitis. In: Seeff L, Lewis JH, ed. Current Prospective

in Hepatology. New York: Plenum Publsihing, 1989.

83. Seeff L, Wright EC, Zimmerman HJ, et al. Post-transfusion hepatitis, 1973-1975: a Veterans Administration cooperative study. In: Vyas G, Cohen SN, Schmid R, ed. Viral Hepatitis. Philadelphia: Franklin Institute Press, 1978.

84. Dienstag J. Non-A, non-B hepatitis. II. Experimental transmission, putative virus agents and markers, and prevention. Gastroenterology 1983; 85: 743-768.

85. Tabor E. Development and application of the chimpanzee animal model for human non-A, non-B hepatitis. In: Gerety R, ed. Non-A, Non-B Hepatitis. New York: Academic Press, 1981.

86. Purcell R, Gerin JL, Popper H, et al. Hepatitis B virus, hepatitis non-A, non-B virus and hepatitis delta virus in lyophilized antihemophilic factor: relative sensitivity to heat. Hepatology 1985; 5: 1091-1099.

87. Tabor E, Gerety RJ. Inactivation of an agent of human non-A, non-B hepatitis by formalin. J Infect Dis 1980; 142: 677-678.

88. He L, Alling D, Popkin T, et al. Non-A, non-B hepatitis virus: determination of size by filtration. J Infect Dis 1987; 156: 636-640.

89. Choo Q, Kuo G, Weiner AJ, et al. Isolation of a cDNA clone derived from a blood-borne non-A, non-B hepatitis genome. Science 1989; 244: 359-362.

90. Alter M, Kruszon-Moran D, Nainan OV, McQuillan GM, et al. The prevalence of hepatitis C virus infection in the United STates, 1988 through 1994. N Engl J Med 1999; 341: 556-562.

91. Prevention CfDCa. Recommendations for prevention and control of hepatitis C (HCV) infection and HCV-related chronic disease. MMWR 1998; 47: 1-38.

92. Alter M. Epidemiology of hepatitis C in the West. Semin Liver Dis 1995; 15: 5-14.

93. Williams I. Epidemiology of hepatitis C in the United States. Am J Med 1999; 107: 3S-9S.

94. Donahue J, Munoz A, Ness PM, et al. The declining risk of post-transfusion hepatitis C virus infection. N Engl J Med 1992; 327: 369-73.

95. Cerny A, Chisary FV. Immunological aspects of HCV infection. Intervirology 1994; 37: 119-125.

96. Poynard T, Bedossa P, Opolon P. Natural history of liver fibrosis progression in patients with chronic hepatitis C. Lancet 1997; 349: 825-832.

97. Tong M, El-Farra NS, Reikes AR, Co RL. Clinical outcomes after transfusion-associated hepatitis C. N Engl J Med 1995; 332: 1463-1466.

98. Schiff R. Transmission of viral infections through intravenous immune globulin. N Engl J Med 1994; 331: 1649-1650.

99. Tremolada F, Casarin C, Alberti A, et al. Long-term follow-up of non-A, non-B (type C) post-transfusion hepatitis. J Hepatol 1992; 16: 273-281.

100. Kenny-Walsh E. Clinical outcomes after hepatitis C infection from contaminated anti-D immune globulin. N Engl J Med 1999; 340: 1228-1233.

101. Niederau C, Lange S, Heintges T, Erhardt A, Buschkamp M, et al. Prognosis of chronic hepatitis C: results of a large prospective cohort study. Hepatology 1998; 28: 1687-1695.

102. Tsukiyama-Kohara K, Iiauka N, Kohara M, et al. Interanl ribosome entry site within hepatitis C virus RNA. J Virol 1992; 66: 1476-1483.

103. Choo Q-L, Richman KH, Han J, et al. Genetic organization and diversity of the hepatitis C virus. Proc Natl Acad Sci USA 1991; 88: 2451-2455.

104. Takamizawa A, Mori C, Fuke I, et al. Structure and organization of the hepatitis C virus genome isolated from human carriers. J Virol 1991; 1991: 1105-1113.

105. Pileri P, Uematsu Y, Campagnoli S, Galli G, et al. Binding of hepatitis C virus to CD81. Science

1998; 282: 938-941.

106. Honda M, Ping LH, Rijnbrand RC, et al. Structural requirements for initiation of translation by internal ribosome entry withing genome-length hepatitis C virus RNA. Virology 1996; 222: 31-42.

107. Lo S, Masiarz F, Hwang SB, Lai MM, et al. Differential subcellular localization of hepatitis C virus core gene products. Virology 1995; 213: 455-461.

108. Grakoui A, McCourt DW, Wychowski C, et al. Characterization of the hepatitis C virus-encoded serine proteinase: determination of proteinase-dependent polyprotein cleavage sites. J Virol 1993; 67: 2832-2843.

109. Gonzalez-Peralta R, Davis GL, Lau JY. Pathogenetic mechanisms of hepatocellular damage in chronic hepatitis C virus infection. J Hepatol 1994; 21: 255-259.

110. Rice C, Walker CM. Hepatitis C virus-specific T lymphocyte responses. Curr Opin Immunol 1995; 7: 532-538.

111. Cooper S, ERickson AL, Adams EJ, et al. Analysis of a successful immune response against hepatitis C virus. Immunity 1999; 10: 439-449.

112. Kao J, Chen PJ, Lai MY, et al. Superinfection of heterologous hepatitis C virus in a patient with chronic type C hepatitis. Gastroenterology 1992; 105: 583-587.

113. Kato N, Ootsuyama Y, Tanka T, et al. Marked sequence diversity in the putative envelope proteins of hepatitis C viruses. Virus Res 1992; 22: 107-123.

114. Krawczynski K, Alter MJ, Tankersley DL, et al. Effect of immune globulin on the prevention of experimental hepatitis C virus infection. J Infect Dis 1996; 173: 822-828.

115. Statement NIoHCDCP. Management of hepatitis C. Hepatology 1997; 26: 25-105.

116. Hoofnagle J, Mullen KD, Jones DB, et al. Treatment of chronic non-A, non-B hepatitis with recombinant human alpha interferon: a preliminary report. N Engl J Med 1986; 315: 1575-1578.

117. Shindo M, DiBisceglie AM, Cheung L, et al. Decrease in serum hepatitis C viral RNA during alpha-interferon therapy for chronic hepatitis C. Ann Intern Med 1991; 115: 700-704.

118. Shindo M, DiBisceglie AM, Hoofnagle JH. Long-term follow-up of patients with chronic hepatitis C treated with alpha-interferon. Hepatology 1992; 15: 1013-1016.

119. Davis G, Balart LA, Schiff ER, et al. Treatment of chronic hepatitis C with recombinant interferon alfa: a multicenter randomized, controlled trial. N Engl J Med 1989; 1989: 501-506.

120. DiBisceglie A, Martin P, Kassianides C, et al. Recombinant interferon alfa therapy for chronic hepatitis C: a randomized, double-blind, placebo-controlled trial. N Engl J Med 1989; 321: 1506-1510.

121. Poynard T, Leroy V, Cohard M, et al. Meta-analysis of interferon randomized trials in the treatment of viral hepatitis C: effects of dose and duration. Hepatology 1996; 24: 778-789.

122. Craxi A, DiMarco V, Lo Iacono O, et al. Lymphoblastoid (alpha)-interferon for post-transfusion chronic hepatitis C: a randomized trial of 6 vs 12 months treatment. J Hepatol 1992; 16: Suppl 1: S8.

123. Poynard T, Bedossa P, Chevallier M, et al. A comparison of three interferon alfa-2b regimens for the long-term treatment of chronic non-A, non-B hepatitis. N Engl J Med 1995; 332: 1457-1462.

124. Lin R, Roach E, Zimmerman M, Strasser S, Farrell GC. Interferon alfa-2b for chronic hepatitis C: effects of dose increment and duration of treatment on response rates: results of the first multicentre Australian trial. J Hepatol 1995; 23: 487-496.

125. Chemello L, Bonetti P, et al. Randomized trial comparing three different regimens of alpha-2a-interferon in chronic hepatitis C. Hepatology 1995; 22: 700-706.

126. Bacon B, Farrell G, Benhamou JP, et al. Lymphoblastoid interfeon improves long-term response to a six month course of treatment when compared with recombinant interferon alfa 2b: results of an international trial. Hepatology 1995; 22: Suppl: 152A.

127. Tong M, Blatt LM, Klein M, Manyak C, et al. Long-term follow-up of chronic hepatitis C virus infected patients treated with consensus interferon. Gastroenterology 1995; 108: Suppl: A1188.

128. Habersetzer F, Marcellin P, Boyer N, et al. Recombinant interferon beta for the treatment of chronic hepatitis C. Hepatology 1995; 22: Suppl: 119A.

129. Reichard O, Andersson J, Schvarcz R, Weiland O. Ribavirin treatment for chronic hepatitis C. Lancet 1991; 337: 1058-1061.

130. DiBisceglie A, Conjeevaram HS, Fried MW, Sallie R, et al. Ribavirin as therapy for chronic hepatitis C. Ann Intern Med 1995; 123: 897-903.

131. McHutchison J, Gordon SC, Schiff ER, Shiffman ML, et al. Interferon alfa-2b alone or in combination with ribavirin as inital treatment for chronic hepatitis C. N Engl J Med 1998; 339: 1485-1492.

132. Davis G, Esteban-Mur R, Rustgi V, Hoefs J, et al. Interferon alfa-2b alone or in combination with ribavirin for the treatment of relapse of chronic hepatitis C. N Engl J Med 1998; 339: 1493-1499.

133. Poynard T, Marcellin P, Lee SS, Niederau C, et al. Randomised trial of interferon alfa-2b plus ribavirin for 48 weeks or for 24 weeks *versus* interferon alfa-2b plus placebo for 48 weeks for treatment of chronic infection with hepatitis C virus. Lancet 1998; 352: 1426-1432.

134. Poynard T, McHutchinson J, Goodman Z, Ling M-H, et al. Is an "a la carte" combination interferon alfa-2b plus ribavirin regimen posible for the first line treatment in patients with chronic hepatitis C. Hepatology 2000; 31: 211-218.

135. Welch P, Yei S, Barber JR. Ribozyme gene therapy for hepatitis C virus infection. Clin Diagn Virol 1998; 10: 163-171.

136. Zeuzem S, Feinman SV, Rasenack J, Heathcoate EJ, et al. Peginterferon Alfa-2a in Patients with Chronic Hepatitis C. N Engl J Med 2000; 343: 1666-1672

137. Glue P, Rouzier-Panis R, Raffanel C, Sabo R, Gupta S, et al. A dose-ranging study of pegylated interferon alfa-2b and ribavirin in chronic hepatitis C. Hepatology 2000; 32: 647-653.

138. Manns MP, McHutchison JG, Gordon S, Rustgi V, Shiffman ML, Lee WM, et al. Peginterferon alfa-2B plus ribavirin compared to interferon alfa-2B plus ribavirin for the treatment of chronic hepatitis C: 24 week treatment analysis of a multicenter, multinational phase III randomized controlled trial. Hepatology 2000; 32: 297

CHAPTER 10

RESPIRATORY VIRUSES

JOHN TREANOR and DOUGLAS FLEMING

Table of Contents

Introduction

Acute respiratory disease, including the common cold, influenza-like illness, croup, bronchiolitis, and viral pneumonia, can be caused by a wide variety of viral and non-viral agents. Among the viruses, those with RNA genomes tend to play a more prominent role, particularly among immunologically intact individuals. DNA viruses are also associated with respiratory disease, these agents are described elsewhere in this text. The characteristics of the viruses most often associated with respiratory disease are described briefly below.

Practical Guidelines in Antiviral Therapy Ed. by Charles A.B. Boucher and George J. Galasso. 223 — 256
© 2002 *Elsevier Science. Printed in the Netherlands.*

Descriptions of Viruses

Influenza Virus

Three distinct types of influenza viruses are recognized, influenza A virus, influenza B virus, and influenza C virus, based on antigenic differences in the nucleoprotein and matrix proteins. All three viruses share certain characteristics including the presence of a viral envelope containing glycoproteins important for viral entry and egress from cells, and a segmented genome. The standard nomenclature for influenza viruses includes the influenza type, place of initial isolation, strain designation, and year of isolation.

The hemagglutinin (HA) of influenza virus mediates attachment of virus to susceptible cells and fusion of the viral envelope with the cell membrane. Antibody to the HA neutralizes viral infectivity and is the main protective mechanism induced by infection or immunization. The neuraminidase (NA) is also an envelope glycoprotein and plays an important role in release of virus from cells. Antibody to the NA also inhibits viral replication, and the NA is an important target for antiviral therapy. A third membrane protein, the M2, is present in small quantities on virions, and is inhibited by amantadine and rimantadine. Finally, viral structural proteins such as the matrix (M) and nucleoprotein (NP) are important targets for cytotoxic T lymphocytes (CTL).

Parainfluenza Virus

Parainfluenza viruses are also enveloped viruses, but with a linear single-stranded RNA genome. Four distinct human serotypes are recognized, termed types 1, 2, 3, and 4. Viral envelope glycoproteins include HN, which serves as both the viral hemagglutinin and neuraminidase, and F, which mediates fusion of the viral envelope with the cell membrane. Antibody to either HN or F neutralize infectivity, but only antibody to F prevents cell to cell fusion. Antibody to both the HN and F proteins play a role in resistance to infection. Passive transfer of monospecific antisera to either F or HN can protect animals, and vaccinia viruses expressing either F or HN induce protective immunity in experimental animals.

Respiratory Syncytial Virus

Another enveloped, single-stranded RNA virus of importance to the respiratory tract is respiratory syncytial (RS) virus. The RS genome encodes 10 distinct proteins, including the envelope glycoproteins F and G. The G or attachment protein mediates binding of the virus to the host cell, while the F or fusion protein allows entry of the virus into the cell and promotes cell to cell spread. Only the F and G viral surface glycoproteins appear to play a role in the induction of neutralizing antibody. Monoclonal antibodies to both the F and G protein neutralize infectivity *in vitro*, but while the majority of monoclonal antibodies to F neutralize virus, only a small proportion of G monoclonal antibodies do so. Two antigenic subgroups of RS virus, denoted A and B, have been recognized primarily due to differences in the G glycoprotein between subgroup A and B. Both subgroups circulate in the population, with some indication of a general predominance of one or the other in alternate years. It has been suggested that infections with subgroup A viruses may be somewhat more severe, with a greater frequency of hospitalizations with RS virus in years in which subgroup A viruses predominate compared to subgroup B.

Rhinovirus

Rhinoviruses are members of the picornavirus family of viruses, non-enveloped viruses with a linear, single stranded genome of positive polarity. Rhinoviruses are differentiated from the related enteroviruses by their relative acid lability and thermal stability. In addition, rhinoviruses replicate most efficiently in cell culture at lower than body temperature. Humans are the only known natural host. To date, over 100 distinct neutralization serotypes of rhinovirus have been identified. This antigenic diversity is the result of amino acid sequence variation in four recognized antigenic sites, which surround the receptor binding site. The majority of human rhinoviruses utilize intracellular adhesion molecule-1 (ICAM-1) as the receptor. This "major binding group" accounts for 91 of 102 known rhinovirus serotypes. Rhinovirus serotypes which do not bind to ICAM-1 are referred to as the minor receptor group viruses.

Illnesses

Acute respiratory infections are one of the commonest problems prompting medical consultation. Data from the United States, collected in the 1992 National Health Interview Survey, suggest that such illnesses are experienced at a rate of 85.6 illnesses per 100 persons per year, and account for 54% of all acute conditions exclusive of injuries. In the national morbidity survey in England and Wales conducted in general practice in 1991/92, acute respiratory infections accounted for 14% of all consultations and approximately 25% of the entire population consulted at least once in the survey year because of acute respiratory infection: in pre-school children these figures were 28% and 60% respectively. From a clinical perspective, the distinction between upper and lower respiratory illness is particularly important because the potential for complications is higher and more serious in lower respiratory disease. Nevertheless, some complications of upper respiratory illness can be serious, for example, acute sinusitis. Damage to the cells lining the lower respiratory tract results in impairment of the oxygenation of the blood and thus persons with pre-existing respiratory or cardiac disease are at particular risk from such infections.

In the assessment of patients presenting to doctors with respiratory infections, cough is a critical symptom. While a minimal cough associated with post nasal drip can be accepted as part of an upper respiratory illness, any significant degree of coughing is indicative of illness at the level of the larynx or major airways. Fever, respiratory rate and pule are useful markers of the severity of illness, although an absence of fever in an older person does not exclude serious respiratory illness. In older persons, lower respiratory infection can prompt disturbances in cardiac rhythm (particularly atrial fibrillation) and drive patients into heart failure.

The diagnostic terminology applied to respiratory viral infections is largely syndrome driven, reflecting the pattern of symptoms and signs observed. These terms are then often used to determine treatment. However, it is important first to consider the likely causes. There is a poor match between the diagnostic terms in common use and the etiological agent, although for some syndromes there is a stronger link (for example, between croup and parainfluenza virus). For most, the link is more tenuous and disease management must take into account the likely specific etiology. The association between clinical syndromes and viruses is described in the following paragraphs.

Common Cold

There is really no single definition of the syndrome of the common cold, but generally this term is taken to mean an acute illness with rhinitis and variable degrees of pharyngitis. Predominant associated symptoms include nasal stuffiness, sneezing, runny nose, and sore throat. Patients often report chills, but true fever is unusual. The presence of lower respiratory tract signs and symptoms indicate the possibility of some complication. Headache and mild malaise may be reported. Although a multitude of viruses may be associated with this syndrome, the pattern of symptoms associated with colds does not appear to vary significantly between agents. Physical findings are non-specific and most commonly include nasal discharge and pharyngeal inflammation. More severe disease, with higher fever, may be seen in children. Colds are generally self-limited, with a total duration of illness of approximately 7-14 days in adults. Recognized complications of colds include secondary bacterial infections of the paranasal sinuses and middle ear, and exacerbations of asthma, chronic bronchitis, and emphysema.

The differential diagnosis of individuals presenting with typical signs and symptoms is not extensive. However, in the presence of additional signs or symptoms which are not part of this clinical description, such as high, persistent fever, signs of respiratory distress, or lower respiratory tract disease, alternative diagnoses should be sought. Allergic causes should be considered in individuals who present with recurrent symptoms restricted to the upper respiratory tract.

The evaluation of patients who present predominantly with pharyngitis centers upon the differentiation of bacterial from viral or other non-bacterial etiologies. The presence of nasal symptoms or of conjunctivitis favors a viral etiology, as does pharyngitis in children less than 3 years of age. The presence of exudate is suggestive of bacterial etiology, but exudates may also be seen with adenovirus or infectious mononucleosis. The presence of tender, palpable cervical lymph nodes is also indicative of a bacterial cause. A rapid test for group A streptococci may be indicated in cases of significant illness where the etiology is uncertain, but routine studies for other bacterial and non bacterial pathogens are usually not obtained.

Otitis Media

Otitis media is commonly thought of as a complication of upper respiratory tract infections, though many children present with a combination of upper respiratory symptoms with concurrent earache at the outset. Infection of the upper respiratory tract is associated with mucosal edema which interferes with the normal function of the Eustachian tube. Pressure in the middle ear increases and gives rise to pain. This can be relieved by tympanic paracentesis though this procedure is rarely adopted since most such illnesses resolve spontaneously with or without rupture of the tympanic membrane. There has been much debate about the usefulness of antibiotics in the treatment of acute otitis media. The critical factor is whether any secondary bacterial infection is established or not. Any virus causing acute respiratory infection predisposes to otitis media, and many viruses can be recovered from middle ear fluid.

Croup

Croup is a clinically distinct illness affecting children under the age of three. The illness typically begins with upper respiratory tract symptoms of rhinorrhea and sore throat, often with a mild cough. After two or three days, the cough deepens and develops a characteristic brassy, barking quality, which is similar to a seal's bark. Fever is usually present, generally between 38° and 40°C. The child may appear apprehensive, and most comfortable sitting forward in bed. The respiratory rate is elevated, but in contrast to bronchiolitis is usually not over 50 breaths per minute.

The characteristic physical finding of croup is inspiratory stridor. Inspiration is prolonged and chest wall retractions may be observed. Children with this finding on presentation have a higher risk of hospitalization or of requiring ventilatory support. Rales, rhonchi, and wheezing may be heard on physical examination. These signs, including the barking cough and inspiratory stridor, arise mostly from inflammation occurring in the larynx and trachea, which is greatest at the subglottic level, the least distensible part of the airway. It is important to recognize inflammatory changes are noted throughout the respiratory tract in croup and hypoxemia is detected in about 80% of children hospitalized with this illness. A fluctuating course is typical for viral croup, and the child may appear to worsen or improve within an hour.

Overall, viruses can be recovered from croup cases more frequently than from other types of respiratory illnesses. The parainfluenza viruses, particularly types 1 and 2, are the most common viruses responsible for croup, accounting for about 75% of cases. Other viral causes of croup include respiratory syncytial virus, influenza A or B viruses, rhinoviruses, and adenoviruses. Although no longer endemic in the United States, measles has long been recognized as a cause of severe croup. Parainfluenza virus type 2, and influenza A viruses are associated with more severe disease, but generally the clinical presentation of the croup syndrome due to individual agents is similar..

It is important when evaluating children with stridor to distinguish the croup syndrome from other, potentially more serious causes of airway obstruction such as bacterial epiglottitis and tracheitis. Epiglottitis is an acute cellulitis of the epiglottis and surrounding structures. Patients present with acute respiratory distress and drooling, but the barking cough of croup is absent. Bacterial tracheitis is a relatively rare syndrome that mimics croup, but abundant purulent sputum is often present. Other infectious causes of stridor include peritonsillar or retropharyngeal abscess and diphtheria. Non-infectious causes of stridor such as trauma or aspiration of a foreign body, should also be considered.

Acute Bronchitis

Acute bronchitis is characterized by cough often with expectoration of sputum and accompanied by wheeze and rales on auscultation. The distinction from asthma can be difficult, though the link with a recent cold or other respiratory symptoms in a person not subject to recurring asthma provides the basis for diagnosis. Persons with chronic obstructive pulmonary disease experience exacerbations of their illness which may be precipitated by virus infections, but may often be complicated by secondary bacterial infection.

Acute bronchitis affects persons of all ages though its effects are greater in young children and elderly persons. It is predominantly a winter illness and incidence increase when respiratory viruses such as RSV and influenza are circulating in the community. The early stages of the illness may primarily relate to the upper respiratory tract but the development and persistence of cough three or four days later is often the reason that prompts consultation. It is not particularly linked to any specific virus but there has only been limited research into the causes of such respiratory exacerbations.

Bronchiolitis

Bronchiolitis is a form of acute bronchits particularly experienced by young children in which the main focus of the infection is in the small peripheral airways. The syndrome is characterized by wheezing and other symptoms due to obstruction to expiratory air flow. The onset of lower respiratory symptoms is usually preceded by rhinitis, often with nasal congestion and discharge, with more severe symptoms characteristically occurring 2-3 days later. Cough may not be prominent initially but when present may be paroxysmal in nature. The presence or absence of cyanosis is not a reliable indicator of the degree of oxygenation. Physical findings are generally confined to musical or moist rales. Fever is frequently present at the beginning of the illness, but one-third or more of hospitalized infants are afebrile. The hospital course is variable, but most infants will show improvement in 3 to 4 days.

The peak age incidence of bronchiolitis is between two and 6 months of age, with over 80% of cases occurring in the first year of life. The risk of hospitalization and severe bronchiolitis is particularly high in infants with congenital heart disease, chronic lung disease, or immunodeficiency. In addition, infants born prematurely, and those who are less than 6 weeks of age at the time of presentation are also at risk.

Respiratory syncytial virus causes the majority of cases of bronchiolitis, and during the RS virus epidemic season, generally between November to February in the Northern hemisphere, essentially all cases are due to this virus. Overall, RS virus is recovered from about three-fourths of all infants admitted to the hospital with bronchiolitis. Several other respiratory viruses are be associated with bronchiolitis, including rhinoviruses, parainfluenza viruses, influenza virus and mumps. Adenoviruses types 3, 7, and 21 are relatively uncommon causes, but may be associated with more severe disease, including the development of a more chronic form of bronchiolitis referred to as bronchiolitis obliterans. The differential diagnosis of diseases characterized by expiratory airflow obstruction in infants is relatively small. Pertussis can occasionally be confused with bronchiolitis, however, more frequent vomiting and more paroxysmal cough would be clues to the diagnosis. Differentiation of acute infectious bronchiolitis from the initial presentation of allergic asthma is difficult, and contributes to the difficulty in assessing therapeutic interventions in this disease. Anatomic defects such as vascular rings can cause obstruction of the airway. Foreign bodies should be considered strongly especially in young infants. Gastroesophageal reflux is an additional consideration.

Influenza-like Illness

The onset of influenza is typically abrupt, and the illness is characterized by the predominance of systemic symptoms, including fever, prostration, myalgias, and malaise. Non-productive couch tends to predominate late in the illness. Other respiratory symptoms may be relatively minimal, particularly early in the course, and include nasal complaints, sore throat, and hoarseness. The presence of fever and cough on presentation are significantly associated with a higher likelihood of isolation of influenza virus from nasopharyngeal secretions. Because of the involvement of tracheal epithelium in infection, complaints of burning throat and substernal pain may be seen. Other than fever, there are usually few findings on physical exam. Individuals with influenza may exhibit rhinitis, pharyngitis, conjunctival injection, and tracheal tenderness. The chest is usually clear in uncomplicated cases. Most acute symptoms resolve in 3-5 days, but complete recovery may take weeks, with malaise and easy fatigability being among the most prolonged symptoms. The clinical features of influenza A and B virus infection are similar. It has been estimated that in the course of an intense influenza epidemic, 70% to 80% of healthy adults who present with the above symptoms will have laboratory evidence of influenza virus infection.

Influenza is also an important cause of acute febrile illness in children during epidemics. Generally symptoms of influenza are similar to those in adults, although children may have higher fever with febrile seizures. In addition, some complaints, such as myalgias, may be less common in children because of their inability to communicate such symptoms. However, parents may note lack of activity or lethargy. Influenza is associated with otitis media, and influenza virus can be isolated from middle ear fluid in affected children.

The impact of influenza on elderly populations is well recognized, and this age group contributes disproportionately to hospitalizations and deaths during influenza epidemics. However, the clinical presentation of influenza in the elderly may be somewhat blunted, with relatively lower fever and a more subtle onset of symptoms. Particularly in elderly individuals who are not very verbal, the only signs of influenza may be low grade fever and lethargy.

Other acute respiratory viral illnesses may present initially with an influenza-like picture, including infections of adults with parainfluenza and respiratory syncytial viruses. In addition to influenza virus, acute infection with respiratory syncytial virus may completely mimic the clinical picture of influenza in this age group. The initial stages of many bacterial infections may resemble influenza, so that the clinician must be aware that individuals initially diagnosed as having acute influenza may have bacterial illnesses such as meningitis.

Viral Pneumonia

Overall, pneumonia represents on end of a spectrum of viral infections of the lower respiratory tract which includes croup, bronchiolitis, tracheobronchitis, and reactive airways changes. The development of pneumonia is defined by the development of abnormalities of alveolar gas exchange accompanied by inflammation of the lung parenchyma, often associated with visible changes on chest xray or abnormalities of other radiologic studies such as gallium scanning. Although there can be considerable variety to the presentation of this syndrome depending on the age and immunologic competence of the host and the specific viral pathogen, there are certain general features.

The clinical features of primary viral pneumonia in adults include cough which is generally non-productive, although production of frothy, pink-tinged sputum is seen in some severely ill individuals. Cyanosis and hypoxemia are typical of severe primary viral pneumonia. Physical findings are often non-specific, and variety of chest xray patterns have been described, including lobar infiltrates, but most typically primary viral pneumonia presents with diffuse, bilateral interstitial infiltrates. The clinical course of primary influenza virus pneumonia is often progressively downhill, and most patients died in the era prior to the availability of mechanical ventilation, but mortality in healthy adults in the non-pandemic era is low.

The basic presentation of viral pneumonia in children is similar, if somewhat milder. The clinical presentation varies considerably with the specific causative agent, but typically includes fever and lower respiratory tract signs and symptoms, such as difficulty breathing, non-productive cough, and physical findings of wheezing or increased breath sounds. Young infants may present with apneic episodes with minimal fever. The clinical presentation may be dominated by the associated croup or bronchiolitis, which are frequently present.

The majority of cases of viral pneumonia in healthy adults are due to or associated with influenza viruses. In addition, adenoviruses have been described as causes of significant outbreaks of atypical pneumonia in military recruits. Other viral cause of pneumonia in otherwise healthy adults include varicella, RSV, and parainfluenza virus. In certain geographic regions clinicians may encounter the hantavirus pulmonary syndrome (HPS) characterized by severe pulmonary dysfunction after a 2 to 3 day prodrome of non-specific influenza-like symptoms, accompanied by increased hematocrit due to hemoconcentration, and thrombocytopenia with coagulopathy.

In children, respiratory syncytial virus has been associated with the largest proportion of viral pneumonia in young children, particularly if accompanied by bronchiolitis. Parainfluenza viruses, particularly type 3, are the second most common viral cause followed by influenza A and B viruses, especially during periods of epidemic prevalence. Other viral etiologies in children include adenoviruses, measles, and more rarely, rhinoviruses, enteroviruses, rubella virus, and herpes simplex virus.

Bacterial superinfection is a common complication of viral lower respiratory tract infection, particularly in adults. The classic history is that of a typical episode of viral illness with more or less complete recovery, followed 2 to 14 days later by a recurrence of fever and development of cough and dyspnea. CXR reveals lobar infiltrates, and the clinical course is typical of bacterial pneumonia. In addition, combined bacterial and viral pneumonia, with clinical features of each, are common in adults and with certain viruses in children. Bacterial superinfection of viral pneumonia can occur with many bacteria, but the most common bacteria responsible for bacterial pneumonia complicating influenza is *Streptococcus pneumoniae*. There are also increases in the relative frequency of Staphylococci and *Hemophilus influenzae*. Differentiation between viral and bacterial forms of pneumonia in children on clinical grounds can be difficult, and radiologic criteria do not always distinguish these entities well. However, in normal infants and children with RS or parainfluenza virus pneumonia, bacteria do not appear to play an important role, and routine addition of antibacterial agents is not useful. The exception to this observation is in developing countries, where mixed viral and bacterial pneumonias in children are frequent and severe.

Individuals with diminished host immunity may develop severe, life-threatening pulmonary infections with the entire spectrum of RNA and DNA viruses, including both viruses that are typical causes of lower respiratory tract disease in normal hosts, and other, more opportunistic viral pathogens. DNA viruses, including cytomegalovirus (CMV), herpes simplex viruses (HSV), varicella zoster virus (VZV) and adenoviruses have received the most recognition in this regard. Antiviral agents for these pathogens are described elsewhere in this book.

RNA viruses have also received increasing recognition as potential causes of significant morbidity and mortality in the immune compromised. RS virus has been well recognized as a cause of pneumonia in recipients of bone marrow and solid organ transplantation. In the typical presentation, an initial upper respiratory infection becomes relentlessly progressive, with involvement of the lower respiratory tract, significant hypoxia, and oftentimes death. Clinical features have been non-specific, but mortality of over 50% has been reported despite treatment with aerosolized ribavirin. Parainfluenza viruses (PIV) have also been reported as an infrequent lower respiratory tract pathogen in both solid organ and bone marrow transplantation. PIV-3 has been most frequently seen, but all four serotypes have been implicated. Influenza may also cause severe disease in transplant recipients, but most subjects have survived.

Laboratory Diagnosis

Generally, the gold standard for specific etiologic identification has been isolation in cell culture. Most of the viruses responsible for respiratory disease can be readily detected in such cell culture systems, provided appropriate care is exercised in the collection and transportation of the specimens. The specific types of cells used depends on the spectrum of viruses being sought, and will vary both with the specific clinical situation and the season during which the cultures are obtained. For example, a laboratory might routinely inoculate respiratory cultures into Hep-2, RhMK, and MRC-5 cells year round, and add LLC-MK2 cells for isolation of parainfluenza viruses for cultures obtained during the spring and fall, while adding MDCK cells to facilitate isolation of influenza viruses during the winter months.

Viral culture is highly sensitive and specific, and also has the advantage that after isolation the virus is available for further characterization. However, under the best of circumstances, the results of such tests are not available during the time when decisions regarding management and therapy of an individual case must be made. Thus, there has been considerable interest in the development of rapid tests for respiratory viral diagnosis.

The most widely used tests are based on immunologic detection of viral antigen in respiratory secretions. For influenza, such tests include the Directigen Flu A (Becton-Dickenson), Flu OIA (Biostar), and QuickVue Influenza A/B test (Quidel Corporation). In addition, the Zstat Flu (ZymeTx) test detects the presence of the viral neuraminidase enzymatically. With the exception of the Directigen test, all of the tests are designed to detect both influenza A and B, and a modification of the Directigen test to allow detection of both types is in clinical development.

The reported sensitivities of each test in relationship to cell culture has varied between 70% and 100% and is somewhat dependent on the nature of the samples tested and the patients from whom they were derived. There is no published comparative data currently available that conclusively demonstrates superiority of one of the tests over another, thus decisions regarding a specific test are generally made on the basis of convenience, cost, and the familiarity of the operator with the specific technique.

Direct antigen detection in respiratory secretions has also been used extensively for rapid diagnosis of respiratory syncytial virus. Direct or indirect immunoflorescent techniques have been used for many years. This technique has an advantage in that microscopic examination of the sample for exfoliated nasopharyngeal cells allows a rapid judgment as to the quality of the sample. However, the techniques are labor intensive and require specialized equipment and highly experienced staff to be performed accurately. For this reason, many laboratories now use ELISA based technologies for rapid detection. Several test kits are currently available with reported sensitivities of 80% to 95% compared to culture. Antigen detection tests for parainfluenza virus or rhinoviruses are not currently commercially available.

A variety of approaches to direct detection of viral nucleic acids in clinical specimens have also been explored for rapid diagnosis, including nucleic acid hybridization and polymerase chain reaction amplification (PCR). PCR in particular has the advantage of potentially being more sensitive than cell culture, and possibly detecting virus in samples in which the virions have lost viability. In addition, it is possible to devise multiplex techniques such that a single test can detect a number of different agents. However, PCR techniques are more labor intensive and technically demanding, and also require the availability of specialized laboratory equipment. Thus, they have generally not supplanted antigen detection for rapid diagnosis.

Treatment Algorithms

Influenza

Amantadine and Rimantadine

The antiviral drugs amantadine and rimantadine belong to the class of M2 inhibitors, and their antiviral effect is primarily manifested in cell culture as inhibition of virus uncoating. Although influenza B viruses use a similar replication strategy, a different protein, the NB protein, appears to serve the role of ion channel for this virus. Therefore, M2 inhibitors are active only against influenza A viruses.

The antiviral activities of the two members of the class, amantadine and rimantadine, are similar. Both drugs are active against all strains of influenza A virus in a variety of cell culture systems and animal models [1]. In cell culture, inhibitory levels for influenza A virus range from 0.2-0.4 ug/mL for amantadine, and from 0.1-0.4 ug/mL for rimantadine [2], most strains are inhibited at concentrations of 0.1 ug/mL or less.

Several studies to evaluate the effectiveness of amantadine in the treatment of H3N2 influenza A viruses were initiated during the 1968 pandemic. In these studies, therapy within the first 48 hours of illness was associated with decreases in the duration of fever by about 24 hours, and a greater proportion of subjects considered to be "rapid resolvers" [3, 4]. In addition, treated individuals had more rapid decreases in individual symptoms of cough, sore throat, and nasal obstruction [5]. The effect of treatment on recovery of virus from the nasopharynx was minimal in these studies. In an additional study conducted in non-institutionalized adults and children infected with the A/Hong Kong/68 virus, treated subjects had an approximately 24 hour reduction in the duration of fever, but no change in other symptoms [6]. Treatment with amantadine has resulted in significantly more rapid improvement in small airways dysfunction in healthy adults with uncomplicated H3N2 influenza [7, 8].

Additional trials of amantadine therapy were performed when H1N1 viruses reappeared in the late 1970's, with similar results. Early therapy of influenza A/USSR/77 in otherwise healthy adults with amantadine was shown to result a more rapid decrease in fever, and in a higher frequency of subjects reporting improved symptoms at 48 hours compared to placebo [9]. In addition, treated subjects were less likely to shed virus at 48 hours. In a second study conducted in young adults infected with A/Brazil/78, amantadine therapy was associated with a more rapid decrease in symptoms compared to aspirin therapy [10]. Amantadine treated subjects also had decreased virus shedding in this study.

Studies of the therapy of acute influenza in adults with rimantadine have shown levels of benefit essentially identical to those seen with amantadine. Treatment of adults with H1N1 [9] and H3N2 [11] influenza A resulted in improved symptoms, decreased fever, and reduced virus shedding compared to placebo. When rimantadine and amantadine were directly compared in a randomized trial of early therapy [9], the efficacy of the two drugs was essentially identical.

Rimantadine has also been evaluated in the treatment of influenza A in children, and shown to reduce the level of virus shedding early in infection when compared to acetaminophen [12, 13]. More variable effects on clinical symptom scores have been seen, with one study showing a slight decrease in scores and fever compared to acetaminophen [12], and the other, in which illness was relatively mild, showing no significant difference [13]. In both studies, virus shedding was relatively prolonged in those receiving rimantadine, and resistant virus was shed late in the course of illness.

Neither amantadine or rimantadine has been subjected to extensive efficacy evaluation in high-risk subjects. One placebo-controlled study carried out in nursing home residents showed more rapid reduction in fever and in symptoms in rimantadine recipients.

Furthermore, physicians who were caring for these patients, but who were blinded to study drug status, prescribed significantly fewer antipyretics, antitussives, and antibiotics and obtained fewer chest x-rays for the rimantadine recipients [14].

Antiviral drug resistance has been one factor which has limited the more widespread use of these agents. Amantadine and rimantadine resistant viruses emerge fairly frequently in treated individuals [15, 16], although resistance is infrequent in unexposed individuals [17]. Resistant virus retain full pathogenic potential in experimental animals and can cause disease in susceptible contacts [15, 16, 18].

Neuraminidase Inhibitors

The influenza virus neuraminidase is a membrane protein whose major function is to remove terminal sialic acid residues from viral receptors on the host cell, thereby releasing virus to spread to other cells. Two neuraminidase inhibitors, zanamivir and oseltamivir, have been licensed for therapy of acute influenza. Both agents are broadly active against all 9 of the known neuraminidase subtypes of influenza A virus as well as against influenza B viruses. Inhibitory levels against most clinical isolates range from 2 to 20 nmol/L in cell culture [19]. The two agents are similar in many respects, but differ in that zanamivir is administered by inhalation (see below), while oseltamivir is administered orally.

Inhaled zanamivir was initially demonstrated to be effective for the treatment of uncomplicated influenza in otherwise healthy adults [20]. In an initial study conducted in Europe and North America, treatment of individuals with laboratory evidence of influenza virus infection within 48 hours of symptom onset was associated with a 0.9-day reduction in the duration of illness, from 6.3 days in the placebo group to 5.4 days in the inhaled zanamivir group. More striking differences were seen when the analysis was restricted to individuals with fever (T ≥ 37.8°F) on enrollment, or those enrolled within 30 hours of onset of symptoms, in whom the difference between treated and placebo groups was approximately 2 days. Treatment within 30 hours of symptom onset was also associated with a significantly more rapid return to normal activities, by approximately 1.5 days. In this study, there was no difference in the level of clinical efficacy between subjects infected with influenza A and influenza B viruses [20].

In a second study conducted in the Southern Hemisphere, treatment of individuals aged 12 and older within 36 hours of symptom onset was associated with a 1.5-day difference in the duration of illness among these infected subjects, from 6 days in the placebo group to 4.5 days in the treated group [21]. Similar to the earlier study, there was no significant difference in the effect on influenza A and B virus, and treatment was associated with an earlier return to work or normal activities. Zanamivir was also of benefit in the small number of subjects enrolled in the study who were considered to be at relatively higher risk for influenza-related complications, and the rate of respiratory complications among such subjects was reduced from 46% in the placebo group to 14% in the treated group. Recently, a third study of zanamivir therapy conducted in Europe showed a 2.5-day reduction in duration, from 7.5 days in placebo recipients to 5 days in zanamivir recipients [22].

To date, results from two trials of oral oseltamivir therapy of acute influenza have been published. In the first trial, treatment of adults 18 and older within 36 hours of symptom onset resulted in a 30% decrease in the duration of illness (from 4.7 days to 2.5 days) and a 40% decrease in the severity of illness [23]. In addition, early therapy was associated with a significantly earlier return to work or other normal activities, and with reductions in the rate of complications, primarily sinusitis and bronchitis. The overall rate of any complication in the placebo group was 17%, this was reduced to 8% in those receiving oseltamivir [23]. The majority of cases of influenza in this study were due to influenza A (H3N2) viruses. Similar results were reported from a treatment study performed concurrently in Canada and Northern Europe [24]. In that study, early therapy was associated with a 25% reduction in the duration of illness among infected subjects, and a 37% reduction in duration among those treated within 24 hours.

Studies of neuraminidase inhibitor therapy in other populations have been reported in abstract form. Early treatment with inhaled zanamivir is associated with reductions in the duration of illness in elderly and high-risk subjects [25], slight reductions in the frequency with which patients require additional prescriptions or health care contacts [26], and an approximately 28% reduction in the rate of complications [27]. Use of oseltamivir in this same type of patient was also reported to result in reductions in the duration of illness and fever, and reductions in the rate of complications [28]. When used for treatment of othewise healthy children aged 5-12 years, zanamivir reduced the duration of illness by 1.25 days, and showed benefits in the severity of illness and use of ancillary medications [19]. More recently, administration of a liquid formulation of oseltamivir at a dose of 2 mg/kg b.i.d. resulted in a 38% reduction in the median duration of illness in children aged 1 to 10. Oseltamivir also resulted in a 40% reduction in the frequency of complications, primarily otitis media, for which antibiotics were prescribed [29].

Because the neuraminidase inhibitors interact with highly conserved residues within the influenza virus neuraminidase, it has been hypothesized that antiviral resistance will be a relatively limited problem. Viruses resistant to the *in vitro* antiviral activity of these agents have been isolated after passage in cell culture [19]. Analysis of these viruses has revealed two basic mechanisms of resistance, and illustrate the interactive roles of the viral HA and NA in binding to and release from infected cells. Mutations within the catalytic framework of the NA which abolish binding of the drugs have been described. Resistance mutations in the NA may be associated with altered characteristics of the enzyme with significantly reduced activity. A second type of mutation associated with cell culture resistant viruses involve mutations in the receptor binding region of the hemagglutinin. HA mutations associated with resistance to neuraminidase inhibitors reduce the affinity of the HA for its receptor, allowing cell to cell spread of virus in the absence of NA activity. Resistant viruses with HA mutations exhibit cross resistance to these drugs in cell culture, but may retain susceptibility in animal models. Many of these viruses also exhibit reduced virulence in animals. However, resistant viruses have been rarely isolated from humans treated with neuraminidase inhibitors in clinical trials to date [30]. The most well characterized resistant virus reported so far was recovered from an immunosuppressed child receiving Zanamivir [31]. Preliminary results from clinical trials in immunologically intact individuals suggest that resistant viruses arise very infrequently during treatment.

Strategies For Treatment

Antiviral therapy of influenza can be considered in any adult who seeks treatment within the first 48 hours of onset of illness. There is clinical experience with the use of M2 inhibitors, and very extensive data from randomized, controlled trials of neuraminidase inhibitors, that leave little doubt that both classes of drugs are effective for this indication, with the exception that only the neuraminidase inhibitors have activity against influenza B virus. To summarize the data presented earlier, the benefits that can be expected include an approximately 1 to 2 day reduction in the duration of symptoms, a return to work or usual activities about 1 day sooner, and possibly, a reduction in rates of complications. The decision about whether to treat any individual patient involves balancing the impact of these benefits on the individual against the cost of therapy, since for the most part, the drugs are without significant risk.

The effectiveness of treatment initiated beyond the 48 hours window after onset of symptoms has not been determined, but is likely to be very low in healthy adults, in whom influenza is generally self-limited. This poses a significant hurdle to the effective use of antiviral therapy for influenza, in that patients must correctly identify their illness, seek medical attention, interact with the medical system and achieve some form of diagnosis, and be prescribed and obtain drug within a very short time frame. For physicians, the issue may balance on the level of comfort in making a clinical diagnosis of influenza, since it may not be practical to confirm each case microbiologically, at the current state of technology. Certainly the evidence from randomized trials of neuraminidase inhibitors suggest that with appropriate epidemiologic support, a clinical diagnosis of influenza can be made with some confidence, since in these trials subjects who met a clinical case definition had a 60-70% rate of microbiologically documented influenza. Individual physician practices therefore will need to adapt the strategies that best suit their patient populations.

Less published information is available regarding therapy of high-risk individuals. There are essentially no studies supporting the utility of amantadine or rimantadine in the elderly or in individuals with cardiac or pulmonary conditions, although with appropriate dosage reductions the drugs can be used safely. Studies of therapy with neuraminidase inhibitors have been conducted in much larger populations, and have included high-risk subjects. Preliminary analysis of studies with both zanamivir and oseltamivir suggest that these drugs also provide benefit to high risk adults, resulting in more rapid recovery of illness, again by about 1 to 2 days. However, these studies have not been able to demonstrate convincingly that early treatment of influenza in such individuals would lead to reductions in subsequent hospitalizations or deaths. It may never be possible to organize prospective randomized controlled trials to demonstrate such an effect, since even in high-risk subjects such events occur rarely.

There is also little information on use of any antiviral therapy for influenza in immunosuppressed individuals or in individuals with severe influenza who are seen beyond 48 hours after the onset of symptoms. Because immunosuppressed patients may exhibit prolonged replication of influenza virus, it is reasonable to imagine that there may be a greater window of opportunity to intervene with antiviral drugs in this situation, but there is no data on which to base this speculation. Similarly, it is reasonable to imagine that severely ill patients who are virus positive at the time that therapy is initiated might benefit even if they more than 48 hours into their illness. Since most adults who are hospitalized with influenza are outside the 48 hour window, this is an extremely relevant issue, and in fact many such individuals currently do receive antiviral therapy. However, it has never been possible to successfully complete a study to evaluate this question in a definitive way.

Therapy of acute influenza in children has also received relatively little attention. Only amantadine is licensed for this indication in the U.S., although there is data, summarized earlier, supporting the efficacy of rimantadine as well. However, use of M2 inhibitors is associated with particularly high rates of development of resistance in children. Zanamivir is currently licensed for use in individuals 7 or older, while oseltamivir is licensed for use in individuals 13 years of age and older, although as described earlier, preliminary evidence of efficacy in younger subjects has been reported.

Studies that directly compared amantadine and rimantadine have shown that there is no significant difference in the therapeutic efficacy of these two drugs. However, there are no studies that have directly compared the efficacy of zanamivir with oseltamivir, or of M2 inhibitors with neuraminidase inhibitors. The published results of individual clinical trials suggest that for influenza A virus infections, all of the available drugs have similar efficacy. In addition, the two drugs with activity against influenza B virus, zanamivir and oseltamivir, appear to have similar levels of benefit against influenza generally, although neither drug has been evaluated extensively against influenza B in humans. Therefore,. decisions regarding the choice of an individual agent should be individualized and consider the side effects, ease of use, concern regarding development of resistance, and cost. There is currently no information regarding the potential use of drugs from the two classes in combination, although theoretically this strategy might be synergistic, since they involve two distinct antiviral targets.

RSV

Ribavirin

Ribavirin (1-β-D-ribofuranosyl-1,2,3-triazole-3-carboxamide) is a broad spectrum antiviral agent with structural similarity to guanosine. In cell culture, this agent has antiviral activity against both DNA and RNA viruses, including RSV. The mechanism of action of the drug is unclear and may be multifactorial, including alterations in cellular nucleotide pools [32] and inhibition of viral mRNA formation. Perhaps for this reason, antiviral resistance is rare and has been reported only for Sindbis virus. Ribavirin is inhibitory to RSV in cell culture at levels of 3-10 ug/mL, and in aerosolized form has been demonstrated to be effective for treatment of experimental infection in a variety of animal models, including in cotton rats and primates.

Several randomized placebo-controlled trials of ribavirin small particle aerosol in naturally occurring RS virus lower respiratory tract disease of normal infants [33-37], or infants with high-risk underlying disease [38] have been conducted. While there have been differences in the measures by which outcome was assessed in these studies, each has indicated some beneficial effect of the drug on both virus shedding and clinical illness.

Ribavirin has also been shown to be of benefit when administered to infants requiring mechanical ventilation, with a markedly decreased total duration of ventilation and hospitalization compared to infants receiving placebo [39]. However, other studies, using both randomized prospective as well as retrospective case-control designs, have not shown beneficial effects of the drug [40-43]. The reasons for these disparate results are not clear, but may involve such factors as the choice of placebo, the endpoints used in the studies, and the specific patient populations involved. However, doubts about the efficacy of ribavirin have lead to reduced enthusiasm for its use among practitioners.

Strategies For Treatment

The variable results of treatment trials and the expense of the drug has recently prompted a reconsideration of recommendations for use of this drug [44]. Current recommendations regarding the treatment of RSV limit such treatment to selected infants and young children who are at high risk for serious RSV disease [45]. Specifically, these indications include infants with congenital heart disease, bronchopulmonary dysplasia, cystic fibrosis, and other chronic lung condition, premature infants, children with immunodeficiency, recent transplant recipients, patients undergoing chemotherpay for malignancy, and severely ill infants such as those receiving mechanical ventilation, and those at high risk of progression.

The optimal treatment of RSV infection in immunocompromised individuals is unclear. Ribavirin therapy of RSV pneumonia in these patients is usually not successful. Use of RSV-IGIV (see below) has been reported to be useful in uncontrolled trials [46, 47], but the doses required are generally not practicable in adults. Because severe RSV lower respiratory tract infections in transplant recipients are usually preceded by several days of upper respiratory tract symptoms, one option would be preemptive therapy before the development of severe disease. Preliminary results with the use of preemptive ribavirin aerosol or ribavirin plus RSV-IGIV have been encouraging [48, 49], but need to be confirmed in controlled trials.

Dosing Schemes, Drug Interactions, Side Effects

Amantadine

The usual dose of amantadine for treatment in healthy adults is 100 mg orally twice a day for 5 days. Amantadine is absorbed readily from the gastrointestinal tract and is excreted unchanged in the urine, with an average plasma elimination half-life of approximately 16 hours in young adults and over 25 hours in the elderly. Consequently, lower doses (100 mg per day) are indicated for older adults in order to minimize the risk of toxicity, although this dose has also been associated with excess side effects in nursing home residents [50].

The major side effects of amantadine are minor, reversible, CNS side effects such as insomnia, dizziness, or difficulty in concentrating. These side effects may be more troublesome in the elderly. In addition, amantadine use has been associated with seizures in individuals with prior seizure disorder [51]. Minor gastrointestinal complaints have also been reported.

Because the elimination of amantadine is almost exclusively renal, significant dosage reductions must be made in the presence of renal impairment. In individuals with complete renal failure, the serum half life can be as long as 30 days [52]. Only small amounts of amantadine are removed during hemodialysis.

The CNS side effects of amantadine are increased when these drugs are co-administered with anticholinergics or antihistamines [52]. In addition, trimethoprim-sulphfamethoxazole may inhibit tubular secretion of amantadine and increase the potential for CNS toxicity. There are no other known significant drug interactions with amantadine. However coadministration of amantadine with other drugs having CNS side effects could conceivably exacerbate these effects.

Rimantadine

The usual therapeutic dose of rimantadine is also 100 mg orally twice a day for 5 days. Rimantadine undergoes extensive metabolism in the liver prior to excretion of the inactive metabolites via the kidney. There is relatively little effect of moderate renal or hepatic insufficiency of serum levels of rimantadine. However, reductions to about one-half of the normal daily dose is recommended in the presence of severe dysfunction. There are no known drug interactions that significantly affect the levels or metabolism of rimantadine.

Rimantadine is associated with a considerably reduced rate of CNS side effects compared to amantadine, and in comparative studies of long term administration, the rate of CNS side effects was not significantly different than placebo [53]. However, it is recommended that the dose of rimantadine should be reduced to 100 mg per day in the elderly, similar to the recommendations for amantadine in this population.

Oseltamivir

Based data showing no difference in clinical trials between the 75 mg and 150 mg bid doses, the recommended dose of oseltamivir for treatment is 75 mg of oseltamivir phosphate twice a day for 5 days. Administration of the drug with food may improve tolerability without impacting drug levels. Oseltamivir is rapidly absorbed from the gastrointestinal tract and is converted in the liver by hepatic esterases to the active metabolite, oseltamivir carboxylate (GS4107). The metabolite is excreted unchanged in the urine by tubular secretion, with a serum half live of 6-10 hours [19].

The dose of oseltamivir should be reduced to 75 mg once daily in individuals with renal impairment, ie., with creatinine clearance of less than 30 mL/min. No data are available regarding the use of the drug in individuals with more significant levels of renal impairment. Likewise, no information is available regarding the use of oseltamivir in individuals with hepatic impairment. Preliminary results of an ongoing study in elderly but otherwise healthy subjects suggests that no dosage adjustment is necessary in this group.

Clinically significant drug interactions are felt to be unlikely with oseltamivir. Competition for hepatic esterases has not been extensively reported in the literature. In addition both oseltamivir phosphate and its carboxylate metabolite exhibit low protein binding. Oseltamivir is a poor substrate for the CYP isoenzymes and hepatic glucuronyl transferases. Because the drug is eliminated by tubular secretion, probenecid increases serum levels of the active metabolite approximately two-fold. However, dosage adjustments are not necessary in individuals taking probenecid. Co-administration of cimetidine, amoxacillin, or acetaminophen has no effect of serum levels of oseltamivir or its metabolite.

Zanamivir

Zanamivir is not bioavailable by the oral route, and must be administered topically in order to be effective. Studies evaluating various modes of administration have determined that the optimal dose for therapeutic use is 10 mg bid x 5 days. The drug is supplied is supplied in blister packs in which each blister contains 5 mg of zanamivir and 20 mg of lactose carrier. The standard dose is therefore two inhalations twice a day. Using the Diskhaler it is estimated that approximately 4 mg of drug are actually delivered with each inhalation.

Studies with radiolabeled carrier suggests that when the Diskhaler device is used by healthy adults, the drug would be distributed throughout the respiratory tract, with relatively little initial distribution into the oropharynx. Approximately 4% to 17% of the inhaled dose is adsorbed systemically, where it is eliminated by the kidneys with a serum half life of from 2.5 to 5.1 hours. The fate of drug that remains in the respiratory tract is unclear. Presumably it remains in the respiratory tract until it is expectorated or swallowed, and excreted in the feces. Although significant increases in serum half life are seen in the presence of renal failure, the small amounts of the drug that are absorbed systemically suggest that dosage adjustments would not be necessary. Studies of the pharmacokinetics of the drug in the presence of impaired hepatic function have not been reported.

Zanamivir has exhibited an excellent safety profile in the majority of studies performed to date. The most commonly reported symptoms in individuals treated with the drug have included diarrhea, nausea, and nasal signs and symptoms which have occurred at essentially the same rate in zanamivir as in placebo recipients. In one study in which zanamivir was used in influenza-infected subjects with asthma or COPD, the frequency of significant changes in FEV_1 or peak flow rates was higher in zanamivir than in placebo recipients. For this reason, individuals with these pulmonary conditions should have ready access to a rapidly acting bronchodilator when using zanamivir, in the event that the drug precipitates bronchospasm.

Because of the low systemic exposure to drug, significant drug-drug interactions would not be expected. In addition, zanamivir does not interact with the CYP series of hepatic microsomal enzymes.

Ribavirin

Ribavirin is significantly more effective for treatment of RSV when delivered topically than when administered systemically. Therefore, the drug is typically administered as a small particle aerosol, designed to generate particles of 1-2 um in diameter. The normal dose is 20 mg/mL in 300 mL of water, administered over 12-20 hours. Treatment duration is usually for 3 to 5 days depending on the patient's clinical course, with a longer duration of therapy sometimes needed in immunodeficient individuals [54]. A higher dose, shorter duration mode of therapy in which the drug is concentrated to 60 mg/mL and administered for a 2-hour period three times daily, appears to be of equal efficacy [55]. At the standard dose, plasma levels vary with the duratin of exposure, varying from 0.5 to 3.3 ug/mL in pediatric patients. In contrast, levels in respiratory secretions are much higher, as high as 1,000 ug/mL [52].

Generally, the drug is extremely well tolerated. Reversible bronchospasm has been reported very rarely. In addition, the drug can precipitate in ventilator tubing, which may create mechanical difficulties depending on the ventilator system. When administered systemically, ribavirin can result in anemia, and in preclinical studies, has been shown to be terotogenic and mutagenic. In addition, possibly because of alteration of intracellular metabolic pools, ribavirin has immunosuppressive effects in experimental antimals [52]. Under most circumstances of use, it is possible to detect ribavirin in the environment of the hospital room. Although evaluation of exposed health care workers have generally not detected significant levels of ribavirin in blood, the drug has been detected in the urine of exposed nurses [54]. Therefore, it is recommended that pregnant women should be advised not to care directly for patients who are receiving ribavirin, and the drug should be administered in well-ventilated rooms.

Prophylaxis and Vaccination strategies

Influenza

Vaccination

Currently, inactivated influenza vaccines, consisting of either whole virus, detergent treated "split-product", or subunit HA/NA vaccines are licensed for the prevention of influenza. Because disease due to influenza A (H1N1), A (H3N2) and influenza B viruses may all occur in a single season, a trivalent vaccine is currently used. Inactivated vaccine is generated by growth of influenza viruses in embryonated hen's eggs. The virions are harvested from the egg allantoic fluid and inactivated by treatment with a chemical agent such as beta-propriolactone, and partially purified. Three preparations are licensed for use: whole virion vaccines; split-product or subvirion vaccines generated by treatment of the virions with detergent, or purified subunit vaccines that predominantly contain HA and NA protein. The safety and immunogenicity of each of these types of vaccines appears to be comparable in adults.

Randomized, placebo-controlled trials of modern influenza vaccines have demonstrated these vaccines to be well tolerated in all age groups. One-quarter to one-half of vaccine recipients feel some discomfort at the vaccine site 8 to 24 hours after vaccination, but only about 5 percent have moderately severe transient local pain and swelling. Systemic symptoms, such as malaise, headache, or myalgias, occur at a low rate similar to placebo. Systemic complaints may be more common in individuals with low levels of prevaccination antibody. Guillain-Barre syndrome has been reported after receipt of influenza vaccine in some years. During the 1976 National Immunization Program against swine influenza the estimated risk of acquiring GBS was 1 in 100,000 vaccinations [56]. National surveillance conducted since 1976 has generally not identified increased rates of this syndrome following vaccination. However, very slight increases in the risk of GBS were seen following the 1992-93 and 1993-94 vaccines, representing an excess of approximately 1 case per million persons vaccinated [57].

Inactivated influenza vaccine has been shown to be effective in the prevention of influenza A in both randomized cohort studies conducted in young adults, with levels of protection of 70 to 90% when there is a good antigenic match between vaccine and epidemic viruses [58]. However, when the antigenic relatedness of the vaccine strain and epidemic strain is low the effectiveness of inactivated vaccine effectiveness is considerably lower. Studies suggest that vaccines reduce the frequency of severe illness to a greater degree than the frequency of infection, in both young adults and in the elderly [59, 60]. Vaccination of healthy adults in the US was associated with decreased absenteeism from work or school and is significantly cost saving [61].

Relatively few prospective trials of protective efficacy have been conducted in high risk populations. In one recent randomized placebo controlled trial in an elderly population, inactivated vaccine was approximately 58% effective in preventing laboratory documented influenza [62]. In addition, numerous retrospective case-control studies are available which have documented the effectiveness of inactivated influenza vaccines in these individuals. A recent meta-analysis of published cohort observational trials derived a very similar estimate of 56% for the level of vaccine efficacy against influenza respiratory illness in the elderly [63]. Vaccine is protective against influenza and pneumonia related hospitalization in the elderly, and is even accompanied by a decrease in all-cause mortality [64]. A recently conducted Medicare demonstration project indicated that vaccine usage had a beneficial effect on reduction of hospital admissions associated with laboratory-documented influenza A or B infection [65]. It has been estimated that among elderly persons in the US, influenza vaccination is associated with a direct savings of $117 per year per person vaccinated [66]. It has also been suggested that vaccination of staff in chronic care facilities can have a major impact on mortality in elderly residents of these institutions [67].

Antiviral Prophylaxis

Prophylactic administration of amantadine has also been shown to prevent influenza due to H1N1, H2N2 and H3N2 influenza A viruses. The majority of studies have utilized a seasonal prophylaxis study design, in which subjects begin the drug at the beginning of influenza epidemic activity and continue prophylaxis for the duration of the epidemic, generally for from 4 to 8 weeks. The levels of protection against illness in adults associated with microbiologically documented influenza A virus infection have been reported as 70% [68] to 90% [53] against H1N1 viruses, and 68% against H3N2 viruses [69]. Seasonal prophylaxis has also been effective in children, in whom an approximately 90% reduction in laboratory confirmed illness due to influenza A H2N2 was reported [70, 71].

Amantadine has also been evaluated for the prevention of influenza in individuals exposed to an index case. These studies have been carried out in the family setting, in which members of a family receive prophylaxis for 10 days after exposure to an index case within the family. In studies where the index case was not treated with amantadine, protection of family contacts was noted [72]. However, if the index case was treated with amantadine at the same time as contacts received prophylaxis, no protection was seen [73], presumably because of the generation and transmission of amantadine-resistant virus in this setting.

Prophylaxis of contacts with amantadine has also been recommended in institutional settings such as nursing homes. There have never been controlled clinical trials documenting the efficacy of this approach, but anecdotal reports of significant decreases in the rate of influenza A cases after initiation of prophylaxis support the concept of outbreak-initiated prophylaxis [51, 74, 75]. Key features that contribute to the success of this strategy include rapid recognition and response to outbreaks, and isolation of individuals who are receiving treatment with amantadine from those who are receiving prophylaxis. Similar to the findings in the family setting, failure to adhere to this practice is associated with the development and transmission of resistant viruses within the institution [18, 76].

Significantly fewer studies of prophylaxis with rimantadine have been performed. However, when rimantadine and amantadine were directly compared in seasonal prophylaxis in healthy adults, the level of protection was approximately equal [53]. Rimantadine has also been evaluated in contact prophylaxis in the family setting, with results similar to those described for amantadine. When only contacts received prophylaxis, rimantadine resulted in significant protection [77, 78], but when the index case also received therapy with rimantadine, no protection was seen, and rimantadine-resistant viruses were recovered from prophylaxis failures [15]. Controlled studies of the prophylactic use of rimantadine in elderly or high-risk subjects have not been reported.

Neuraminidase inhibitors have also been shown to be effective in the prevention of influenza infection and illness. The first studies evaluated the use of zanamivir for seasonal prophylaxis [79], similar to the strategy used in evaluation of M2 inhibitors. In this study, adults were randomized to receive either zanamivir 10 mg once daily by inhalation, or placebo, beginning when an increase in influenza activity was documented at the study sites, and continuing for the next 4 weeks. The frequency of respiratory illness associated with microbiological documentation of influenza infection was reduced from 6% in the placebo group to 2% in the zanamivir group, resulting in 67% protective efficacy against this endpoint. The overall rates of all febrile respiratory illness, irrespective of the results of laboratory tests, were reduced by 43%, from 10% in the placebo group, to 6% in the zanamivir group. Oseltamivir has also been assessed in the seasonal prophylaxis model, where administration of oseltamivir at 75 mg once daily to healthy adults during the duration of the influenza season (6 weeks) was associated with a 74% reduction in the overall rate of respiratory illness associated with laboratory confirmed influenza infection, from 4.8% in the placebo group to 1.2% in those receiving oseltamivir [80]. In a recent study, oseltamivir was also reported to result in a 91% reduction in laboratory confirmed influenza in a vaccinated elderly population living in nursing homes or chronic care facilities [81].

These drugs have also been evaluated for prophylaxis of influenza in individuals after exposure to an index case have also been reported. In one study, [82] families in which one individual had acute influenza-like illness of 36 hours duration or less were randomized to either receive zanamivir (treatment of the index case with 10 mg bid x 5 days and prophylaxis of other family members with 10 mg qd. x 10 days) or placebo. Zanamivir prophylaxis was associated with a 79% reduction in the frequency with which one or more contacts developed influenza in the family, from 19% in families receiving placebo to 4% in families receiving zanamivir. Oseltamivir has also been tested for family prophylaxis with similar results. In this study, the index case did not receive treatment. However, prophylaxis of family members resulted in an 89% reduction in families experiencing illness [83].

The most frequent use of contact prophylaxis currently is for the termination of outbreaks within chronic care facilities. There have been several anectdotal reports of success when using zanamivir in this fashion [84]. In addition, zanamivir and rimantadine were recently compared in a prospective randomized trial of outbreak initiated prophylaxis [85]. In this study, use of zanamivir resulted in 61% fewer cases than seen in individuals randomized to receive either rimantadine (influenza A outbreaks) or no therapy (influenza B outbreaks). Of note, the majority of instances of failure of rimantadine prophylaxis were associated with infection with rimantadine resistant viruses.

Strategies For Prevention

The most efficient approach to prevention of influenza is the yearly administration of inactivated influenza vaccine. Influenza vaccine should be administered as a dose of 0.5 mL by intramuscular injection, to those 3 years of age and older, while younger children should receive 0.25 mL. Adults and older children should receive vaccine in the deltoid, while younger children are generally vaccinated in the anterolateral aspect of the thigh. Only a single dose of vaccine is required in individuals who been previously vaccinated or who have experienced prior infection with a related subtype, but a two dose schedule is required in children less than 9 who are receiving influenza vaccine for the first time and in other unprimed individuals [86, 87]. Use of a second dose of vaccine otherwise does not provide any additional benefit [88]. Whole virus vaccines should be avoided in children under 12 years of age as they are associated with relatively higher rates of fever in this age group.

It is possible to identify certain individuals who are at particularly high risk of influenza related hospitalizations and deaths, and towards whom programs of vaccination should be particularly directed. The currently recommended target groups for influenza vaccination are summarized in Table 5. Specific recommendations regarding target groups are reviewed each year and updated [89]. Additional individuals in whom vaccination is recommended include individuals such as health care workers, who can transmit virus to others at high risk, individuals infected with HIV, and high-risk individuals who will be traveling to an area where influenza epidemics are occurring. While it is relatively easy to identify such individuals, it is not always easy to deliver vaccine to them. Rates of influenza immunization in individuals 65 and older in the U.S. have risen dramatically, and now exceed the 60% "healthy people 2000" goal in all 50 states. However, the vaccine coverage rate in high-risk individuals under 65 is considerably lower, estimated to be approximately 30% to 35%.

Antiviral drugs could also be considered for prevention in certain limited circumstances. At the moment, only amantadine and rimantadine are licensed for the prevention of influenza, so that currently licensed antiviral strategies currently would be effective only for prevention of influenza A. In, individuals are administered the antiviral drug for the duration of potential exposure. As reviewed earlier, the seasonal prophylaxis strategy has been the basis for multiple clinical trials demonstrating the prophylactic activity of the M2 and neuraminidase inhibitors. In this is fairly obviously not a practical solution for the general use, but seasonal prophylaxis should be considered in particularly high-risk individuals who cannot be vaccinated or would not be expected to respond to vaccination at all. In addition, seasonal prophylaxis would be one method of dealing with a situation in which the vaccine did not include the prevalent epidemic strain, such as during a pandemic. However, there might be expected to be significant logistic and supply difficulties with the use of antiviral prophylaxis on such a large scale.

Antiviral drugs can also be used for short-term prevention. One scenario is the individual who is not vaccinated until influenza epidemic activity has already begun. Under these circumstances, it is reasonable to use antivirals until vaccine immunity has been established. Because immunity develops quite rapidly following inactivated vaccine in adults, generally 2 weeks of prophylaxis after vaccination is recommended. The other form of short-term prophylaxis that is commonly employed is after exposure, either in the family or institutional setting. As described above, there is good evidence to support the effectiveness of a 7-10 day administration of antivirals to contacts after a family member develops acute influenza. For the most part, this strategy would be appropriate in the setting of a high-risk individual within the family, but under unusual circumstances (e.g., a vacation or other important life event) such a strategy could be considered in healthy persons. Because of the possibility of generation and transmission of resistant influenza viruses, the success of this strategy when M2 inhibitors are utilized depends on not also using M2 inhibitors to treat the index case. It is not clear whether such a proscription would be important for neuraminidase inhibitors as well.

The more common use of short term prophylaxis is after potential exposure in the institutional setting. In this situation, the recipients have generally already been vaccinated, but constitute a group in whom vaccine efficacy may not be ideal, and in whom the potential consequences of influenza demand that every additional effort be taken to prevent infection. There is surprisingly little placebo-controlled data to support the use of outbreak-initiated prophylaxis with any antiviral, but the experience with family studies and various anecdotal reports suggest that there may be some benefit to this approach. If outbreak initiated prophylaxis is to be used, it is essential that it be instituted promptly to be most effective, since influenza can spread rapidly in the institutional setting, and the peak of the outbreak may occur only a few days after recognition of the index case. Therefore, programs that utilize standing orders are generally more successful. Rapid diagnostic tests for detection of influenza may also be quite useful in this regard, since the clinical presentation of influenza in this population can be muted and difficult to differentiate from other respiratory viruses such as RSV and rhinovirus. Although these tests may have lower sensitivity than culture, the aggregate sensitivity in detecting at least one positive out of several samples should be adequate to allow early recognition and response to influenza outbreaks. For any individual outbreak, the recommended duration of prophylaxis is from 2 to 3 weeks, or for one week beyond the last documented case. For the same reasons as described for family prophylaxis, isolation of individuals receiving treatment with M2 inhibitors from individuals receiving prophylaxis with M2 inhibitors is important to reduce the generation and spread of resistant viruses. Alternatively, one could consider treatment with one class of agent (e.g., neuraminidase inhibitors) and prophylaxis with the other class (e.g. M2 inhibitors).

Respiratory Syncytial Virus

Passive Antibody

Passive immunization has received considerable attention for both the treatment and prevention of respiratory syncytial virus infection. This strategy is based on early observations that passively transferred antibody to either the F or G protein prevented infection in experimental animals and was also effective therapeutically. Although therapeutic administration of antibody has not resulted in clinical benefit in humans [90], prophylaxis with passive antibody has been successful in selected infants. Initial studies utilized selected pools of immunoglobulin screened for high titers of RS virus neutralizing antibody, referred to as RSV-IGIV (RespiGam) [91]. When administered intravenously at monthly intervals during RSV seasonal activity, RSV-IGIV was shown to reduce the incidence of RSV-related respiratory hospitalizations in infants with prematurity or bronchopulmonary dysplasia [92, 93]. The currently recommended dose of RSV-IVIG is 750 mg/kg IV monthly during the RSV season. However, administration of this agent involves administration of large volumes of fluid, and children with cyanotic congenital heart disease who received RSV-IGIV had a higher incidence of severe adverse events, and those that went on to have cardiac surgery had enhanced mortality [94]. Thus, this product is considered to be contraindicated in infants with cyanotic congenital heart disease [45].

One approach to circumventing the problem of the large volumes of RSV-IVIG that must be administered is the use of humanized monoclonal antibodies with very high RS virus neutralizing titers [95]. Paluvizumab (Synagis) is a humanized monoclonal antibody directed against a conserved region of the F protein with high-titered neutralizing activity against RSV. When administered intramuscularly at monthly intervals to premature infants or infants with chronic lung disease, paluvizumab was shown to result in a 55% reduction in RSV hospitalizations, as well as in reductions in total days of RSV hospitalization, O_2 requirements, and ICU admissions [96].

The recommended dose of this agent is 15 mg/kg intramuscularly once monthly during the RSV season [97]. Of note, although this product is a humanized, rather than human, monoclonal, development of antibody to paluvizumab has not been reported in infant recipients, and its use has not been associated with significant adverse events.

Vaccines

The success of passive antibody approaches suggests that under the right circumstances, prevention of severe disease due to RS virus by active immunization is a reasonable goal. The traumatic experience of enhanced disease with inactivated RS virus vaccine remains a major obstacle to further vaccine development. Initial attempts to develop a vaccine for RS virus involved use of formalin inactivated virus. However, this vaccine failed to provide protection in field trials carried out in the 1960s, despite inducing high levels of RS virus antibodies. Instead, subjects who received vaccine experienced enhanced disease with subsequent RS virus infection, compared to others who received control vaccines. The mechanism of this enhancement remains unknown. At the moment there is no commercially available vaccine for the prevention of RSV, although several are in clinical development.

Strategies For Prevention

The cornerstone of prevention of RSV remains the institution of appropriate infection control practices, as vaccination is not currently available, and immunoglobulin prophylaxis is currently only recommended for limited categories of patients. Immunoglobulin prophylaxis should be considered for infants and children less than 2 years of age with chronic lung disease who are receiving medical management on a long-term basis (e.g., have required medical therapy within the previous 6 months) [97]. The benefit for this group has mostly been shown for the first RSV season, and there are limited data on the effectiveness of prophylaxis during a second season of exposure. Another group to consider for prophylaxis are infants born at 32 weeks of gestation or earlier. Because such children generally have low levels of maternal antibody, they are at higher risk for severe disease. Children with congenital cyanotic heart disease or with immunodeficiencies could also theoretically benefit from prophylaxis, but data supporting the efficacy of either preparation in these conditions are not available.

There are several potential advantages of paluvisumab over RSV-IVIG for the prevention of RSV infection, including the relative ease and convenience of IM compared to IV administration, the considerably smaller volumes of fluid administered, and the fact that paluvisumab is not a human blood-derived product. For this reason, paluvisumab is generally favored for most clinical circumstances. In addition, RSV-IVIG is contraindicated in children with cyanotic congenital heart disease. However, RSV-IVIG, likely because it contains polyclonal antibodies to a variety of pathogens, is associated with decreased rates of non-RSV respiratory hospitalizations. Thus, this product might be a consideration for infants in whom fluid considerations are not paramount and who already have IV access, for example infants with severe combined immunodeficiency disease or other recipients of chronic immunoglobulin therapy.

Table 1.   Viral respiratory syndromes

Disease Syndrome	Age group	Modifying circumstances	Predominant etiologies
Common cold	Any	Any	Rhinovirus, coronavirus, RSV, parainfluenza viruses
Otitis media	Children	Any	Respiratory syncytial virus, influenza, others
Croup	Children	Any	Parainfluenza, influenza, measles
Acute bronchitis	Any	Any	None established
Bronchiolitis	Infants and children	Any	Respiratory syncytial virus, influenza, measles
Influenza-like illness	Any	Any	Influenza virus, RSV, parainfluenza
Viral pneumonia	Children	Healthy	RSV, parainfluenza, measles, influenza
	Adults	Healthy	Influenza, adenovirus
		Immunocompromised	CMV, HSV, RSV

Table 2.   Diagnostic tests for viral respiratory diseases

Test	Application	Examples	Advantages	Disadvantages
Cell culture	All viruses	MDCK (influenza), Hep2 (RSV)	Gold standard for diagnosis High sensitivity Virus available for study	Requires cell culture Time consuming
Antigen detection	Influenza RSV	Directigen Flu OIA Directigen	Very rapid Least amount of operator skill	Somewhat insensitive compared to cell culture
Genome detection	All viruses	Nucleic acid hybridization PCR	Highly sensitive Adaptable for all viruses	Technically complex Expensive Takes longer than antigen detection

Table 3. Treatment strategies

Virus	Modifying circumstances	Primary therapy	Alternate therapy
Influenza A	Healthy adults < 48 hours	Amantadine/Rimantadine[1]	Zanamivir/Oseltamivir
	Immunocompromised	Zanamivir/Oseltamivir[2]	
	Children[3]	Amantadine	Rimantadine, Oseltamivir, Zanamivir
	Elderly	Rimantadine[4]	Oseltamivir, zanamivir
	Institutional outbreak[5]	Oseltamivir, zanamivir	Rimantadine, amantadine
Influenza B	Any	Oseltamivir, zanamivir	
RSV	Severely ill[6]	Ribavirin	
	Immunocompromised	Ribavirin (?+IG)[7]	
	All others	Supportive care	
Parainfluenza	All[8]	Supportive care	
Rhinovirus	All[8]	Supportive care	

1 – All licensed drugs appear to have equivalent efficacy, so choice is often made on basis of cost.

2 – Use of M2 inhibitors in immunocompromised individuals is associated with high rates of development of resistant virus and treatment failure

3 – Only amantadine currently licensed for treatment of children, zanamivir licensed to age 7, oseltamivir application for use in children 1 year of age and older is pending review

4 – Amantadine is associated with frequent CNS toxicity in this age group

5 – Consider use of NI for treatment if other individuals in institution are receiving prophylaxis with M2 inhibitor

6 – See American Academy of Pediatrics guidelines [44]

7 – IG = immunoglobulin. No data from randomized controlled trials support use, but success rate with ribavirin alone is poor

8 – There is no approved therapy available at this time

Table 4.   Doses and side effects

Agent	Modifying circumstances	Dose	Adverse effects
Amantadine	Children 1-9 years	5 mg/kg/day upt to 150 mg/day in two divided doses	CNS, GI
	Ages 10 to 64	100 mg bid	
	≥65 yrs	100 mg qd	
	Cr Cl ≤ 50 mL/min	See package insert	
Rimantadine	Children	Not licensed for this application	GI, CNS (rare)
	Aged 14-64	100 mg bid	
	≥65	100 mg or qd or bid	
	Cr Cl ≤ 10 mL/min	100 mg qd	
	Severe hepatic dysfunction	100 mg qd	
Zanamivir	Ages 7 and above	2 inhalations (10 mg) bid	Bronchospasm (rare)
	Renal and hepatic impairment	Limited data, dose reduction does not appear to be needed	
Oseltamivir	Ages 18 and above	75 mg bid	Nausea and vomiting
	Cr Cl < 30 mL/min	75 mg qd	
	Hepatic dysfunction	Not studied	
Ribavirin	Infants with severe RSV	20 mg/mL continuous small particle aerosol for 12-20 hours per day	Reversible bronchospasm (rare)

Derived from [89]

Table 5.   Groups at increased risk of influenza complications, for whom annual vaccination is recommended [89].

- Persons aged 50 years or greater
- Residents of nursing homes or other chronic care facilities
- Adults and children with chronic disorders of the pulmonary or cardiovascular systems, including asthma
- Adults and children with chronic metabolic diseases (including diabetes mellitus), renal dysfunction, hemoglobinopathies, or immunosuppression (including HIV).
- Children and teenagers receiving long-term aspirin therapy.
- Women who will be in the second or third trimester of pregancy

References

1. Dolin R. Antiviral chemotherapy and chemoprophylaxis. Science 1985; 227: 1296-1303
2. Douglas RG, Jr. Prophylaxis and treatment of influenza. N Engl J Med 1990; 322: 443-450
3. Togo Y, Hornick RB, Felitti VJ, et al. Evaluation of the therapeutic efficacy of amantadine in patients with naturally occurring A2 influenza. JAMA 1970; 211: 1149-1156
4. Hornick RB, Togo Y, Mahler S, Iezzoni D. Evaluation of amantadine hydrochloride in the treatment of A2 influenzal disease. Bull WHO 1969; 41: 671-676
5. Knight V, Fedson D, Baldini J, Douglas RG, Jr., Couch RB. Amantadine therapy of epidemic influenza A2/Hong Kong. Antimicrob Agents Chemother 1969: 370-371
6. Galbraith AW, Oxford JS, Schild GC, Potter CW, Watson GI. Therapeutic effect of 1-adamantanamine hydrochloride in naturally occurring influenza A2/Hong Kong infection. Lancet 1971; 1: 113-115
7. Little J, Hall W, Douglas RG, Jr., Hyde RW, Speers DM. Amantadine effect on peripheral airways abnormalities in influenza. Ann Intern Med 1976; 85: 177-182
8. Little JW, Hall WJ, Douglas RG, Jr., Mudholkar GS, Speers DM, Patel K. Airway hyperreactivity and peripheral airway dysfunction in influenza A infection. Am Rev Respir Dis 1978; 118: 295-303
9. Van Voris LP, Betts RF, Hayden FG, Christmas WA, Douglas RG, Jr. Successful treatment of naturally occurring influenza A/USSR/77 H1N1. JAMA 1981; 245: 1128-1131
10. Younkin SW, Betts RF, Roth FK, Douglas RG, Jr. Reduction in fever and symptoms in young adults with influenza A/Brazil/78 H1N1 infection after treatment with aspirin or amantadine. Antimicrob Agents Chemother 1983; 23: 577-582
11. Hayden FG, Monto AS. Oral rimantadine hydrochloride therapy of influenza A virus H3N2 subtype infection in adults. Antimicrob Agents Chemother 1986; 29: 339-341
12. Hall CB, Dolin R, Gala CL, et al. Children with influenza A infection: treatment with rimantadine. Pediatrics 1987; 80: 275-282
13. Thompson J, Fleet W, Lawrence E, Pierce E, Morris L, Wright P. A comparison of acetaminophen and rimantadine in the treatment of influenza A infection in children. J Med Virol 1987; 21: 249-255
14. Betts RF, Treanor J, Braman P, Bentley D, Dolin R. Antiviral agents to prevent or treat influenza in the elderly. J Respir Dis 1987; 8: S56-S59
15. Hayden FG, Belshe RB, Clover RD, Hay AJ, Oakes MG, Soo W. Emergence and apparent transmission of rimantadine-resistant influenza A virus in families. N Engl J Med 1989; 321: 1696-1702
16. Hayden FG, Sperber SJ, Belshe RB, Clover RD, Hay AJ, Pyke S. Recovery of drug-resistant influenza A virus during therapeutic use of rimantadine. Antimicrob Agents Chemother 1991; 35: 1741-1747
17. Belshe RB, Burk B, Newman F, Curruti RL, Sim I. Resistance of influenza A virus to amantadine and rimantadine: results of one decade of surveillance. J Infect Dis 1989; 159: 430-435
18. Degelau J, Somani SK, Cooper SL, Guay DRP, Crossley KB. Amantadine-resistant influenza A in a nursing facility. Arch Intern Med 1992; 152: 390-392
19. Gubareva LV, Kaiser L, Hayden FG. Influenza virus neuraminidase inhibitors. Lancet 2000; 355: 827-835
20. Hayden FG, Osterhaus ADME, Treanor JJ, et al. Efficacy and safety of the neuraminidase inhibitor zanamivir in the treatment of influenzavirus infections. N Engl J Med 1997; 337: 874-880
21. MIST. Randomised trial of efficacy and safety of inhaled zanamivir in treatment of influenza A and B virus infections. Lancet 1998; 352: 1877-1881
22. Makela MJ, Pauksens K, Rostila T, et al. Clinical efficacy and safety of the orally inhaled neuraminidase inhibitor zanamivir in the treatment of influenza: a randomized, double-blind, placebo-controlled

European study. J Infect 2000; 40: 42-48

23. Treanor JJ, Hayden FG, Vrooman PS, et al. Efficacy and safety of the oral neuraminidase inhibitor oseltamivir in treating acute influenza: a randomized, controlled trial. JAMA 2000; 283: 1016-1024

24. Nicholson KG, Aoki FY, Osterhaus ADME, et al. Efficacy and safety of oseltamivir in treatment of acute influenza: a randomized controlled trial. Lancet 2000; 355: 1845-1850

25. Lalezari J, Elliott M, Keene O. The efficacy and safety of inhaled zanamivir in the treatment of influenza A and B in 'high-risk' individuals - results of phase II and III clinical studies. [Abstr]: 39th Interscience Conference on Antimicrobial Agents and Chemotherapy. San Francisco, CA: , 1999

26. Lalezari J, Griffin AD, Edmundson S. The impact of zanamivir on resoruce use in the treatment of influenza. [Abstr]: 37th Annual Meeting of the Infectious Diseases Society of America. Philadelphia, PA: , 1999

27. Kaiser L, Hayden FG, Hammond JMJ, Keene O. Efficacy of inhaled zanamivir in reducing complications and antibiotic use in influenza - results of phase II and III clinical studies. [Abstr]: 39th Annual Interscience Conference on Antimicrobial Agents and Chemotherapy. San Francisco, CA: , 1999

28. Martin C, Mahoney P, Ward P. Oral oseltamivir reduces febrile illness in patients considered at hihg risk of influenza complications. [Abstr]: Options for the Control of Influenza IV. Crete: , 2000

29. Hayden FG, Reisinger KS, Whitley R, et al. Oral oseltamivir is effective and safe in children for the treatment of acute influenza A and B. [Abstr]: Options for the Control of Influenza IV. Crete: , 2000

30. Barnett JM, Cadman A, Gor D, et al. Zanamivir susceptibility monitoring and characterization of influenza virus clinical isolates obtained during phase II clinical efficacy studies. Antimicrob Agents Chemother 2000; 44: 78-87

31. Gubareva LV, Matrosovich MN, Brenner MK, Bethell RC, Webster RG. Evidence for zanamivir resistance in an immunocompromised child infected with influenza B virus. J Infect Dis 1998; 178: 1257-1262

32. Gilbert BE, Knight V. Biochemistry and clinical applications of ribavirin. Antimicrob Agents Chemother 1986; 30: 201-205

33. Hall CB, McBride JT, Walsh EE, et al. Aerosolized ribavirin treatment of infants with respiratory syncytial viral infection: a randomized double-blind study. N Engl J Med 1983; 308: 1443-1447

34. Taber LH, Knight V, Gilbert BE, et al. Ribavirin aerosol treatment of bronchiolitis associated with respiratory syncytial virus infection in infants. Pediatrics 1983; 72: 613-618

35. Barry W, Cockburn F, Cornall R, Price JF, Sutherland G, Vardag A. Ribavirin aerosol for acute brochiolitis. Arch Dis Child 1986; 61: 593-597

36. Conrad DA, Christenson JC, Waner JL, Marks MI. Aerosolized ribavirin treatment of respiratory syncytial virus infection in infants hospitalized during an epidemic. Pediatr Infect Dis J 1987; 6: 152-158

37. Rodriguez WJ, Kim HW, Brandt CD, al e. Aerosolized ribavirin in the treament of patients with respiratory syncytial virus diseases. Pediatr Infect Dis J 1987; 6: 159-163

38. Hall CB, McBride JT, Gala CL, Hildreth SW, Schnabel KC. Ribavirin treatment of respiratory syncytial viral infection in infants with underlying cardiopulmonary disease. JAMA 1985; 254: 3047-3051

39. Smith DW, Frankel LR, Mathers LH, Tang ATS, Ariagno RL, Prober CG. A controlled trial of aerosolized ribavirin in infants receiving mechanical ventilation for severe respiratory syncytial virus infection. N Engl J Med 1991; 325: 24-29

40. Wheeler JG, Wofford J, Turner RB. Historical cohort evaluation of ribavirin efficacy in respiratory syncytial virus infection. Pediatr Infect Dis J 1993; 12: 209-213

41. Meert KL, Sarnaik AP, Gelmini MJ, Lich-Lai MW. Aerosolized ribavirin in mechanically ventilated children with respiratory syncytial virus lower respiratory tract disease: a prospective, double-blind,

randomized trial. Crit Care Med 1994; 22: 566-572

42. Law BJ, Wang EE, MacDonald N, et al. Does ribavirin impact on the hospital course of children with respiratory syncytial virus (RSV) infection? An analysis using the pediatric investigators collaborative network on infections in Canada (PICNIC) RSV database. Pediatrics 1997; 99: E7

43. Guerguerian AM, Gauthier M, Lebel MH, Farrell CA, Lacroix J. Ribavirin in ventilated respiratory syncytial virus bronchiolitis. A randomized, placebo-controlled trial. Am J Resp Crit Care Med 1999; 160; 829-34

44. American Academy of Pediatrics. Reassessment of the indications for ribavirin therapy in respiratory syncytial virus infections. Pediatrics 1996; 97: 137-140

45. American Academy of Pediatrics. Respiratory syncytial virus. In: Peter G, ed. 1997 Red Book: Report of the committee on infectious diseases. 24 ed. Elkgrove Village, IL: American Academy of Pediatrics, 1997; 443-447

46. Sable CA, Hayden FG. Orthomyxoviral and paramyxoviral infections in transplant recipients. Infect Transplant 1995; 9: 987-1003

47. DeVincenzo JP, Hirsch RL, Fuentes RJ, Top Jr FH. Respiratory syncytial virus immune globulin treatment of lower respiratory tract infection in pediatric patients undergoing bone marrow transplantation - a compassionate use experience. Bone Marrow Transpl 2000; 25: 161-165

48. Adams R, Christenson J, Petersen F, Beatty P. Pre-emptive use of aerosolized ribavirin in the treatment of asymptomatic pediatric marrow transplant patients testing positive for RSV. Bone Marrow Transpl 1999; 24: 661-4

49. Ghosh S, Champlin RE, Englund J, et al. Respiratory syncytial virus upper respiratory tract illnesses in adult blood and marrow transplant recipients: combination therapy with aerosolized ribavirin and intravenous immunoglobulin. Bone Marrow Transpl 2000; 25: 751-755

50. Degelau J, Somani S, Cooper SL, Irvine PW. Occurrence of adverse effects and high amantadine concentrations with influenza prophylaxis in the nursing home. J Am Geriatr Soc 1990; 38: 428-432

51. Atkinson WL, Arden NH, Patriarca PA, Leslie N, Lui K-J, Gohd R. Amantadine prophylaxis during an institutional outbreak of type A (H1N1) influenza. Arch Intern Med 1986; 146: 1751-1756

52. Hayden FG. Antiviral drugs (other than antiretrovirals). In: Mandell GL, Bennett JE, Dolin R, eds. Mandell, Douglas, and Bennett's Principles and Practice of Infectious Diseases. 5 ed. Philadelphia: Churchill Livingstone, 2000: 460-490

53. Dolin R, Reichman RC, Madore HP, Maynard R, Linton PN, Webber-Jones J. A controlled trial of amantadine and rimantadine in the prophylaxis of influenza A in humans. N Engl J Med 1982; 307: 580-584

54. American Academy of Pediatrics. Use of ribavirin in the treatment of respiratory syncytial virus infection. Pediatrics 1993; 92: 501-504

55. Englund JA, Piedra PA, Ahn YM, Gilbert BE, Hiatt P. High-dose, short-duration ribavirin aerosol therapy compared with standard ribavirin therapy in children with suspected respiratory syncytial virus infection. J Pediatr 1994; 125: 635-41

56. Schonberger LB, Bregman DJ, Sullivan-Bolyai JZ, et al. Guillan-Barre syndrome following vaccination in the national influenza immunizaiotn program, United States, 1976-1977. Am J Epidemiol 1979; 110: 105-123

57. Lasky T, Tarracciano GJ, Magder L, et al. The Guillan-Barre syndrome and the 1992-1993 and 1993-1994 influenza vaccines. N Engl J Med 1998; 339: 1797-1802

58. Meiklejohn G, Eickhoff TC, Graves P, I J. Antigenic drift and efficacy of influenza virus vaccines, 1976-1977. J Infect Dis 1978; 138: 618-624

59. Gross PA, Quinnan GV, Rodstein M, et al. Association of influenza immunization with reduction in mortality in an elderly population: a prospective study. Arch Intern Med 1988; 148: 562-565

60. Keitel WA, Cate TR, Couch RB. Efficacy of sequential annual vaccination with inactivated influenza virus vaccine. Am J Epidemiol 1988; 127: 353-64

61. Nichol KL, Lind A, Margolis KL, et al. The effectiveness of vaccination against influenza in healthy, working adults. N Engl J Med 1995; 333: 889-893

62. Govaert TM, Thijs CT, Masurel N, Sprenger MJ, Dinant GJ, Knottnerus JA. The efficacy of influenza vaccination in elderly individuals. A randomized double-blind placebo-controlled trial. JAMA 1994; 272: 1956-1961

63. Gross PA, Hermogenes AW, Sacks HS, Lau J, Levandowski RA. The efficacy of influenza vaccine in elderly persons: a meta-analysis and review of the literature. Ann Intern Med 1995; 123: 518-527

64. Fedson DS, Wajda A, Nicol JP, Hammond GW, Kalser DL, Roos LL. Clinical effectivenss of influenza vaccination in Manitoba. JAMA 1993; 270: 1956-1961

65. Bennett NM, Lewis B, Doniger AS, et al. A coordinated, community wide program in Monroe County, New York, to increase influenza immunization rates in the elderly. Arch Intern Med 1994; 154: 1741-1745

66. Nichol KL, Margolis KL, Wuorenma J, Von Sternberg T. The efficacy and cost effectiveness of vaccination against influenza among elderly persons living in the community. N Engl J Med 1994; 331: 778-784

67. Potter J, Stott DJ, Roberts Ma, et al. Influenza vaccination of health care workers in long-term-care hospitals reduces the mortality of elderly patients. J Infect Dis 1997; 175: 1-6

68. Monto AS, Gunn RA, Bandyk MG, King CL. Prevention of Russian influenza by amantadine. JAMA 1979; 241: 1003-1007

69. Oker-Blom N, Hovi T, Leinikki P, Palosuo T, Pettersson R, Suni J. Protection of man from natural infection with influenza A2 Hong Kong virus by amantadine: a controlled field trial. Br Med J 1970; 3: 676-678

70. Quilligan JJ, Harayama M, Baernstein HD, Jr. The suppression of A2 influenza in children by the chemoprophylactic use of amantadine. J Pediatr 1966; 69: 572-575

71. Finklea JF, Hennessy AV, Davenport FM. A field trial of amantadine prophylaxis in naturally occurring acute respiratory illness. Am J Epidemiol 1967; 85: 403-412

72. Galbraith AW, Oxford JS, Schild GC. Protective effect of 1-adamantanamine hydrochloride on influenza A2 in the family environment. Lancet 1969; 2: 1026-1028

73. Galbraith AW, Oxford JS, Schild GC, Watson GI. Study of 1-adamantanamine hydrochloride used prophylactically during the Hong Kong influenza epidemic in the family environment. Bull WHO 1969; 41: 677-682

74. Arden NH, Patriarca PA, Fasano MB, et al. The roles of vaccination and amantadine prophylaxis in controlling an outbreak of influenza A(H3N2) in a nursing home. Arch Intern Med 1988; 148: 865-868

75. Patriarca PA, Arden NH, Koplan JP, Goodman RA. Prevention and control of type A influenza infections in nursing homes: benefits and costs of four approaches using vaccination and amantadine. Ann Intern Med 1987; 107: 732-740

76. Mast EE, Harman MW, Gravenstein S, et al. Emergence and possible transmission of amantadine-resistant viruses during nursing home outbreaks of influenza A(H3N2). Am J Epidemiol 1991; 134: 988-997

77. Clover RD, Crawford SA, Abell TD, Ramsey CN, Jr., Glezen WP, Couch RB. Effectiveness of

rimantadine prophylaxis of children within families. Am J Dis Child 1986; 140: 706-709

78. Crawford SA, Clover RD, Abell TD, Ramsey CR, Jr., Glezen WP, Couch RB. Rimantadine prophylaxis in children: a follow-up study. Pediatr Infect Dis J 1988; 7: 379-383

79. Monto AS, Robinson DP, Herlocher ML, Hinson JM, Jr., Elliot MJ, Crisp A. Zanamivir in the prevention of influenza among healthy adults: a randomized controlled trial. JAMA 1999; 282: 31-35

80. Hayden FG, Atmar RL, Schilling M, et al. Use of the selective oral neuraminidase inhibitor oseltamivir to prevent influenza. N Engl J Med 1999; 341: 1336-1346

81. de Bock V, Peters P, T-A vP, et. al. Prophylaxis of influenza infection in the frail elderly by oseltamivir. [Abstr]: ECCMID. Stockholm 2000

82. Hayden FG, Gubareva LV, Monto AS, et al. Inhaled zanamivir for the prevention of influenza in families. N Engl J Med 2000; 343: 1282-1289

83. Oxford J. Short term prophylaxis with oseltamivir effectively prevents the spread of influenza A and B. [Abstr]: Second International Symposium on Influenza and Other Respiratory Viruses. Cancun, Mexico: , 1999

84. Lee C, Loeb M, Phillips A, et al. Use of zanamivir to control an outbreak of influenza A. [Abstr]: 39th Interscience Conference on Antimicrobial Agents and Chemotherapy. San Francisco, CA: , 1999

85. Gravenstein S, Drinka P, Osterweil D, et al. A multicenter prospective double-blind randomized controlled trial comparing the relative safety and efficacy of zanamivir to rimantadine for nursing home influenza outbreak control. [Abstr]: Options for the Control of Influenza IV. Crete: , 2000

86. Wright PF, Thompson J, Vaughn WT, Folland DS, Sell SHW, Karzon DT. Trials of influenza A/New Jersey/76 virus vaccine in normal children: an overview of age-related antigenicity and reactogenicity. J Infect Dis 1977; 136: S731-S741

87. Wright PF, Cherry Jd, Foy HM, et al. Antigenicity and reactogenicity of influenza A/USSR/77 virus vaccine in children - a multicentered evaluation of dosage and toxicity. Rev Infect Dis 1983; 5: 758-764

88. Gross PA, Weksler ME, Quinnan GVJ, Douglas RG, Jr., Gaerlan PF, Denning CR. Immunization of elderly people with two doses of influenza vaccine. J Clin Microbiol 1987; 25: 1763-1765

89. CDC. Prevention and control of influenza: recommendations of the advisory committee on immunization practices (ACIP). MMWR 2000; 49 (RR-3): 1-30

90. Rodriguez WJ. Management strategies for respiratory syncytial virus infections in infants. J Pediatr 1999; 135: 45-50

91. Siber GR, Leszczynski J, Pena-Cruz V, et al. Protective activity of a human respiratory syncytial virus immune globulin prepared from donors screened by microneutralization assay. J Infect Dis 1992; 165: 456-463

92. Groothuis JR, Simoes EAF, Levin MJ, et al. Prophylactic administration of respiratory syncytial virus immune globulin to high-risk infants and young children. N Engl J Med 1993; 329: 1524-1530

93. Connor E, and the PREVENT study group. Reduction of respiratory syncytial virus hospitalization among premature infants and infants with bronchopulmonary dysplasia using respiratory syncytial virus immune globulin prophylaxis. Pediatrics 1997; 99: 93-99

94. Simoes EA, Sondheimer HM, Top FH, Jr., et al. Respiratory syncytial virus immune globulin for prophylaxis against respiratory syncytial virus disease in infants and children with congenital heart disease. The Cardiac Study Group. J Pediatr 1998; 133: 492-9

95. Johnson S, Oliver C, Prince GA, et al. Development of a humanized monoclonal antibody (MEDI-493) with potent *in vitro* and *in vivo* activity against respiratory syncytial virus. J Infect Dis 1997; 176: 1215-1224

96. IMPACT RSV Study Group. Paluvizumab, a humanized respiratory syncytial virus monoclonal antibody,

reduces hospitalization from respiratory syncytial virus infection in high-risk infants. Pediatrics 1998; 102: 531-537

97.   American Academy of Pediatrics. Prevention of respiratory syncytial virus infections: Indications for the use of palivizumab and update on the use of RSV-IGIV. Pediatrics 1998; 102: 1211-12116

CHAPTER 11

PAPILLOMAVIRUSES

RICHARD REICHMAN and MARGARET STANLEY

Table of Contents

General Introduction

Human papillomaviruses (HPV) infect epithelial tissues of skin and mucous membranes, producing both benign and malignant neoplasms [1]. Alternatively, infection may be asymptomatic, leading to a latent state and the possible development of disease after prolonged periods of time. HPV are members of the Papillomavirus genus of the family Papovaviridae. They are nonenveloped viruses, 50 to 55 nm in diameter, and have

Practical Guidelines in Antiviral Therapy Ed. by Charles A.B. Boucher and George J. Galasso. 257 — 278 icosahedral capsids containing a double-stranded, circular DNA genome. HPV types are highly tissue specific and are distinguished from one another by degree of nucleic acid sequence homology. More than 100 HPV types are recognized, and individual types are associated with specific clinical manifestations [2] (Table 1). For example, the vast majority of plantar warts are caused by HPV-1 and most common warts are caused by HPV-2. HPV-6 and HPV-11 account for most anogenital warts, and HPV 16 DNA can be detected in approximately one half of all cervical cancers [3]. HPVs are also highly species specific, and have not been propagated in common experimental animals or in routine tissue culture systems. However, some HPV types have been grown in human tissues implanted in immunodeficient mice [4-6].

Table 1.   Human papillomavirus (HPV) diseases and associated virus types

Disease	Age Group	Principal HPV Type (s)
Common warts	Children	2, 1
Plantar warts	Adolescents	1, 2
Flat warts	Children	3, 10
Anogenital warts	Young adults	6, 11, 42, 43, 44
Intraepithelial dysplasias, cancers	Adults	16, 18, 31, 33, 35, 45
Respiratory papillomatosis	Children, adults	11, 6
Epidermodysplasia verruciformis	Life long	5, 8, many others

Few good studies have been performed to determine the incidence or prevalence of HPV disease in well-defined populations [7, 8]. Common warts (verruca vulgaris) are most prevalent among young children, occurring in as many as 25 percent of some groups. Plantar warts (verruca plantaris) occur most often among adolescents and young adults. Condyloma acuminatum (pl. condylomata acuminata, anogenital warts) is one of the most common sexually transmitted diseases worldwide, and HPV infections of the uterine cervix produce the most frequently detected abnormalities on Papanicolaou smears [9].

Most genital HPV infection is transmitted through sexual contact with infectious lesions. Intimate personal contact is assumed also to play a major role in the transmission of most cutaneous warts; the importance of fomites is not clear. Inapparent or minor trauma at the site of inoculation may facilitate transmission. Recurrent respiratory papillomatosis in young children is acquired from maternal genital tract infection but is an uncommon disease. Orogenital sexual contact may transmit the disease among adults.

Throughout the world, infection with oncogenic or high risk HPV types produces the vast majority of cancer of the uterine cervix [3], although most cervical HPV infections are self-limited. More than 95 percent of cervical cancers contain oncogenic HPV DNA, and HPV DNA is also present in cervical intraepithelial neoplasias (CIN), the precursor lesions of cervical cancer. Infection with HPV has also been associated with squamous cell carcinomas and dysplasias of the penis, anus, vagina, and vulva [2, 10, 11].

In patients with epidermodysplasia verruciformis, a rare dermatologic disease character-ized by extreme susceptibility to HPV infection, squamous cell cancers develop frequently, particularly in sun exposed areas [12].

Clinical Diagnosis

Most warts that can be easily seen can be diagnosed correctly on the basis of a carefully performed medical history and physical examination. Colposcopy is an essential component of the evaluation of vaginal and cervical disease and can also be helpful in the assessment of oral and cutaneous lesions.

Most cutaneous warts are easily recognized [13]. Common warts occur most frequently on the hands as flesh-colored to brown, exophytic, hyperkeratotic papules. Plantar warts can be painful and may be confused with calluses. However, when the surface is pared, thrombosed capillaries can be observed at the base of warts. Flat warts are usually observed among children and occur on the face, neck, chest, and flexor surfaces of forearms and legs. Seborrheic keratoses, nevi, and a variety of less common lesions may be confused with cutaneous warts.

Molluscum contagiosum may be mistaken for condyloma acuminatum, or anogenital warts. However, the lesions of molluscum tend to occur primarily over the pubis and are rarely pedunculated, whereas anogenital warts develop on the skin and mucosal surfaces of external genitalia and perianal areas and generally have an identifiable stalk. Sites of lesions among men vary according to whether individuals are circumcised or not. Among circumcised men, warts are most commonly found on the penile shaft, whereas among uncircumcised men, lesions are most commonly observed in the coronal sulcus. In either case, lesions may also be seen at the urethral meatus and may extend proximally. Perianal warts are most common among men who have sex with men, but develop in heterosexual men as well. Among women, warts usually appear first at the posterior introitus and adjacent labia. Other parts of the vulva then become involved, and lesions often develop in the vagina and on cervix as well. Internal lesions may be present without external warts. In men, a normal anatomic variant of the corona called hirsutoid papillomatosis or pearly coronal papules, may be difficult to distinguish from small warts. A similar anatomic variant may appear in women at the vulvar introitus and be confused with HPV disease. In addition, some HPV lesions may be small and round and difficult to distinguish from lichen planus and a variety of less common dermatologic conditions. Condyloma latum of syphilis is also in the differential diagnosis of anogenital warts.

Symptoms of respiratory compromise may appear in patients with respiratory papillomatosis, a disease produced by growth in the upper respiratory tract of lesions caused primarily by HPV types 6 and 11 [14]. In young children, the syndrome may be life threatening; in adults, it is generally more mild.

Immunosuppressed patients may develop extensive, severe HPV disease that is often difficult to treat (see below). Recipients of organ transplants frequently develop pityriasis versicolor-like lesions containing HPV DNA. These skin lesions may become malignant. Patients with underlying HIV disease appear to be at high risk for cervical and anal malignancies. Disease in these patients often recurs despite therapy.

An unusual dermatologic condition, epidermodysplasia verruciformis, is characterized by extreme susceptibility to cutaneous HPV infection [15]. Unusual virus types have been detected in specimens of skin obtained from these patients, who frequently develop squamous cell malignancies, particularly in sun-exposed areas. Lesions are similar to those of pityriasis versicolor.

Itching and bleeding may complicate the course of warts. Superinfection is rare. Large lesions may produce mechanical problems such as birth canal obstruction. Dysplasias of the uterine cervix and anus are generally asymptomatic until frank carcinoma develops. Patients with anogenital HPV disease may develop serious psychological symptoms.

Cutaneous lesions of unusual appearance that are suspected of being of HPV origin should be biopsied. Examples of lesions where histological examination should be considered include those of the external genitalia that are pigmented, appear as plaques, bleed, or are unusually large in size. A clinical diagnosis of warts in the oral cavity or upper airways should be confirmed histologically.

Patients with perianal warts should undergo anoscopy; sigmoidoscopy is usually not required to define the extent of intra-anal disease [16, 17].

Routine cytological examinations of cervical smears (Pap smear) is an essential part of routine health care for women. Those in whom HPV disease is suspected should undergo colposcopy and acetic acid application.

Laboratory Diagnosis

HPVs cannot be grown efficiently in tissue culture or in animal models. Diagnosis of HPV infection in the genital tract relies therefore on the direct detection of HPV genomes and/or gene products in fresh or fixed tissue biopsies, tissue scrapings and exfoliated cells. HPV detection and typing are not tests routinely available in diagnostic laboratories and the technologies referred to below are those used, at the present, in research studies.

Genome Detection

Direct detection of HPV DNA is achieved by molecular hybridization procedures usually preceded by nucleic acid amplification. Two methods are widely used in epidemiologic and natural history studies, the Hybrid Capture Assay (HC-II, Digene Co., Gaithersburg, Md) and the polymerase chain reaction (PCR) with generic primers. These technologies have equivalent sensitivities and specificities [18]. The hybrid capture assay detects 18 of the most prevalent and clinically relevant genital HPV types in a relatively simple and robust assay [19] which may be suitable for diagnostic laboratories. Consensus PCR is potentially capable of detecting all mucosal HPVs [20] and the generic PCR protocols widely used in epidemiological studies make use either of the consensus primers GP5/GP6 [21], GP5+/GP6+ [22] or the degenerate primers MYO9/11 [23]. HPV typing of the detected DNA can then be achieved by various hybridization strategies [24, 25]. Both HC [19] and PCR [26, 27] can provide an estimate of viral copy number by quantitating HPV DNA, although the accuracy of this has been questioned, and real time PCR is probably the methodology of choice to address that issue [28]. Other molecular hybridization procedures can be used to address specific questions in different clinical research contexts. Southern blot hybridization is the gold standard for HPV genome analysis but requires relatively large amounts of highly purified DNA and full length DNA molecules. It is not, therefore, suitable for the analysis of archival paraffin wax embedded wax material. PCR protocols can be applied with reasonable success to the latter [29]. DNA: DNA and DNA: RNA *in situ* hybridization are also suitable for archival material although the sensitivity of detection is highly dependent upon both fixation time and the fixative used.

Electron microscopy of lesions can reveal virus particles in the superficial keratinocytes of condyloma. Immunohistochemistry using specific monoclonal antibodies against the capsid protein L1 or the E4 protein, which is highly abundant, have been used in research studies [30] but are not a diagnostic tool.

Serology

Individuals infected with genital HPVs do make a type specific serum antibody response to the major viral capsid protein L1 [31]. Virions are generally not available for ELISA since HPVs cannot be grown in tissue culture. However, geometrically correct virus like particles (VLPs) can be synthesized *in vitro* by expression of the L1 gene in recombinant vectors and these have been used widely as the target antigen in ELISA in sero-epidemiologic studies [32]. Unfortunately due to the highly variable interval between infection, lesion development and sero-conversion plus the relatively low sensitivity of the assay, detection of anti-capsid serum antibody is not useful for diagnosis in the individual patient.

HPV Testing In Cervical Cancer Screening Programs

There is at present substantial debate about the role of HPV testing in population based screening programs. In brief, infection with the high risk HPVs is the major risk factor for the subsequent development of cervical cancer. HPV DNA is readily detectable in the specimens collected for PAP smears using either HC-II or PCR and is an obvious candidate for screening [33]. There are 3 potential clinical settings for such a test.

As Part of Primary Screening To Improve Sensitivity

Genital HPV infection is common in young sexually active women and is detectable in about 20% of 20-25 year old women with a cytologically normal PAP smear [34]. In most women this is a transient infection and is cleared [35, 36]. The prevalence in women in the 30-55 age group is about 3% and it is speculated that this represents persistent infection [34]. Natural history studies show clearly that viral persistence is a key factor in progressive cervical intra-epithelial disease [35, 37]. Persistent infection with high risk HPV types in the older age group is of clinical importance [38, 39] and there is a strong argument for HPV testing as an adjunct to cytology in this group [40] but HPV testing in the younger group may not give results of clinical utility.

Triage of ASCUS or AGUS

There is very strong evidence that HPV testing markedly increases sensitivity of detection of HGSIL (CIN2/3) in the highly contentious ASCUS/AGUS patient group [41-43]. This effect is particularly marked in the 35+ age group. The argument for HPV testing in these groups of patients seems overwhelming.

Post Treatment Surveillance To Detect Incomplete Excision or Ablation of HGSIL or Recurrence of Disease

HPV testing has a better sensitivity for detecting CIN2/3 and this argues for its use in this setting.

When To Treat

In general, treatment of non-malignant HPV disease is symptomatic. Highly effective systemic therapy is not available, and eradication of infection is not a reasonable objective. In addition, treatment of disease has not been shown to reduce rates of transmission. Thus, the primary goal of therapy is to eliminate or reduce the size of clinically apparent lesions. Decisions regarding initiation of treatment should be made after the patient has been thoroughly advised of the therapeutic objectives and the likelihood of success. Because non-malignant HPV disease is rarely fatal or associated with major morbidity, and because many lesions will regress spontaneously, withholding therapy is a reasonable alternative. Symptomatic respiratory papillomatosis is an exception, and close monitoring and expectant therapy may avoid potentially life-threatening situations.

Management of malignant HPV disease is discussed below, and requires the participation of a surgical subspecialist.

Treatment Algorithms For Warts

Most treatments for warts involve physical or chemical destruction of infected tissue, or removal. In addition, several interferon preparations and the immunomodulator imiquimod have some efficacy in treatment of HPV disease. Less success has been achieved with antiviral drugs.

Cutaneous Warts

A variety of treatment modalities are available for treatment of cutaneous warts, such as hand warts and plantar warts [44]. These treatments include salicylic and lactic acid paint preparations (SAL), glutaraldehyde, 5-fluorouracil, and podophyllin resin. Cryotherapy may also be used in this setting. Localized heat therapy using a radiofrequency generator has also been employed for treatment of cutaneous warts [45]. Curettage or resection may be performed, and several methods of electrosurgery can be used to remove these lesions. Flat warts generally do not need to be treated. Eyelid, nasal, and periungual warts are usually managed with cryotherapy [46, 47].

Anogenital Warts

Condyloma acuminatum is an extremely common manifestation of sexually transmitted HPV infection, and treatment of anogenital warts (condylomata acuminata) has been studied extensively [48-53]. Nevertheless, optimal methods of treatment have not been established. There are few data to suggest that currently available therapies can eradicate infection, alter the rare progression to malignancy, or decrease transmission [54-56]. Thus, as noted above, the primary goal of therapy is to decrease symptoms, including the adverse psychological impact of this common sexually transmitted disease [57]. When considering treatment, it should be remembered that within about 4 months, 10-20 percent of patients will experience spontaneous resolution of disease [58-60].

In most settings, cryotherapy, administered with liquid nitrogen or cryoprobe, is the treatment of first choice [61-65]. Rates of complete lesion resolution average around 75% and side effects, primarily burning for a few hours, are tolerable.

Podophyllin resin, an extract from the rhizome of Podophyllum peltatum or P. emodi, has been a mainstay of treatment for anogenital warts for many years. However, initial reports of high rates of efficacy have not been confirmed by more recent studies, and the drug has been associated with a variety of local and systemic toxicities including neurologic, hematologic, and febrile complications, occasionally leading to death [66-68]. Podophyllotoxin (podofilox), a purified preparation of the most active component of podophyllin resin, has significant advantages over the parent compound. It is chemically uniform and of standardized potency, and also appears to be more efficacious and less toxic [69, 70]. In addition, it does not need to be washed off, and can be easily self-administered by patients. Clinical trials have demonstrated that podofilox produces rates of complete response of about 55% [70-72]. Side-effects are similar in nature to those of podophyllin, but more mild. Relapse is not uncommon; application of podofilox to prevent recurrence is effective but the long term outcome is unknown [73].

Several other compounds have been used to treat anogenital warts including 5-fluorouracil (5FU), trichloracetic acid (TCA), and bichloracetic acid. 5FU in a topically applied 5% cream has been used to treat intraurethral warts in men and to prevent recurrence of vulvar warts in women [74, 75]. Use of the drug has been limited by side effects of pain and ulceration. Like podophyllin, 5FU is contraindicated during pregnancy.

TCA is painful and can produce ulcers. Studies have shown it to have rates of efficacy and recurrence similar or inferior to those of cryotherapy [76].

Conventional surgery and electrosurgery have also been used to treat anogenital warts [77-79]. Conventional surgery has been used primarily to remove anal warts.

Electrosurgery has produced high rates of complete response. Scarring and recurrence may occur following surgical removal.

High rates of lesion resolution have also been reported with CO2 laser therapy, although results may be no better than those obtained with conventional techniques [80-82]. The success of laser therapy may be highly operator dependent. The procedure often requires general anesthesia and may be associated with significant discomfort and scarring.

Several different interferon preparations have been studied in the treatment of anogenital warts, and some are useful in selected clinical situations. Best results have been obtained when interferons are injected directly into individual warts. [83-86]. When administered subcutaneously at a remote site, interferons are less effective [59, 87]. Several of these preparations have also been administered in combination with conventional modes of therapy with contradictory results [88-92].

Imiquimod is a chemical inducer of interferon and other cytokines which has been shown to have efficacy in the treatment of anogenital warts. The drug is administered as a 5% cream and may be associated with burning, itching, erythema, and swelling. In some patients, erosions may develop. In most studies, women have benefitted from imiquimod more than men [93-96].

Treatment Algorithms For Intra-epithelial Genital HPV Disease

Infection of the genital mucosae with HPV results in a cytologically and histologically distinct spectrum of intra-epithelial lesions. In the cervix these are graded on the degree to which they have lost cytoplasmic maturation with 3 classes, mild (cervical intra-epithelial neoplasia CIN 1), moderate (CIN2) and severe (CIN 3) recognized in Europe [97]. The Bethesda classification used in the USA recognizes 2 classes, low grade and high grade squamous intra-epithelial lesions, LGSIL (CIN 1) and HGSIL (CIN 2 and 3) [98]. Most SIL will regress if left untreated, but a fraction infected with oncogenic HPV types have the potential to progress to invasive carcinoma. The risk of progression is highest with HSIL but at least 10% of LGSIL will progress [99].

HGSIL (CIN2 and 3)

HGSIL is a precancerous condition and all high grade lesions are treated with ablative therapy by gynecologists. They are not treated as HPV infections. Treatment modalities are summarized below.

Methods of Treatment for SIL [100]
    Local destruction (must destroy tissue to a depth of 6-7mm)
        Cryotherapy, anaesthesia not usually required
        Cold coagulation, with local anaesthesia
        Electrodiathermy, local or general anaesthesia
        Carbon dioxide laser evaporation, local anaesthesia

Excisional techniques (general anaesthesia)
  Cold knife cone biopsy
  Laser cone biopsy
  Large loop diathermy and cone biopsy
  Hysterectomy

Doubts have been cast on the efficacy of superficial ablative techniques [101] and many authors consider that excision should be the primary technique for HGSIL [102-104]. Loop diathermy and cone biopsy, a widely used and proven technique [105] provides a tissue specimen suitable for the histopathological assessment which will confirm that the lesion has been completely excised and exclude invasive cancer. Hysterectomy in the primary management of HGSIL is rarely indicated and the criteria have been clearly defined [100].

Follow up is traditionally by cytology and colposcopy and this is an area where HPV testing will be of value [39]. Long term complications of treatment are mainly cervical stenosis and scarring. Effects on subsequent fertility and pregnancy seem to be minimal [100].

LGSIL (CIN 1)

The treatment of LGSIL is a clinical problem [100]. Treatment approaches can be categorized as:

1. Surveillance by cytology – this risks missing the small number of women who harbor HGSIL and are at risk for progression

2. Routine treatment - this over treats since most LGSIL are self limiting HPV infections which will naturally regress with time

3. Selective treatment – the ideal management situation but presumes that those at risk for progression can be identified

The predictive value of HPV testing in patients with mildly abnormal smears has been shown in several studies [42, 106, 107]. HPV testing should become a component of the treatment algorithm for these patients [36, 108].

There is a high prevalence of CIN/SIL in HIV infected women with more frequent and rapid progression to high grade disease [109] and increased recurrence rates post treatment [110]. Treatment algorithms are the same for immunosuppressed women but monitoring and follow up post therapy is more frequent.

Vaginal Intra-epithelial Neoplasia (VAIN)

VAIN is rare and accounts for 0.4% of genital intra-epithelial disease. Women at risk include those who:

1. Have been treated for CIN/SIL

2. Have received radiation therapy for cervical cancer

3. Are immunosuppressed either post transplant or as a consequence of HIV infection.

HPV infection is probably the etiologic factor in many cases but the extent of this association is not known. There is a wide range of therapies most of which are ablative.

Treatment options for VAIN
    Local excision (biopsy)
    Intravaginal 5 Fluorouracil, 5FU)
    Local Destruction
    Carbon dioxide laser
    Cryosurgery
    Electrocautery
    Vaginectomy

Before treatment the lesion should be submitted to vaginoscopy and biopsy and treatment decisions based on the biopsy results.

Vulval Intra-epithelial Neoplasia (VIN)

VIN encompasses a range of conditions previously described as Bowen's disease, leukoplakia, Bowenoid papulosis, squamous cell carcinoma, carcinoma in situ and hyperplastic dystrophy [111]. VIN is graded in a similar way to its cervical counterpart as VIN 1(mild) VIN2 (moderate) and VIN 3 (severe). There is a clear association with HPV infection although the prevalence of HPV varies with different series. Several reports show an association between warty basaloid lesions in younger women and HPV infection but not in Bowenoid lesions in older women [112, 113] but this correlation was not found by others [114]. The natural history of VIN is poorly understood and the relationship to vulvar carcinoma is far from clear. There is a debate about whether VIN 1 and 2 are truly pre-cancerous or self limiting HPV infections which will regress with time. VIN 3 is frequently multi-focal with a peak age incidence of 35 years. The potential for progression to vulvar carcinoma is uncertain with rates as low as 2-4% reported in some studies [115]. This contrasts with retrospective studies in which an incidence of 10-22% of invasive disease was found at excisional treatment when the initial diagnosis was VIN 3 [116-118]. Overall because of these uncertainties the optimal management for VIN still has to be determined. Certainly before any treatment option is undertaken vulvoscopy and biopsy are necessary to define the extent of disease and exclude invasive cancer. Treatment options are varied.

Treatment options for VIN
  Conservative – observation and monitoring
  Medical
    5 Fluorouracil
    Interferon-a
    Dinitrochlorobenzene (DNCB) cream
  Photodynamic (photochemical destruction of cells sensitized with a light activator)
  Wide local excision with knife or laser
  Laser treatment
  Skinning vulvectomy with skin grafting
  Simple vulvectomy

Medical therapies are limited in number and of low efficacy and surgical procedures are potentially mutilating in these women. Furthermore, after all therapies, even extensive surgical procedures, recurrences are common particularly with multifocal disease. The emotional trauma associated with vulval surgery, particularly in younger women is considerable and there is the risk of the development of psychosexual disease.

New and effective therapies for VIN are a priority and this is a condition where treatment of HPV infection either by immunotherapy or specific anti-viral therapies may significantly improve management if only by identifying those patients in whom extensive surgical procedures are necessary.

Immunobiology of HPV and Prospects For Immunotherapy of Intra-epithelial Genital HPV Disease

A Th1 biased cell mediated immune response is critical for successful clearance of HPV infections [119]. Antibody plays no role in established HPV infections but prevents re-infection with the same HPV type. A defective host response almost certainly underpins viral persistence and progressive HPV lesions seem to be associated with partial tolerance to viral antigens [120]. Successful immunotherapies against established infections will need to induce a strong virus specific cell mediated immune response of the appropriate type.

Immunomodulators

Interferons a and b have been used both topically and intra-lesionally but in double blind placebo controlled trials no obvious beneficial effects were observed and side effects were pronounced [121, 122].

The central importance of the innate immune system in the form of dendritic cells and macrophages in activating the appropriate antigen specific immune response is now clearly recognized. Pharmacological agents which modulate dendritic cell and macrophage function could therefore have therapeutic value. Imiquimod, formulated as the self applied topical therapy AldaraTM is such a molecule inducing macrophages to release IFN-a and other pro-inflammatory cytokines [123]. It has shown efficacy and safety in clinical trials for treatment of external HPV infected genital warts [93]. It is feasible that Imiquimod will have a therapeutic effect on intra-epithelial disease but no placebo controlled trials on LGSIL, HGSIL or VIN have been reported to date and the drug is not licensed for this use. Immunomodulators such as Imiquimod which induce the production of proinflammatory cytokines have the potential to induce potent local inflammatory side effects and their use on mucosal lesions in the upper genital tract will require caution.

Gene therapy approaches in which cytokine genes are transduced into tumor cells enhancing anti-sense gene therapies [124] or HPV immunization are under test.

Therapeutic Vaccines

HPV early proteins (E6, E7, E1 and E2) do not evoke strong responses during the natural infection but experimental infections in cattle [125] and rabbits [126] indicate that deliberate immunization with them could be effective therapeutically. Vaccines in which HPV early proteins are used as immunogens are all currently either in Phase I/II clinical trials or in pre-clinical evaluation (Table 2).

Table 2.   Therapeutic vaccines for human papillomavirus (HPV)-associated intraepithelial dysplasias and cancers

Antigen	Delivery	Development Status
HPV 6 L2/E7	Protein + alum	Phase IIa [128]
HPV 16 E7	Protein + alum	Phase I
HPV 16 E7	Peptides	Phase I [129]
HPV 16 E7	Protein bound to Mycobacterium bovis Hsp 65	Phase I
HPV 16/18 E6/E7	Recombinant vaccinia virus vector	Phase I [130]
CRPV E1, E2, E6	DNA	Preclinical
HPV 16 E7	DNA	Preclinical

Phase I and IIa trials of a recombinant HPV 6 protein vaccine comprising a fusion L2/E7 protein bound to allhydrogel for treatment of genital warts have been reported. The preparation was safe well tolerated and immunogenic and showed efficacy in prevention of recurrence [127, 128]. DNA vaccines encoding papillomavirus early antigens have been shown to be effective in animal models such as the rabbit, but no clinical trials using HPV polynucleotide vaccines have been reported.

A live recombinant vaccinia virus encoding modified HPV 16 and 18 E6 and E7 sequences, has been used in a Phase I trial in 8 patients with late stage cervical cancer [131]. Follow up studies using this live vector are in progress in HGSIL and cancer patients and the results are awaited with interest. Vaccinia virus vaccines have well documented adverse effects and there is substantial research into replication defective or attenuated vaccinia viruses (fowlpox and modified vaccinia virus Ankara) as vaccine vectors encoding both HPV E6 and E7 and cytokines such as IL-2. These viruses have shown promise in experimental tumor models and elicit strong immune responses (Balloul JM personal communication). Recombinant replication defective adenoviruses expressing E6 and E7 also show promise in mouse tumor models but no clinical trials have been reported. VLPs can be engineered to include both the L1 protein and an early protein such as E7 so that E7 is directed to the class I pathway during processing by dendritic cells and CTL responses are elicited [132] providing both prophylaxis and therapy.

Some or all of these strategies may prove to be effective in benign or low grade disease and decisions about which vaccine modality to use will be dictated by cost, safety and acceptability. In HGSIL and cervical cancer the question remains as to whether tumor immune evasion mechanisms, such as the down regulation and loss of MHC class I, will prevent successful therapeutic vaccination. It seems likely in any event that immunomodulators and/or therapeutic vaccines will not be primary therapies for HGSIL and cervical cancer but used in combination with ablative and chemotherapies to prevent recurrent disease.

Dosing Schemes, Drug Interactions, Side Effects (Excepting Immunotherapies)

Details regarding specific methods of therapy are described above under Treatment algorithms and in the associated references. As noted previously, modes of therapy for HPV diseases are directed primarily at physical or chemical destruction of infected tissue and the majority of side effects are local in nature. Exceptions include excessive doses of podophyllin preparations, which may produce a variety of systemic effects, and interferons, which commonly produce an influenza-like syndrome consisting of fever, malaise, and myalgias [59]. Interferon can also produce neutropenia and other laboratory abnormalities, although with the doses generally used for anogenital warts, these effects are rarely if ever of clinical significance. Prolonged interferon therapy can produce chronic fatigue, which resolves upon cessation of treatment.

Special Considerations For Subgroups of Patients

Patients with epidermodysplasia verruciformis need to be followed frequently for the development of cutaneous malignancies. Individual lesions can be treated with conventional modes of treatment [133].

Patients with recurrent respiratory papillomatosis should be managed primarily by a surgeon with expertise in the treatment of these patients [134-138]. The primary mode of therapy is endoscopic surgical destruction or removal with laser, cryotherapy, and/or photodynamic therapy. In general, tracheostomy should not be performed because of the risk of distal spread of disease. Radiotherapy has been associated with the development of malignancy and is contraindicated [139]. Interferons may be of some help in the management of this disease by decreasing the need for surgery or possibly by inducing long lasting remissions in some patients [140, 141]. Intralesionally administered cidofovir may be of benefit in some patients [142].

Patients with intraoral warts are usually treated with cryotherapy or surgical excision. [143].

Some groups of immunosuppressed patients are prone to develop HPV disease that may be atypical in appearance, extensive, caused by unusual HPV types, and difficult to manage. For example, renal allograft recipients have high rates of pityriasis versicolor-like skin disease caused by multiple HPV types [144-148]. Patients with HIV infection often develop large anogenital warts which are refractory to conventional therapy. In addition, these individuals are at high risk for the development of both anal and cervical dysplasias. When cervical cancer develops in HIV-infected women, the disease appears to be unusually difficult to control. Surgical removal of warts in the setting of HIV infection has produced inconsistent results [149-151]. Interferon therapy has been less effective in patients with HIV infection than in immunocompetent individuals [152, 153].

Prophylaxis and Vaccination Strategies

The induction of serum neutralizing antibody to the L1 capsid protein protects against virus challenge in natural papillomavirus infections in animals [32] suggesting that prophylactic vaccination should be effective in humans. VLPs are obvious candidate immunogens for prophylactic vaccination and at least 4 Phase I and Phase I/II trials using HPV 11 and 16 L1 VLPs are in progress with large placebo controlled Phase II trials in planning. The end point in Phase II trials with HPV 16 VLPs is likely to be the development of cervical intra-epithelial disease over the 5 year period post vaccination. Immunization of volunteers in Phase I trials with HPV 11 and 16 L1 VLPs induces good serum antibody responses [154, Schiller personal communication]. The key issues are whether the antibodies generated will be protective and how long the protection will last. Neutralizing antibody responses to L1 are type specific and polyvalent vaccines will be required to protect against the spectrum of oncogenic HPVs. Although the data from the animal models, is very encouraging for human vaccination, none of these model genital infection and the effectiveness of serum IgG at protecting against HPV infection at the genital mucosal surface remains in question and will only be answered by field trials in humans.

References

1. Bonnez W, Reichman RC. Papillomaviruses. In: Principles and Practice of Infectious Diseases, 5th Edition. GL Mandell, JE Bennet, R Dolin, Eds. Churchill Livingstone, New York, NY. 2000.
2. Bonnez W. Papillomavirus. In: Richman DD, Whitley RJ, Hayden FG, eds. Clinical Virology. First ed. New York, NY: Churchill Livingstone 1997: 569-611.
3. Bosch, FX, Manos, MM; Munoz, N; et al. Prevalence of human papillomavirus in cervical cancer: a worldwide perspective. International biological study on cervical cancer (IBSCC) Study Group [see comments]. JNCI 1995; 87: 796-802.
4. Brown DR et al: Nucleotide sequence and characterization of human papillomavirus type 83, a novel

genital papillomavirus. Virology 1999; 260(1): 165.

5. Bonnez W, DaRin C, Borkhuis C, de Mesy Jensen K, Reichman RC, Rose RC. Isolation and propagation of human papillomavirus type 16 in human xenografts implanted in the severe combined immunodeficiency mouse. J Virol 1998; 72: 5256-5261.

6. Howett MK, Christensen ND, Kreider JW. Tissue xenografts as a model system for study of the pathogenesis of papillomaviruses. Clin Dermatol 1997; 15: 229-36.

7. Massing AM, Epstein WL. Natural history of warts. A two year study. Arch Dermatol 1963; 87: 306-10.

8. Williams HC, Pottier A, Strachan D. The descriptive epidemiology of warts in British schoolchildren. Br J Dermatol 1993; 128: 504-11.

9. de Villiers E-M, Schneider A, Miklaw H, et al. Human papillomavirus infections in women with and without abnormal cytology. Lancet 1987; 2: 703-6.

10. Northfelt DW et al: Anal neoplasia. Pathogenesis, diagnosis, and management. Hematol Oncol Clin North Am 1996; 10: 1177-87.

11. Okagaki T. Inmpact of human papillomavirus research on the histopathologic concepts of genital neoplasms. Curr Topics Pathol 1992; 85: 273-307.

12. Majewski S, Jablonska S. Epidermodysplasia verruciformis as a model of human papillomavirus-induced genetic cancer of the skin. Arch Dermatol 1995; 131: 1312-8.

13. Jablonska S; Orth G; Obalek S; et al. Cutaneous warts. Clinical, histologic, and virologic correlations. Clinics in Dermatology 1985; 3: 71-82.

14. Derkay CS. Task Force on recurrent respiratory papillomatosis. A preliminary report. Arch Otolaryngol Head Neck Surg 1995; 121: 1386-91.

15. Grussendorf-Conen E-I. Papillomavirus-induced tumors of the skin: cutaneous warts and epidermodysplasia verruciformis. In: Syrjänen K, Gissmann L, Koss LG, eds. Papillomaviruses and Human Disease. Berlin: Springer Verlag, 1987: 158-81.

16. McMillan A. Sigmoidoscopy - a necessary procedure in the routine investigation of homosexual men? Genitourin Med 1987; 63: 44-6.

17. Parker BJ, Cossart YE, Thompson CH, Rose BR, Henderson BR. The clinical management and laboratory assessment of anal warts. Med J Austral 1987; 147: 59-63.

18. Peyton CL, Schiffman M, Lorincz AT et al. Comparison of PCR- and hybrid capture-based human papillomavirus detection systems using multiple cervical specimen collection strategies. J Clin Microbiol 1998; 36: 3248-54.

19. Reid R, Lorincz AT. Human papillomavirus tests. Baillieres Clin Obstet Gynaecol 1995; 9: 65-103.

20. Bernard HU, Chan SY, Manos MM et al. Identification and assessment of known and novel human papillomaviruses by polymerase chain reaction amplification, restriction fragment length polymorphisms, nucleotide sequence, and phylogenetic algorithms [see comments]. J Infect Dis 1994; 170: 1077-85.

21. Van Den Brule AJ, Snijders PJ, Gordijn RL, Bleker OP, Meijer CJ, Walboomers JM. General primer mediated polymerase chain reaction permits the detection of sequenced and still unsequenced human papillomavirus genotypes in cervical scrapes and carcinomas. Int J Cancer 1990; 45: 644-9.

22. de Roda Husman AM, Walboomers JM, van den Brule AJ, Meijer CJ, Snijders PJ. The use of general primers GP5 and GP6 elongated at their 3' ends with adjacent highly conserved sequences improves human papillomavirus detection by PCR. J Gen Virol 1995; 76: 1057-62.

23. Gravitt PE, Manos MM. Polymerase chain reaction based methods for the detection of human papillomavirus DNA. IARC Sci Publ 119. 1992: 121-33.

24. Bauer HM, Ting Y, Greer CE et al. Genital human papillomavirus infection in female university students as determined by a PCR based method [see comments]. JAMA 1991; 265: 472-7.

25. Gravitt PE, Peyton CL, Apple RJ, Wheeler CM. Genotyping of 27 human papillomavirus types by using L1 consensus PCR products by a single-hybridization, reverse line blot detection method. J Clin Microbiol 1998; 36: 020-7.

26. Caballero OL, Villa LL, Simpson AJ. Low stringency PCR (LS PCR) allows entirely internally standardized DNA quantitation. Nucleic Acids Res 1995; 23: 192-3.

27. Jacobs MV, Walboomers JM, van Beek J et al. A quantitative polymerase chain reaction-enzyme immunoassay for accurate measurements of human papillomavirus type 16 DNA levels in cervical scrapings. Br J Cancer 1999; 81: 114-21.

28. Josefsson A, Livak K, Gyllensten U. Detection and quantitation of human papillomavirus by using the fluorescent 5' exonuclease assay. J-Clin-Microbiol 1999; 37: 490-6.

29. Unger ER, Vernon SD, Lee DR, Miller DL, Reeves WC. Detection of human papillomavirus in archival tissues. Comparison of *in situ* hybridization and polymerase chain reaction. J Histochem Cytochem 1998; 46: 535-40.

30. Doorbar J, Foo C, Coleman N et al. Characterization of events during the late stages of HPV16 infection *in vivo* using high-affinity synthetic Fabs to E4. Virology 1997; 238: 40-52.

31. Nonnenmacher B, Hubbert NL, Kirnbauer R et al. Serologic response to human papillomavirus type 16 (HPV 16) virus like particles in HPV 16 DNA positive invasive cervical cancer and cervical intraepithelial neoplasia grade III patients and controls from Colombia and Spain. J Infect Dis 1995; 172: 19-24.

32. Stanley MA. Genital papillomaviruses - prospects for vaccination. Curr Opin Infect Dis 1997; 10: 55-61.

33. Herrero R, Hildesheim A, Bratti C et al. Population-based study of human papillomavirus infection and cervical neoplasia in rural Costa Rica. J Natl Cancer Inst 2000; 92: 464-74.

34. Melkert PW, Hopman E, Van Den Brule AJ et al. Prevalence of HPV in cytomorphologically normal cervical smears, as determined by the polymerase chain reaction, is age dependent. Int J Cancer 1993; 53: 919-23.

35. Ho GY, Burk RD, Klein S et al. Persistent genital human papillomavirus infection as a risk factor for persistent cervical dysplasia [see comments]. J Natl Cancer Inst 1995; 87: 1365-71.

36. Nobbenhuis MA, Walboomers JM, Helmerhorst TJ et al. Relation of human papillomavirus status to cervical lesions and consequences for cervical-cancer screening: a prospective study. Lancet 1999; 354: 20-5.

37. Remmink AJ, Walboomers JM, Helmerhorst TJ et al. The presence of persistent high risk HPV genotypes in dysplastic cervical lesions is associated with progressive disease: natural history up to 36 months. Int J Cancer 1995; 61: 306-11.

38. Londesborough P, Ho L, Terry G, Cuzick J, Wheeler C, Singer A. Human papillomavirus genotype as a predictor of persistence and development of high-grade lesions in women with minor cervical abnormalities. Int J Cancer 1996; 69: 364-8.

39. ter Harmsel B, Smedts F, Kuijpers J, van Muyden R, Oosterhuis W, Quint W. Relationship between human papillomavirus type 16 in the cervix and intraepithelial neoplasia. Obstet-Gynecol 1999; 93: 46-50.

40. Cuzick J, Beverley E, Ho L et al. HPV testing in primary screening of older women. Br J Cancer 1999; 81: 554-8.

41. Cox JT, Lorincz AT, Schiffman MH, Sherman ME, Cullen A, Kurman RJ. Human papillomavirus testing by hybrid capture appears to be useful in triaging women with a cytologic diagnosis of atypical squamous cells of undetermined significance. Am J Obstet Gynecol 1995; 172: 946-54.

42. Manos MM, Kinney WK, Hurley LB et al. Identifying women with cervical neoplasia: using human

papillomavirus DNA testing for equivocal Papanicolaou results [see comments]. JAMA 1999; 281: 1605-10.

43. Sherman ME, Tabbara SO, Scott DR et al. "ASCUS, rule out HSIL": cytologic features, histologic correlates, and human papillomavirus detection. Mod-Pathol 1999; 12: 335-42.

44. Bunney MH, Nolan MW, William DA. An assessment of methods of treating viral warts by comparative treatment trials based on a standard design. Br J Dermatol 1976; 94: 667-9.

45. Stern P, Levine N. Controlled localized heat therapy in cutaneous warts. Arch Dermatol 1992; 128: 945-8.

46 Bunney MH. Viral Warts: Their Biology and Treatment. 1st ed. Oxford: Oxford University Press, 1982.

47. Rees RB. The treatment of warts. Clin Dermatol 1985; 3(4): 179-84.

48. Ling MR. Therapy of genital human papillomavirus infection. Part II: Methods of treatment. Int J Dermatol 1992; 31: 769-76.

49. Stone KM. Human papillomavirus infection and genital warts: update on epidemiology and treatment. Clin Inf Dis 1995; 20(Suppl. 1): S91-7.

50. Mayeaux EJ Jr, Harper MB, Barksdale W, Pope JB. Noncervical human papillomavirus genital infections. Am Fam Phys 1995; 53: 19.

51. Reid R. The management of genital condylomas, intraepithelial neoplasia, and vulvodynia. Obstet Gynecol Clin North Am 1996; 23: 917-91.

52. Baker GE, Tyring SK. Therapeutic approaches to papillomavirus infections. Dermatol Clin 1997; 15: 331-40.

53. Anon. 1998 guidelines for the treatment of sexually transmitted diseases. MMWR 1998; 47(RR-1): 1-116.

54. Evans TG, Bonnez W, Rose RC, Koenig S, Demeter L, Suzich J, O'Brien D, Campbell M, White WI, Balsley J, Reichman RC. A phase I study of a recombinant virus-like particle vaccine against human papillomavirus type 11 in healthy adult volunteers. J. Inf. Dis. 183: 1485-1493. 2001.

55. Krebs H-B, Helmkamp BF. Does the treatment of genital condylomata in men decrease the treatment failure rate of cervical dysplasia in the female sexual partner? Obstet Gynecol 1990; 76: 660-3.

56. Sigurgeirsson B, Lindelöf B, Eklund G. Condylomata acuminata and risk of cancer: an epidemiological study. BMJ 1991; 303: 341-4.

57. Reitano M. Counseling patients with genital warts. Am J Med 1997; 102(Suppl. 4S): 38-43.

58. Schonfeld A, Nitke S, Schattner A, et al. Intramuscular human interferon-_ injections in treatment of condylomata acuminata. Lancet 1984; i: 1038-42.

59. Reichman RC, Oakes D, Bonnez W, et al. Treatment of condyloma acuminatum with three different alpha interferon preparations administered parenterally: A double-blind, placebo-controlled trial. J Infect Dis 1990; 162: 1270-6.

60. Condylomata International Collaborative Study Group. Recurrent condylomata acuminata treated with recombinant interferon alfa-2a. A multicenter double-blind placebo-controlled clinical trial. J Am Med Assoc 1991; 265: 2684-7.

61. Godley MJ, Bradbeer CS, Gellan M, Thin RNT. Cryotherapy compared with trichloracetic acid in treating genital warts. Genitourin Med 1987; 63: 390-2.

62. Bashi SA. Cryotherapy *versus* podophyllin in the treatment of genital warts. Int J Dermatol 1985; 24: 535-6.

63. Stone KM, Becker TM, Hadgu A, Kraus SJ. Treatment of external genital warts: a randomised clinical trial comparing podophyllin, cryotherapy, and electrodessication. Genitourin Med 1990; 66: 16-9.

64. Berth-Jones J, Hutchinson PE. Modern treatment of warts: cure rates at 3 and 6 months. Br J Dermatol 1992; 127: 262-5.

65. Simmons PD, Langlet F, Thin RNT. Cryotherapy *versus* electrocautery in the treatment of genital warts. Br J Vener Dis 1981; 57: 273-4.

66. Miller RA. Podophyllin. Int J Dermatol 1985; 24: 491-8.

67. Simmons PD. Podophyllin 10% and 25% in the treatment of ano-genital warts. A comparative double-blind study. Br J Vener Dis 1981; 57: 208-9.

68 Beutner KR. Podophyllotoxin in the treatment of genital human papillomavirus infection: a review. Sem Dermatol 1987; 6: 10-8.

69. Edwards A, Atma-Ram A, Thin RN. Podophyllotoxin 0.5% v podophyllin 20% to treat penile warts. Genitourin Med 1988; 64: 263-5.

70. Beutner KR, Friedman-Kien AE, Artman NN, et al. Patient-applied podofilox for treatment of genital warts. Lancet 1989; i: 831-4.

71. Kirby P, Dunne A, King DH, Corey L. Double-blind randomized clinical trial of self-administered podofilox solution *versus* vehicle in the treatment of genital warts. Am J Med 1990; 88: 465-9.

72. Greenberg MD, Rutledge LH, Reid R, Berman NR, Precop SL, Elswick RK Jr. A double-blind, randomized trial of 0.5% Podofilox and placebo for the treatment of genital warts in women. Obstet Gynecol 1991; 77: 735-9.

73. Bonnez W, Elswick RK Jr, Bailey-Farchione A, et al. Efficacy and safety of 0.5% podofilox solution in the treatment and suppression of anogenital warts. Am J Med 1994; 96: 420-5.

74. de Benedictis JT, Marmar JL, Praiss DE. Intraurethral condylomata acuminata: management and a review of the literature. J Urol 1977; 118: 767-9.

75. Krebs H-B. Prophylactic topical 5-fluorouracil following treatment of human papillomavirus-associated lesions of the vulva and vagina. Obstet Gynecol 1986; 68: 837-41.

76. Abdullah AN, Walzman M, Wade A. Treatment of external genital warts comparing cryotherapy (liquid nitrogen) and trichloracetic acid. Sex Trans Dis 1993; 20: 344-5.

77. Duus BR, Philipsen T, Christensen JD, Lundvall F, Sondergaard J. Refractory condylomata acuminata: a controlled clinical trial of carbon dioxide laser *versus* conventional surgical treatment. Genitourin Med 1985; 61: 59-61.

78. McMillan A, Scott GR. Outpatient treatment of perianal warts by scissor excision. Genitourin Med 1987; 63: 114-5.

79. Bonnez W, Oakes D, Choi A, et al. Therapeutic efficacy and complications of excisional biopsy of condyloma acuminatum. Sex Trans Dis 1996; 23: 273-6.

80. Baggish MS. Improved laser techniques for the elimination of genital and extragenital warts. Am J Obstet Gynecol 1985; 153: 545-50.

81. Reid R. Physical and surgical principles governing expertise with the carbon dioxide laser. Obstet Gynecol Clin North Am 1987; 14: 513-35.

82. Bar-Am A, Shilon M, Peyser MR, Ophir J, Brenner S. Treatment of male genital condylomatous lesions by carbon dioxide laser after failure of previous nonlaser methods. J Am Acad Dermatol 1991; 24: 87-9.

83. Reichman RC, Oakes D, Bonnez W, et al. Treatment of condyloma acuminatum with three different interferons administered intralesionally: A double-blind, placebo-controlled trial. Ann Int Med 1988; 108: 675-9.

84. Eron LJ, Judson F, Tucker S, et al. Interferon therapy for condylomata acuminata. N Engl J Med 1986; 315: 1059-64.

85. Friedman-Kien A, Eron LJ, Conant M, et al. Natural interferon alfa for treatment of condylomata acuminata. J Am Med Assoc 1988; 259: 533-8.

86. Vance JC, Bart BJ, Hansen RC, et al. Intralesional recombinant alpha-2 interferon for the treatment of patients with condyloma acuminatum or verruca plantaris. Arch Dermatol 1986; 122: 272-7.

87. Condylomata International Collaborative Study Group. A comparison of interferon alfa-2a and podophyllin in the treatment of primary condylomata acuminata. Genitourin Med 1991; 67: 394-9.

88. Petersen CS, Bjerring P, Larsen J, et al. Systemic interferon alpha-2b increases the cure rate in laser treated patients with multiple persistent genital warts: a placebo-controlled study. Genitourin Med 1991; 67: 99-102.

89. Condylomata International Collaborative Study Group. Randomized placebo-controlled double-blind combined therapy with laser surgery and systemic interferon-alpha 2a in the treatment of anogenital condylomata acuminatum. J Infect Dis 1993; 167: 824-9.

90. Fleshner PR, Freilich MI. Adjuvant interferon for anal condyloma - A prospective, randomized trial. Dis Colon Rectum 1994; 37: 1255-9.

91. Handley JM, Maw RD, Horner T, Lawther H, Walsh M, Dinsmore WW. A placebo controlled observer blind immunocytochemical and histologic study of epithelium adjacent to anogenital warts in patients treated with systemic interferon alpha in combination with cryotherapy or cryotherapy alone. Genitourin Med 1992; 68: 100-5.

92. Bonnez W, Oakes D, Bailey-Farchione A, et al. A randomized, double-blind trial of parenteral low dose *versus* high dose interferon-_ in combination with cryotherapy for treatment of condyloma acuminatum. Antiviral Res 1997; 35: 41-52.

93. Slade HB, Owens ML, Tomai MA, Miller RL. Imiquimod 5% cream (AldaraTM). Exp Opin Invest Drugs 1998; 7: 437-49.

94. Beutner KR, Spruance SL, Hougham AJ, Fox TL, Owens ML, Douglas JM. Treatment of genital warts with an immune-response modifier (imiquimod). J Am Acad Dermatol 1998; 38: 230-9.

95. Edwards L, Ferenczy A, Eron L, et al. Self-administered topical 5-percent imiquimod cream for external anogenital warts. Arch Dermatol 1998; 134: 25-30.

96. Beutner KR, Tyring SK, Trofatter KF Jr, et al. Imiquimod, a patient-applied immune-response modifier for treatment of external genital warts. Antimicrob Agents Chemother 1998; 42: 789-94.

97. Buckley CH, Butler EB, Fox H. Cervical intraepithelial neoplasia. J Clin Pathol. 35. 1982: 1-13.

98. Anon. National Cancer Institute Workshop. The 1988 Bethesda system for reporting cervical/vaginal cytologic diagnoses. JAMA. 262. 1989: 931-4.

99. Syrjänen KJ. Natural history of genital human papillomavirus infections. In *Papillomavirus Reviews: Current Research on Papillomaviruses*. Lacey, C. (ed.), Leeds, Leeds University Press 1996: 189-206.

100. Singer A, Monaghan JMEditors. Lower Genital Tract Precancer. Colpscopy, Pathology and Treatment. 2nd Edition. Oxford: Blackwell Science. 2000.

101. Wright TC Jr, Richart RM, Ferenczy A, Koulos J. Comparison of specimens removed by CO2 laser conization and the loop electrosurgical excision procedure. Obstet Gynecol. 79. 1992: 147-53.

102 McIndoe GA, Robson MS, Tidy JA, Mason WP, Anderson MC. Laser excision rather than vaporization: the treatment of choice for cervical intraepithelial neoplasia. Obstet Gynecol. 74. 1989: 165-8.

103. Buxton EJ, Luesley DM, Shafi MI, Rollason M. Colposcopically directed punch biopsy: a potentially misleading investigation. Br J Obstet Gynaecol. 98. 1991: 1273-6.

104. Murdoch JB, Crimshaw RN, Morgan PR, Monaghan JM. The impact of loop diathermy on management of early invasive cancer. Int J Gynecol Cancer. 2. 1992: 129-.

105. Prendiville W, Cullimore J, Norman S. Large loop excision of the transformation zone (LLETZ). A new method of management for women with cervical intraepithelial neoplasia. Br J Obstet Gynaecol. 96. 1989: 1054-60.

106. Cuzick J, Terry G, Ho L, Hollingworth T, Anderson M. Type specific human papillomavirus DNA in abnormal smears as a predictor of high grade cervical intraepithelial neoplasia. Br J Cancer. 69. 1994: 167-71.

107. Cuzick J, Terry G, Ho L, Hollingworth T, Anderson M. Human papillomavirus type 16 DNA in cervical smears as predictor of high grade cervical cancer. Lancet. 339. 1992: 959-60.

108. Sigurdsson K, Arnadottir T, Snorradottir M, Benediktsdottir K, Saemundsson H. Human papillomavirus (HPV) in an Icelandic population: the role of HPV DNA testing based on hybrid capture and PCR assays among women with screen-detected abnormal Pap smears. Int J Cancer. 72. 1997: 446-52.

109. Fink MJ, Fruchter RG, Maiman M et al. The adequacy of cytology and colposcopy in diagnosing cervical neoplasia in HIV-seropositive women. Gynecol Oncol. 55. 1994: 133-7.

110. Fruchter RG, Maiman M, Sedlis A, Bartley L, Camilien L, Arrastia CD. Multiple recurrences of cervical intraepithelial neoplasia in women with the human immunodeficiency virus. Obstet Gynecol. 87. 1996: 338-44.

111. Ridley CM, Frankman O, Jones IS et al. New nomenclature for vulvar disease: International Society for the Study of Vulvar Disease. Hum Pathol 20. 1989: 495-6.

112. Park JS, Jones RW, McLean MR et al. Possible etiologic heterogeneity of vulvar intraepithelial neoplasia. A correlation of pathologic characteristics with human papillomavirus detection by *in situ* hybridization and polymerase chain reaction. Cancer. 67. 1991: 1599-607.

113. Toki T, Kurman RJ, Park JS, Kessis T, Daniel RW, Shah KV. Probable nonpapillomavirus etiology of squamous cell carcinoma of the vulva in older women: a clinicopathologic study using *in situ* hybridization and polymerase chain reaction. Int J Gynecol Pathol. 10. 1991: 107-25.

114. Van Beurden M, Ten Kate FJ, Smits HL et al. Multifocal vulvar intraepithelial neoplasia grade III and multicentric lower genital tract neoplasia is associated with transcriptionally active human papillomavirus. Cancer. 75. 1995: 2879-84.

115. Jones RW, McLean MR. Carcinoma *in situ* of the vulva: a review of 31 treated and five untreated cases. Obstet Gynecol. 68. 1986: 499-503.

116. Herod JJ, Shafi MI, Rollason TP, Jordan JA, Luesley DM. Vulvar intraepithelial neoplasia with superficially invasive carcinoma of the vulva. Br J Obstet Gynaecol. 103. 1996: 453-6.

117. Hording U, Junge J, Poulsen H, Lundvall F. Vulvar intraepithelial neoplasia III: a viral disease of undetermined progressive potential. Gynecol Oncol. 56. 1995: 276-9.

118. van Beurden M, van de Vanger N, ten Cate FJW, Lammes F. Restricted surgical management of vulvar intra-epithelial neoplasia 3: focus on invasion and relief of symptoms. Int J Gynecol Cancer. 8. 1998: 73-.

119. Stanley M, Coleman N, Chambers M. The host response to lesions induced by human papillomavirus. In: Mindel, A., ed., title, place, publisher*******. 1994: 21-44.

120. Frazer IH, Thomas R, Zhou J et al. Potential strategies utilised by papillomavirus to evade host immunity. Immunol Rev. 168. 1999: 131-42.

121. Byrne MA, Moller BR, Taylor Robinson D et al. The effect of interferon on human papillomaviruses associated with cervical intraepithelial neoplasia. Br J Obstet Gynaecol. 93. 1986: 1136-44.

122. Frost L, Skajaa K, Hvidman LE, Fay SJ, Larsen PM. No effect of intralesional injection of interferon on moderate cervical intraepithelial neoplasia. Br J Obstet Gynaecol. 97. 1990: 626-30.

123. Arany I, Tyring SK, Stanley MA et al. Enhancement of the innate and cellular immune response in patients with genital warts treated with topical imiquimod cream 5%. Antiviral Res. 43. 1999: 55-63.

124. He YK, Lui VW, Baar J et al. Potentiation of E7 antisense RNA-induced antitumor immunity by co-delivery of IL-12 gene in HPV16 DNA-positive mouse tumor. Gene-Ther. 5. 1998: 1462-71.

125. McGarvie GM, Grindlay GJ, Chandrachud LM, O'Neill BW, Jarrett WFH, Campo MS. T-cell responses to BPV- E7 during infection and mapping of T-cell epitopes. Virology. 206. 1995: 504-10.

126. Selvakumar R, Borenstein LA, Lin Y-L, Ahmed R, Wettstein FO. Immunization with nonstructural proteins E1 and E2 of cotton tail rabbit papillomavirus stimulates regression of virus-induced papillomas. J Virol 69. 1995: 602-5.

127. Thompson HS, Davies ML, Holding FP et al. Phase I safety and antigenicity of TA-GW: a recombinant HPV6 L2E7 vaccine for the treatment of genital warts. Vaccine. 17. 1999: 40-9.

128. Lacey CJ, Thompson HS, Monteiro EF et al. Phase IIa safety and immunogenicity of a therapeutic vaccine, TA-GW, in persons with genital warts. J Infect Dis. 179. 1999: 612-8.

129. van Driel WJ, Ressing ME, Kenter GG et al. Vaccination with HPV16 peptides of patients with advanced cervical carcinoma: clinical evaluation of a phase I-II trial. Eur J Cancer. 35. 1999: 946-52.

130. Borysiewicz LK, Fiander A, Nimako M et al. A recombinant vaccinia virus encoding human papillomavirus types 16 and 18, E6 and E7 proteins as immunotherapy for cervical cancer [see comments]. Lancet. 347. 1996: 1523-7.

131. Borysiewicz K, Fiander A, Nimako M et al. A recombinant vaccinia virus encoding human papillomavirus types 16 and 18, E6 and E7 proteins as immunotherapy for cervical cancer. Lancet. 347. 1996: 1523-7.

132. Greenstone HL, Nieland JD, de Visser KE et al. Chimeric papillomavirus virus-like particles elicit antitumor immunity against the E7 oncoprotein in an HPV16 tumor model. Proc Natl Acad Sci USA. 95. 1998: 1800-5.

133. Grussendorf-Conen E-I. Papillomavirus-induced tumors of the skin: cutaneous warts and epidermodysplasia verruciformis. In: Syrjänen K, Gissmann L, Koss LG, eds. Papillomaviruses and Human Disease. Berlin: Springer Verlag, 1987: 158-81.

134. Derkay CS. Task Force on recurrent respiratory papillomatosis. A preliminary report. Arch Otolaryngol Head Neck Surg 1995; 121: 1386-91.

135. Kashima HK, Shah K. Recurrent respiratory papillomatosis. Clinical overview and management principles. Obstet Gynecol Clin North Am 1987; 14: 581-8.

136. Bauman NM, Smith RJ. Recurrent respiratory papillomatosis. Ped Clin North Am 1996; 43: 1385-401.

137. Gabbott M, Cossart YE, Kan A, Konopka M, Chan R, Rose BR. Human papillomavirus and host variables as predictors of clinical course in patients with juvenile-onset recurrent respiratory papillomatosis. J Clin Microbiol 1997; 35: 3098-103.

138. Somers GR, Tabrizi SN, Borg AJ, Garland SM, Chow CW. Juvenile laryngeal papillomatosis in a pediatric population: a clinicopathologic study. Pediatric Pathology & Laboratory Medicine 1997; 17: 53-64.

139. Lindeberg H, Elbrond O. Malignant tumours in patients with a history of multiple laryngeal papillomas: the significance of irradiation. Clin Otolaryngol 1991; 16: 149-51.

140. Healy GB, Gelber RD, Trowbridge AL, Grundfast KM, Ruben RJ, Price KN. Treatment of recurrent respiratory papillomatosis with human leukocyte interferon. N Engl J Med 1988; 319: 401-7.

141. Leventhal BG, Kashima HK, Mounts P, et al. Long-term response of recurrent respiratory papillomatosis to treatment with lymphoblastoid interferon alfa-n1. N Engl J Med 1991; 325: 613-7.

142. Snoeck R, van Ranst M, Andrei G, et al. Treatment of anogenital papillomavirus infections with an acyclic nucleoside phosphonate analogue. N Engl J Med 1995; 333: 943-4.

143. Praetorius F. HPV-associated diseases of oral mucosa. Clin Dermatol 1997; 15(3): 399-413.

144. Boyle J, Briggs JD, Mackie RM, Junor BJR, Aitchison TC. Cancer, warts and sunshine in renal transplant patients. A case-control study. Lancet 1984; i: 702-5.

145. Barr BBB, Benton EC, McLaren K, et al. Human papillomavirus infection and skin cancer in renal

allografts recipients. Lancet 1989; 1: 124-8.

146. Alloub MI, Barr BBB, McLaren KM, Smith IW, Bunney MH, Smart GE. Human papillomavirus infection and cervical intraepithelial neoplasia in women with renal allografts. BMJ 1989; 298: 153-6.

147. McGregor JM, Proby CM, Leigh IM. Virus infection and cancer risk in transplant recipients. Trends Microbiol 1996; 4: 2-3.

148. Euvrard S, Kanitakis J, Chardonnet Y, et al. External anogenital lesions in organ transplant recipients. A clinicopathologic and virologic assessment. Arch Dermatol 1997; 133: 175-8.

149. Beck DE, Jaso RG, Zajac RA. Surgical management of anal condylomata in the HIV-positive patient. Dis Colon Rectum 1990; 33: 180-3.

150. Miles AJG, Mellor CH, Gazzard B, Allen-Mersh TG, Wastell C. Surgical management of anorectal disease in HIV-positive homosexuals. Br J Surg 1990; 77: 869-71.

151. Lord RVN. Anorectal surgery in patients infected with human immunodeficiency virus - Factors associated with delayed wound healing. Ann Surg 1997; 226: 92-9.

152. Douglas JM, Rogers M, Judson FN. The effect of asymptomatic infection with HTLV-III on the response of anogenital warts in intralesional treatment with recombinant _2 interferon. J Infect Dis 1986; 154: 331-4.

153. Douglas JM Jr, Eron LJ, Judson FN, et al. A randomized trial of combination therapy with intralesional interferon _2b and podophyllin *versus* podophyllin alone for the therapy of anogenital warts. J Infect Dis 1990; 162: 52-9.

154. Reichman RC, Bonnez W, O'Brien D, Rose R, Koenig S, Suzich J, et al. A phase I study of a recombinant virus like particle vaccine against human papillomavirus type 11 in healthy adult volunteers. 38th ICAAC. San Diego CA, 1998.

CHAPTER 12

OTHER VIRUSES AND EMERGING VIRUSES OF CONCERN

DELIA ENRIA and C. J. PETERS

Table of Contents

Introduction

As the earth is increasingly changed by human activity and the growing human population encroaches on the remaining earth's surface available to us, we will increasingly encounter "new" pathogens. Travel of potentially viremic humans and transport of reservoirs and vectors will move dangerous viruses to new geographic areas. Some of these pathogens will find receptive homes because of ecological alterations, human activity, and the development of particularly susceptible populations such as the immunosuppressed or "monocultures" of hosts. We will be called upon to deal with these challenges and antiviral therapy will assume even more importance in the struggle.

Practical Guidelines in Antiviral Therapy Ed. by Charles A.B. Boucher and George J. Galasso. 279 — 301
© 2002 *Elsevier Science. Printed in the Netherlands.*

This chapter will concentrate on the viral hemorrhagic fevers (VHF) which comprise one syndrome that is caused by members of several RNA virus families which have "emerged" over the last few decades (Table 1). In addition we will review data on selected viruses that have recently been discovered, that are particularly virulent, or that are well-known but which may be newly important because of threats of bioterrorism or their geographic translocation (Table 2).

Viral Hemorrhagic Fevers (VHF)

The Viruses

Four families contain viruses that cause the VHF syndrome (Table 1). They are all RNA viruses with lipid envelopes but have different replication strategies. They are often aerosol hazards, making them dangerous in the laboratory and also potential biological warfare agents [65]; interestingly interhuman transmission is rarely airborne [59]. All the viruses circulate in nature independently of humans and are transmitted to humans by arthropods (ticks or mosquitoes) or seemingly normal but chronically infected rodents [62]. Yellow fever and particularly dengue viruses use humans as regular amplifiers for mosquito infection, but they have primordial cycles involving monkeys.

As would be expected from viruses in such different families, the pathogenesis of disease in humans also varies [63]. The rodent-borne arenaviruses infect cells with relatively little direct cytopathic effect and may well cause most of their effects through direct induction of cytokine secretion with bleeding noted in a setting of thrombocytopenia or ineffective platelet function, as well as alterations in blood coagulation and fibrinolysis [45]. The two arthropod-borne members of the Bunyaviridae family, Rift Valley fever and Crimean Congo HF, have multiple mechanisms of disease causation and are associated with some degree of disseminated intravascular coagulation [53, 75]. The only non-arthropod borne members of Bunyaviridae are the hantaviruses. These rodent-borne viruses cause an immunopathologic disease in the human host (58). The filoviruses are capable of direct cytopathic effects [83], induce cytokine secretion [20, 78], and also damage endothelium with the possibility of DIC [23; 75]. The two mosquito-borne flaviviruses, yellow fever and dengue viruses, have markedly different pathogenesis when they cause HF. Yellow fever virus has several effects with hepatic necrosis being prominent. Dengue virus rarely causes a primary HF but in settings of previous infection with other dengue serotypes may result in an immunopathologic vascular permeability syndrome and HF [25, 56].

Clinical Diagnosis

These diseases can be suspected by the travel history of the subject, the incubation period, and specific epidemiologic risk factors for each disease (Figure 1; Table 1 [62, 64]). Most are rural diseases (exceptions being *Aedes aegypti* transmitted yellow fever and dengue HF or *Rattus norvegicus* transmitted Seoul hantavirus). Generally, there is abrupt onset of fever (exceptions being the gradual onset of arenavirus disease) with a few day's period of fever, myalgia, malaise. As the full-fledged syndrome emerges, dizziness, postural hypotension, abdominal pain with other gastrointestinal symptoms, and a variety of complaints are common, as well as more severe prostration. Flushing over the face and chest and conjunctival injection are common clues [64]. Periorbital edema or proteinuria may signal increased vascular permeability. Early signs of hemorrhage may be manifest as petechiae, often best-visualized in the axillae, or metrorrhagia in women. Hypotension gives way to shock; CNS manifestations may range from tremor to convulsions and coma. Severe cases will generally have extensive hemorrhage, but *hemorrhage is not necessarily present, even in fatal cases*. SGOT elevations are usual in most of the VHF, but jaundice is common only in filovirus diseases, Rift Valley fever, or Crimean Congo HF. Renal failure is proportional to the degree of circulatory compromise except in hemorrhagic fever with renal syndrome (HFRS) which is characterized by acute renal failure and hyposthenuria. Pulmonary involvement is the rule in hantavirus pulmonary syndrome (HPS), and is the main presenting symptom although accompanied by myocardial depression and shock.

Virological Diagnosis

This is only available in specialized biosafety level 4 laboratories, either national or regional. With the exception of hantaviruses, patients are viremic during the acute phase and so virus isolation (special containment usually required), antigen detection, or reverse transcription with polymerase chain reaction (RT-PCR) are most useful in diagnosis. Antibodies appear later, around the time of clinical improvement, and may co-circulate for short periods of time with detectable infectivity or RT-PCR positivity. In Lassa there may be several days during which antibodies and viral infectivity are found simultaneously in blood [36, 2]. Hantavirus diseases such as HPS and HFRS are immunopathologic and IgM antibodies are detectable at the time of presentation for medical care. RT-PCR can detect viral genomic material for 10 days or more after onset of HPS; although it is not needed for diagnosis, it may be useful for defining the genetics of the infecting virus because serological tests are cross-reactive.

Principles of Therapy

With the differences in phylogeny and pathogenesis, it is no surprise that specific and supportive therapy may vary among the different HF viruses, but the principles are quite similar. There is a need for early, careful, and atraumatic transport to a nearby center that can manage a complicated illness. Hypotension and shock should be managed with careful fluid replacement including monitoring of venous pressure or wedge pressure if illness is at all severe. The patients generally have diffuse increase in vascular permeability, including the pulmonary bed, and cardiac impairment. These diseases do not necessarily have the same pathogenesis as septic shock, and in particular the presentation is usually with a low cardiac output and high peripheral vascular resistance [58]. Therefore, pressors are used carefully and cardiotonic drugs chosen. Bleeding should be managed with replacement therapy depending on monitoring; DIC occurs in some of the VHF but should be treated with heparin only if clear laboratory evidence is present

Table 1.   Viral hemorrhagic fevers

Virus	Disease	Incubation (days)	Geography	$\log_{10}$ cases per annum	Case fatality (%)	Treatment
Arenaviridae						
Junin	Argentine HF	7-14	Argentine pampas	2-3	15-30	Convalescent plasma adjusted for neutralizing antibody content is established therapy. IV ribavirin may also be effective. Vaccine available in Argentina.
Machupo	Bolivian HF	7-14	Bolivia, Beni Province	1-2	25	No established therapy. IV ribavirin probably effective and should be used. Junin vaccine may cross-protect.
Guanarito	Venezuelan HF	7-14	Venezuela, Portuguesa State	1-2	40	No established therapy. IV ribavirin probably effective and should be used.
Sabia	-	-	rural area, Sao Paulo State	0-1	1/2	No established therapy. IV ribavirin probably effective and should be used.
Lassa	Lassa fever	5-16	West Africa	4-5	15	IV ribavirin effective and should be used if serum SGOT >150 IU/ml
Bunyaviridae						
Phlebovirus						
Rift Valley fever virus	RVF	2-5	Sub-Saharan Africa	3-5	~50	No established therapy. Experimental use of ribavirin or antibody effective and could be tried. Investigational vaccine exists but availability doubtful.
Nairovirus						
Crimean Congo HF virus	CCHF	3-12	Africa, Asia, Balkans, USSR	2-4	30	No established therapy. IV ribavirin effective in experimental animal and clinical experience suggests useful. Should be used.

Table 1. Continued

Virus	Disease	Incubation (days)	Geography	Log_{10} cases per annum	Case fatality (%)	Treatment
Hantavirus						
Hantaan, Dobrava, etc	HFRS	9-35	World-wide	5-6	5-15	Supportive Rx including dialysis critical and iv ribavirin can be useful.
Sin Nombre, Laguna Negra, Andes, etc	HPS	7-28	Americas	2-4	40	No established therapy. Open label ribavirin showed no effect. Supportive ICU Rx particularly important.
Filoviridae						
Marburg, Ebola	Filovirus HF	3-16	Africa, ?Philippines	1-2?	25-90	No established therapy. Experimental therapies all marginal or ineffective.
Flaviviridae						
Yellow fever	Yellow fever	3-6	Africa, South America	4-5	5-20	No established therapy. Excellent vaccine.
Dengue	DHF/DSS	3-15	Tropic, sub-tropic	5-6	1	No established therapy. Proper fluid management can be particularly important because of massive capillary leak.
Kyasanur Forest disease virus	KFD	3-8	Mysore State, India	2-3	5	No established therapy. Vaccine produced in India.
Omsk HF virus	OHF	3-8	Western Siberia	0-1	5	No established therapy.
Al Kumrah virus	-	-	?Middle East	?1	10	No established therapy.

Table 2. Emerging and other important diseases and their viruses

Disease	Virus	Comments	Possible therapy
Viral hemorrhagic fevers	RNA viruses from four families (see Table 2)	First virus discovered was yellow fever in 1900; new ones continue to appear regularly, including 2000.	Ribavirin, convalescent plasma, vaccination available for most (Table 1)
Arboviral encephalitis	Bunyaviridae	La Crosse virus: commonest cause of childhood encephalitis in US.	La Crosse virus sensitive to ribavirin *in vitro*.
	Togaviridae (*Alphavirus* genus)	Eastern, Western, Venezuelan equine encephalitis	Vaccines for alphaviruses are investigational. No therapy for togaviruses or flaviviruses.
	Flaviviridae	West Nile virus: increased activity in past years, importation into NE US recognized in 1999	Drugs and vaccines under investigation
		Tick borne encephalitis virus: important pathogen in certain areas Europe, Siberia, Asia	Tick borne encephalitis virus: inactivated vaccine, immunoglobulin after tick exposure
Arboviral arthritis	Togaviruses (*Alphavirus* genus) Others	Ross River virus increasing problem in Australia.	No therapy. Developmental vaccines for Ross River and Chikungunya viruses.
Poxvirus diseases	Smallpox, monkeypox, and vaccinia	Protection of vaccinia lab workers	Vaccinia for lab workers every 3 years.
		Terrorist risk of smallpox, continuing activity of monkeypox	Cidofovir has been used in laboratory models of monkeypox with some efficacy.
Encephalitis and respiratory disease in domestic animals and humans	New genus of paramyxoviruses: Hendra and Nipah viruses	Discovered in 1995 and 1998	Ribavirin has been used arbitrarily in Nipah patients, but efficacy not established

Table 3. Properties of the viruses causing the VHF syndrome

Disease syndrome similar although the pathogenesis differs
Aerosol infectivity
Persist transmission in nature, but different survival strategies
Lipid enveloped and acid sensitive
Small RNA viruses, genome molecular weight 1-2x10^6 daltons
Negative, positive, and ambisense replication strategies
Different morphology and morphogenesis
Interactions with cells differ: cytopathic effects, interferon sensitivity
Human immune response differs

---

and close monitoring by experienced clinicians is possible. Hantaviruses will differ in that Hantaan virus and its relatives will cause primary renal failure and Sin Nombre virus and its relatives will cause acute pulmonary edema as major manifestations that will demand attention. In every case, therapy should be given for malaria, rickettsia, leptospira, relapsing fever, and other pathogens that could be confused unless the diagnosis is definitive. In those partially immune to malaria, of course, parasites may circulate in the blood without being a cause of severe illness.

The presence of viremia during the acute course of most of the VHF makes them an obvious target for agents that can interfere with viral replication or can neutralize virus. Arenaviruses are the most vulnerable because of their rather long clinical course. Furthermore, virtually all cases of potentially fatal VHF can be diagnosed within four hours using IgM and antigen detection ELISA's. Postmortem diagnosis should not be over-looked because specific immunohistochemical methods will detect viral antigens in formalin-fixed tissues and also provide valuable information for management of later cases that might appear.

Ribavirin is the most generally useful antiviral drug, and is clinically effective against members of the families Arenaviridae and Bunyaviridae [74]. Flaviviruses and togaviruses are sensitive to the *in vitro* effects of the drug, but effective levels are higher and animal studies have failed to show efficacy [61]. Antibody is also a useful potential modality in human or model diseases such as Argentine HF [14], Bolivian HF [13], and RVF [60]. Some of the viruses are quite sensitive to the antiviral effects of alpha or gamma interferon [53] but generally the disease process is too advanced to expect important clinical effects. Immunomodulators have had some effect in animal models but are not yet clinically relevant [60].

In the virus laboratory or medical care setting, prophylaxis after a high risk exposure is sometimes an issue. There are no useful human data. When dealing with diseases for which there is effective therapy with ribavirin, it is preferable to watch the patient carefully and institute therapy as soon as fever appears. This avoids the risks of treating the large proportion of exposures that never develop disease, the uncertainties of dose and duration, and carries a high expectation of success given the early initiation of treatment.

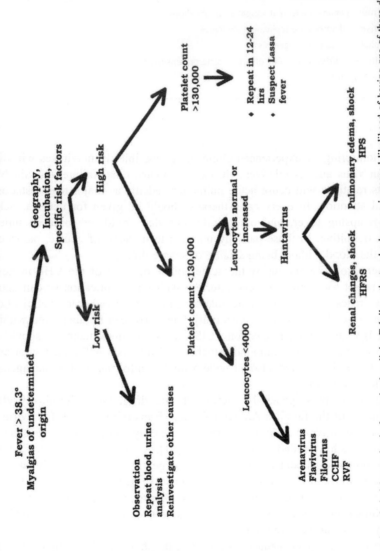

Figure 1. Early detection of viral hemorrhagic fevers in the clinic. Febrile patients who have an increased likelihood of having one of these diseases will have clear antecedents of epidemiological risk factors. They usually develop thrombocytopenia relatively early in their course. Some are strongly (South American arenaviral HF, flavivirus HF) or moderately strongly (CCHF, RVF) associated with leucopenia whereas hantavirus diseases are not. Lassa fever has variable platelet and leucocyte counts. Other findings that may suggest HF include vascular flushing, conjunctival injection, petechiae, proteinuria, or non-dependent edema. VHF patients may also present with increasing prostration and other subjective findings that indicate the severity of the patient's illness.

In animal models, it seems that post-exposure prophylaxis of arenavirus infections with the "static" drug ribavirin may fail to prevent central nervous system involvement and in other situations cessation of drug can be followed by recrudescence of visceral disease [74, 38]. Convalescent plasma with high titered neutralizing antibodies has been given to persons with high risk exposure to Argentine or Bolivian HF viruses.

Specific Hemorrhagic Fevers

Arenaviral HF

Argentine HF

This disease, like other arenaviral HF is characterized by the insidious onset of a prodromal phase lasting about one week, characterized by fever and constitutional signs and symptoms, with minor neurologic and/or hemorrhagic signs. A severe hemorrhagic-neurologic phase, often fatal, is seen in 20-30% of cases during the second week. The specific treatment consists of the transfusion of convalescent plasma in a standardized dose of neutralizing antibodies [14]; to be effective, it should be given within 8 days of onset. A late neurologic syndrome, generally benign and characterized mainly by truncal cerebellar ataxia with fever, is seen in around 10% of cases following this treatment [16]. Intravenous ribavirin in the same dosage as used in Lassa fever has been well-tolerated with some exacerbation of the anemia often associated with Argentine HF [17]. There have been suggestions of utility when patients beyond 8 days of evolution have received the drug [17].

There is an effective live attenuated Junin virus vaccine (Candid #1) which has been administered to more than 175,000 persons in the endemic area, but currently is only accessible to very high risk people because of limited availability [44]. This vaccine is thought to cross-protect against the Bolivian virus based on guinea pig and monkey studies, but has no apparent effect against Guanarito virus.

Other South American HF

Bolivian hemorrhagic fever closely resembles the Argentine disease in its clinical course and the causative viruses are genetically and antigenically closely related. There is no established therapy, but ribavirin is effective in animal models, including non-human primates [74]. Open label treatment of a limited number of human cases suggests the drug is useful and it should be employed in individual cases on a compassionate use basis, using the same regimen as for Lassa fever [40]. Passive antibodies have been used to good effect in animal models but higher doses may result in late encephalitis similar to that seen in the serotherapy of Argentine HF [13]. As in other arenavirus infections, interferon is circulating during the acute disease and exogenous interferon or inducers have either not been useful or have appeared to exacerbate disease [18].

Sabia virus, another human-pathogenic arenavirus, is found in Brazil. A laboratory infection in the US was successfully aborted by intravenous ribavirin given in the same dose as employed for Lassa fever [1]. Within 12-24 hours of drug administration virus could no longer be detected by isolation or RT-PCR. The patient's laboratory parameters became normal and 35 days after infection a humoral immune response was detected.

Lassa Fever

This important endemic disease of West Africa is also the VHF most often exported to Europe, the UK, or the US. Ribavirin is highly effective in animal models of Lassa fever, including macaques [33]. It has been tested in Sierra Leone against severe Lassa fever and found to be life-saving [47]. A randomized double-blind trial was not possible, but retrospective controls were stratified by serum viremia or SGOT, both predictors of a fatal outcome [36]. The intravenous drug (see below for administration) was beneficial in patients with an SGOT indicating an increased risk of dying (>150 IU/ml) (Table 4). The drug had its maximum impact if initiated during the first 6 days of illness but significant improvement in mortality was still evident even if therapy were begun at later time periods. Oral drug (2 g loading dose followed by 1 g/day in three divided doses for 10 days) also decreased mortality, but most experience has been with intravenous ribavirin. Retrospective analysis of uncontrolled data with half the intravenous dose suggests that it may be less effective [5].

In all arenavirus hemorrhagic fevers the fetus is known or thought to be at risk and pregnant patients are at an increased risk of dying. In Lassa fever, one series of 58 pregnancies was successful only in ¼ of cases and including neonatal deaths only 13% of infants survived. The maternal case fatality rate was 30% in the last trimester, compared to the approximately 15% in non-pregnant women [67]. Patients with spontaneous or induced evacuation of the uterus had a lower case fatality rate. This suggests that ribavirin treatment should be carefully considered in pregnant women, in spite of its relative contradiction in pregnancy.

Bunyaviridae: Rift Valley Fever (RVF) and Crimean Congo HF (CCHF)

RVF virus is sensitive *in vitro*, and model diseases in rodents and primates are readily prevented or treated by achievable doses of ribavirin [60]. Because of the unpredictability of Rift Valley fever outbreaks no trial has been carried out in humans. Modern tools may allow us to understand when to expect major epidemics and obtain the relevant data [43]. Even with advance warning, the best strategy is not clear. Treatment of established HF cases, which are a minority, may be too late to achieve a positive result. Another approach would be to give oral drug to all febrile patients in hopes of aborting the expected ~1% of cases of HF.

Although interferon is critical in determining the fate of macaques inoculated with RVF and both alpha and gamma interferon are active in modifying the course of disease, there seems to be a limited role for these compounds in human therapy [53, 52]. Passive neutralizing antibody prevents and treats RVF in macaques in very low doses [60, Morrill, unpublished data], but the logistics suggest that antibody will see limited use.

Table 4. Therapy of Lassa fever: time of initiation. Patients with AST >150 IU/ml at admission

Ribavirin	≤6 days			≥7 days		
	N	Deaths	(%)	N	Deaths	(%)
None	18	11	(61)	42	22	(52)
IV [A]	20	1	(5)	43	11	(26)
Oral [B]	5	1	(20)	9	1	(11)

[A] p = .0002, ≤6 days vs no therapy
  p = .01, ≥7 days vs no therapy
  p = .05, ≤6 days vs ≥7 days
[B] p = .030, ≥7 days vs no therapy

Adapted from (47)

High risk persons such as laboratory or veterinary workers expected to come in contact with the virus can be immunized with a formalin inactivated vaccine [66]. A new live, attenuated vaccine has undergone extensive animal evaluation and found to be safe and effective [51]. Good neutralizing antibody titers were induced, viral challenge was resisted, and no evidence of teratogenicity was seen in pregnant sheep or cattle; even direct inoculation of fetal bovines was without incident. Based on these results as well as extensive other data including very low monkey neurovirulence, the vaccine (MP-12) was inoculated into more than 60 human volunteers. Neutralizing antibody titers developed promptly and side-effects were minimal. Unfortunately, further development of the vaccine candidate is not planned.

CCHF virus is sensitive to ribavirin *in vitro* [80] and the only available animal model, the virus-infected weanling mouse, can be successfully treated with the drug [76]. Open label administration of intravenous drug in South Africa has been interpreted by clinicians as showing prompt clinical improvement, decreased morbidity, and fewer deaths leading to its routine employment there. Efficacy has been supported by comparisons of survival in treated cases to the historic record after stratification by clinical laboratory predictors of fatal outcome [75]. In Pakistan the drug has been given orally (4 g/day in 4 divided doses followed by 2.6 g/day) to CCHF patients but no data on efficacy are available [23].

CCHF vaccine has been produced from mouse brain, but there is little information on its safety and efficacy and its utility remains speculative.

Bunyaviridae: Hantavirus Diseases: Hemorrhagic Fever With Renal Syndrome (HFRS) and Hantavirus Pulmonary Syndrome (HPS)

Like other Bunyaviridae, viruses in the *Hantavirus* genus are inhibited by moderate concentrations of ribavirin in cell culture [Ruo and coworkers, unpublished data]. The only animal model for hantavirus disease, encephalitis in the intracranially inoculated suckling mouse, has also shown a positive effect with the drug [30].

HFRS

Hantaan and Dobrava viruses regularly cause severe HFRS [58] in Asia and the Balkans respectively. This disease pursues a course initiated by fever and constitutional involvement, followed by shock, and culminating in oliguric or anuric renal failure. Insightful supportive care with aggressive renal dialysis are key to survival. Ribavirin has been shown to significantly decrease the duration of oliguria the hemorrhagic manifestations, and mortality in a controlled trial in China [29]. In this study, intravenous drug was initiated within 4-6 days of onset during the early febrile phase of illness. Dialysis was not available so the shortening of oliguria may have been crucial in reducing the mortality from 10/127 (7.9%) to 3/122 (2.5%). Although numbers were small, the decrease in mortality in the treated group was only apparent after 6 days of therapy, suggesting that some time was needed for drug effects to be manifest in HFRS. There was no evident need for dose reduction in renal failure and there has been no requirement for additional dosing during dialysis.

Ribavirin is given by many Chinese clinicians to any patient with suspected HFRS presenting during the febrile phase of illness and could be a useful adjunct even in settings where dialysis is routinely available. The milder form of HFRS caused by Puumala virus in Europe probably would not benefit significantly from the drug, but no data are available.

Steroids may have a role in ameliorating the clinical signs of HFRS. Early reports of clinical improvement during the Korean conflict led to a randomized, placebo controlled trial in 68 patients presenting within 72 hours of onset. There was an improvement in overall well-being including vomiting; but more importantly there were statistically significant decreases in fever, proteinuria, and azotemia. The small groups did not allow an assessment of mortality, but there was a trend toward fewer patients with severe shock in the treated group. Only 1100 mg hydrocortisone was given over a 5 day period with doses of 300 mg the first two days [72]. In contrast, a more recent study in China failed to show any improvement in renal function or survival after receiving prednisone [68]. In light of the over-all poor results obtained in septic shock and ARDS, it is difficult to be enthusiastic about routine therapy of HFRS patients with corticosteroids, but there may well be subsets of patients and dosage regimens that should be subjected to further trials. For example, "stress doses" of hydrocortisone (100 mg iv followed by.18 mg/kg/hr were useful in one study of patients with septic shock [4]. It should not be forgotten that HFRS patients may have pituitary compromise and be functionally hypoadrenal during the course of severe disease [42].

Other attempts to treat the immunopathogenesis of HFRS with cyclophosphamide or to use exogenous interferon in sick patients have failed to show any significant benefit.

HPS

This disease, as the name says, presents with pulmonary signs and symptoms after a febrile prodrome [58]. As in HFRS, supportive care, including the difficult problem of managing shock and myocardial dysfunction in the face of pulmonary vascular permeability increase is critical to survival. Recognition of the disease is difficult during the prodromal period [50]. As pulmonary insufficiency develops, thrombocytopenia provides an important clue and IgM antiviral antibodies will already be present at this time. Most deaths occur within 24-48 hours of admission to the hospital so there is little time to intervene. An open-label experience with ribavirin showed little evidence for toxicity, but there was no evident benefit [9]. A controlled trial to confirm these findings is underway

Because of the likelihood of interpersonal transmission [81, 82] of one of the HPS agents, Andes virus, an open-label trial with intravenous ribavirin is underway in contacts of Andes cases in Argentina. Drug is given at the first signs of febrile disease without waiting for evidence of pulmonary involvement.

In Argentina and Chile some clinicians have a strong impression that HPS patients treated with steroids have a better course than otherwise [77]. In Argentina a placebo-controlled trial of hydrocortisone (200 mg iv q 6 hours for 4 days) is under consideration.

Other approaches such as blocking the cytokines that seem to be the prime movers in the pathogenesis of the pulmonary lesion have not been attempted, at least in part because of the lack of a realistic animal model for preclinical testing and the complexity of the problem as exemplified by the poor results obtained to date in cytokine therapy of septic shock. Salvage therapy with NO inhalation [69] and extracorporeal membrane oxygenation [11] have had anecdotal success, but the over-all case fatality remains 30-40% of hospitalized cases.

Filoviridae: Ebola and Marburg

These viruses cause disease in Africa and the pattern is usually that of uncommon human infection followed by interpersonal transmission or even epidemic disease from nosocomial or needle-borne spread [71]. The viruses can infect hospital workers even in modern hospital settings [73]. This is the only HF for which there is neither vaccine nor investigational human therapy. Studies *in vitro* and in animal models have failed to show efficacy for interferons or ribavirin.

Recovery from filovirus infection is thought to be largely mediated by effector T cells because simple convalescent plasma has had little protective effect [63]. Serum from horses hyperimmunized to the Zaire subtype of Ebola virus has enhanced *in vitro* neutralizing capacity and protects guinea pigs and baboons when given in large quantities shortly after inoculation of small doses of virus, but is only marginally effective when tested in macaques [32, 34]. Bone marrow from survivors of the 1995 Zaire epidemic yielded mRNA coding for antibodies that may have greater activity than the spectrum found in polyclonal convalescent sera and such monoclonals may be exploited therapeutically [46].

During an epidemic in Zaire in 1995 eight Ebola patients were transfused with whole blood from recently convalescent survivors and seven survived [54]. Although this was impressive in an epidemic with an 80% case fatality, closer analysis of the length of survival before transfusion, age, sex, and timing during the epidemic suggested that there may well not have been a real effect on the disease particularly because many recipients were several days in their disease course before treatment [70]. In any case, the phenomenon suggests that we should broaden our perspective to include the possible activities of lymphocytes or soluble factors other than antibody.

In experimental animals, SAAH inhibitors have had some efficacy [31], but as yet there is no additional data to suggest there is a role for them in human therapy.

Flaviviridae

The most important flavivirus is yellow fever virus, which is transmitted in tropical Africa and America among non-human primates by mosquitoes. Travelers to forest areas of those regions should be vaccinated for yellow fever because of the high case fatality rate (20%) and the lack of any effective therapy. Periodically in Africa yellow fever emerges from the forest to circulate in savanna regions. The virus also can be transmitted between humans by the urban-dwelling *Aedes aegypti* which have been vectors of massive epidemics in the past. This cycle functions occasionally in African cities. Today there is great concern for the large cities of South America where intense dengue circulation signals the existence of high *Ae. aegypti* populations and possible receptivity to urban yellow fever epidemics. Preventable deaths continue to occur in residents and travelers [8] in spite of a highly effective vaccine with few contraindications and only rare adverse effects; current detailed geographic recommendations can be obtained from [6].

Dengue fever continues to be a world-wide problem. It is mainly transmitted between humans by *Ae. aegypti*. The four dengue viruses are readily transported around the globe by incubating or viremic humans and often find receptive areas for intensive transmission because of the multiple factors that have allowed the intensive breeding of its mosquito vector throughout tropical and sub-tropical regions of Asia, Africa, and the Americas. Dengue virus infection is often unpleasant and temporarily incapacitating but rarely causes primary hemorrhagic fever. Dengue fever patients may have thrombocytopenia, petechiae, nosebleed, or hemorrhage from preexisting lesions. Sequential infection with different dengue serotypes occasionally (~1%) results in a severe vascular permeability syndrome (dengue shock syndrome, DSS) with hemorrhage and shock. There is no specific antiviral therapy, but supportive care with fluid replacement is usually effective (case fatality probably <1%, although poor ascertainment of fatal and non-fatal cases makes exact figures difficult to come by) [25, 56]. As with other VHF, myocardial dysfunction should be suspected during management decisions [79]. Dengue vaccines are under development and may be available within the next few years for travelers and residents of areas at risk for DSS.

Another phylogenetically distinct group of flaviviruses is transmitted by ticks. The best known are the agents of tick-borne encephalitis, which is a biphasic disease with an initial period of fever, malaise, and thrombocytopenia followed by a second phase of central nervous system invasion. The VHF that belong to this group, such as Omsk HF or Kyasanur Forest disease, have a similar course but the initial manifestations are usually accompanied by hemorrhagic manifestations and shock and the subsequent encephalitic part of the disease is clinically relatively minor. There is no antiviral therapy, but an inactivated vaccine has been used in India to protect against Kyasanur Forest disease with apparent success.

Use of Ribavirin To Treat VHF

The VHF are life-threatening diseases and ribavirin has been used in a relatively small number of cases, so we can anticipate there are as yet undefined side-effects and clinical problems associated with the most commonly used iv dosage.

The intravenous dose used for Lassa fever and other HF is 32 mg/kg loading dose, 16 mg/kg every 6 hours for 4 days and then 8 mg/kg every 8 hours for 6 additional days. The maximum doses given should not exceed 2 g loading dose, 1 g per dose for the next 4 days and 0.5 g per dose for the final 6 days. Episodes of chills and other symptoms may accompany bolus administration [21] so the drug is best given in 100-125 ml of fluid over 30 minutes. No adjustment of the dose has been made for diminished renal function [29]. The basic safety of this regimen for adults appears to be well established [17, 47, 29, 9].

There is a predictable decrease in hematocrit that seems to be a result of both hemolysis and a block in erythropoesis. The anemia has always been reversible and is generally not severe. A mild indirect hyperbilirubinemia is usual. Subjective symptoms are also common, including malaise and nausea, but their relation to drug administration is not well-defined.

Pregnant women have not been treated because of teratogenic effects of ribavirin in rodents. This is moot in the last trimester of pregnancy in Lassa fever when fetal mortality is high and the maternal mortality is 30% [67]. Forthcoming data with lower oral doses inadvertently administered to pregnant women under treatment for hepatitis C may shed additional light on this.

Children have not been included in iv ribavirin studies because of reports of growth retardation in rodents given ribavirin chronically; however, risk-benefit considerations would presumably justify extending treatment to children in certain circumstances. For example, Lassa fever is a virulent pediatric disease in West Africa and would be a candidate for future studies with intravenous drug and appropriate monitoring for adverse effects.

CNS penetration is an important issue in ribavirin use. Some animal studies have shown convincingly that the drug is much less efficacious in CNS involvement [74, 38]. Nevertheless, 73-115% of plasma concentrations have been found in CSF after chronic administration of ribavirin to three HIV-infected patients [12] and there is room for further exploration.

It is frustrating that there is so little hard data on the efficacy of ribavirin in the VHF, as well as its use in special groups such as pregnant women and children. We also need more data on different dosing regimens, particularly the possible utility of mixed regimens with iv loading followed by oral maintenance. Part of the problem relates to poverty, inadequate infrastructure, and sporadic occurrence of some of the diseases. Nevertheless, the risk-benefit equation for serious illnesses caused by Arenaviridae and some Bunyaviridae (RVF, CCHF, and probably Hantaan) favors the drug's use.

Other Viruses

Arboviral Encephalitis

Members of several virus families are responsible for varying morbidity and mortality from central nervous system infections in the US each year. The most common childhood encephalitis in the US is caused by La Crosse virus. The mortality from the disease is very low and obvious sequelae are uncommon. Nevertheless, the morbidity is considerable and behavioral residuals are controversial. The drug is effective against the virus *in vitro* [57] and has been used to treat a severe case of La Crosse encephalitis [48].

Alphaviruses cause Eastern, Western, and Venezuelan encephalitis in the Americas. In the US the number of human cases is generally small, there is no virus specific therapy, and the available human vaccines are experimental and not generally available [37].

The recent reports of West Nile virus epidemics in several areas of Europe [28] coupled with its recognition as having been introduced into the US in 1999 have increased awareness of it as a cause of febrile disease with rash, hepatitis, and encephalitis, however no antiviral therapy or vaccine is available. Related mosquito-borne flaviviruses causing encephalitis are St. Louis encephalitis virus in the US, Murray Valley encephalitis virus in Australia, and the Asian Japanese encephalitis virus. The latter is an important cause of morbidity and mortality in many areas of Asia and a Japanese-manufactured inactivated vaccine is licensed in the US. Summer travel to rural areas of endemic zones may justify the small risk of vaccination [49, 6].

Tick-borne encephalitis (another flavivirus) occurs in Europe and Asia and is particularly dangerous in areas of Far Eastern Russia where a more severe form of the disease is recognized. Travelers expecting to spend time in rural areas of endemic zones hiking, orienteering, etc should consider prophylaxis with one of the European licensed vaccines [49]. There have been rare reports of reactions, but the vaccines have good safety and efficacy records. In addition, virus-specific IgG is sometimes administered after tick-bites in unvaccinated persons. There appears to be efficacy, but the reagent must be given within the first 4 days and later administration may have a risk of enhancement; vaccine can be given simultaneously without suppressing the rate of seroconversion [26].

Arboviral Arthritis

Many mild arboviral illnesses, including dengue fever, are associated with arthralgias, but a few result in true arthritis. Notable among these are epidemic alphavirus disease such as Ross River virus in Australia, Chikungunya virus in Africa and Asia, and Mayaro virus in Central and South America [37]. An incapacitating acute phase may be followed by weeks of residual joint symptoms. There is no chemotherapy available. An inactivated vaccine is under development for Ross River virus and an investigational live-attenuated Chikungunya virus vaccine exists.

Poxvirus Diseases

Several zoonotic poxviruses circulate in nature and may result in localized lesions and systemic symptoms in humans, and of course molluscum contagiosum is a human pathogen that assumes major proportions in immunosuppressed patients [20]. However, there are still three important considerations for poxvirus infections in the general population: monkeypox, smallpox, and vaccinia. Monkeypox virus is thought to be a zoonotic infection of arboreal squirrels in the African tropical forest, which occasionally spills over into humans with consequent interhuman transmission. The classic studies have clearly shown that monkeypox virus has a relatively low mortality in humans (11% in children with virtually no medical care), chains of human transmission die out, and vaccinia protects against the disease [35]. In the absence of vaccine deployment for protection against smallpox, monkeypox transmission has been more pronounced, but widespread use of vaccinia is not indicated to protect against monkeypox. The possibility that the virus might adapt to more efficient interhuman spread or that HIV infection could change transmission dynamics exists but there has been no credible evidence to suggest so. Thus, an antiviral drug to ameliorate the impact of monkeypox or to deal with possible future developments would be useful, but its actual deployment would be unlikely given the economic and political considerations.

Smallpox virus was eliminated from nature in October 1977 and the eradication has been repeatedly confirmed. In spite of this, a smallpox death occurred in August 1978 in a laboratory in the United Kingdom. Today, the World Health Assembly has restricted smallpox stocks and research to two laboratories, one in the US and one in Russia. The chance that the virus would accidentally escape from either of these repositories is very small and could be managed with retained stocks of vaccinia, the same smallpox vaccine that served to eradicate the virus. Unfortunately, there is a widespread concern among officials of the US and other governments that there are stocks of smallpox virus in several other sites and that smallpox could be used as a tool for biological warfare or terrorism. The authors have no objective evidence to evaluate the probability that this might occur, but the proponents are credible and the idea is plausible; if such an incident should occur, the consequences would be very different from a unifocal problem arising from a laboratory incident. The ability to control a multifocal outbreak with current stocks of vaccine would be questionable and the outcome of such an epidemic would be simply impossible to accept [27].

When one examines our options to respond to smallpox, they are remarkably limited. The only credible modality is widespread use of the classical smallpox vaccine in large quantities to stop the spread of smallpox and to provide assurance that the virus would indeed be contained and subsequently eradicated. The development of an alternative vaccine that might be protective and would be less reactogenic may be technologically feasible, but in practice it is impossible to demonstrate before an emergency that we could rely on a "new" vaccine to keep this dangerous virus in check. Antiviral therapy with methisazone and adenine arabinoside during the smallpox era failed whenever properly evaluated [41]. Development of new antiviral agents might seem like a valuable adjunct, but its application is bedeviled by the same problems as improving the vaccine: any proposed remedy cannot be tested against smallpox in humans and its impact on a confused, demanding emergency situation would remain problematic. This being said, there are therapeutic possibilities among drugs that have been developed for other viruses. One of these is cidofovir, which has been shown have some activity in cowpox infection of mice and monkeypox infection of macaques [3].

The area where we can respond meaningfully is with antivirals against vaccinia. If widespread vaccination against smallpox is required, there will be a real enigma as to how to protect the persons immunosuppressed by chemotherapy for malignancy or AIDS who are present in much greater numbers than when the vaccine was used pre-1970. It seems unlikely that a person whose immune system cannot limit the spread of vaccinia could be immunized against smallpox with any vaccine. If by medical oversight or interhuman transmission, immunosuppressed persons are inoculated with vaccinia, we need a modality to effectively protect them. Vaccinia immune globulin was somewhat effective, but the mortality was high even with this treatment and development of an antiviral drug could be extremely useful. It also seems possible to develop an adequate experimental animal database and test the drug against localized vaccinia infections of humans. Ribavirin, a drug that has activity *in vitro* against poxviruses has been used in progressive vaccinia to enhance the effects of vaccinia immune globulin with apparent good effects [39].

Vaccinia itself is widely employed in biomedical research and users of the laboratory strains should be protected from accidental inoculation (particularly ocular) of the laboratory viruses by the standard smallpox vaccine initially and every three years subsequently; this provides a well-characterized vaccinia strain administrated by a standardized dose, site, and route. Major contraindications are immunosuppression, eczema, and pregnancy in the recipient or the likelihood of close contact with someone with those conditions [7].

New Paramyxovirus Diseases

In 1994 Australia encountered the first member of the previously undescribed *Megamyxovirus* (proposed) genus of Paramyxoviridae [55]. Initial findings from infected horses suggested a virus related to measles and the inadequate appellation "equine morbillivirus" was used. Although the horse epizootic was small and self-limited and only three humans were infected, the findings were disturbing. One human with very close horse contact died from an acute respiratory disease and a second human had a brief illness after assisting in an equine necropsy but after more than a year developed progressive, fatal viral encephalitis. The virus, named Hendra after the town in which the first cases were recognized, has only recurred in two horses in 1999, but fruit bats have been implicated as the reservoir.

In 1998 an epidemic of encephalitis was recognized in Malaysia and initially confused with Japanese encephalitis. Eventually, the cause was recognized as Nipah virus, a new paramyxovirus related to Hendra [10, 24]. The virus had entered the pig population and spread among the pigs in a setting of intensive pork production and export. Human cases were virtually all in close contact with swine and massive culling of pigs was associated with cessation of human cases. There were more than 200 human cases with approximately 35% case fatality. Many were treated with ribavirin, but no systematic data were collected so the efficacy remains unknown. The source of the virus may be *Pteropus* bats because antibodies have been found in members of that genus.

It seems likely that these viruses or their relatives will reemerge in the future and chemotherapy for them could become important. Hendra virus has caused a late-relapse encephalitis in one person and thus future treatment for survivors, should they relapse, could potentially be useful as well [55]. In fact, acute cases may be occurring at this time, masquerading as Japanese encephalitis, but not being diagnosed for lack of adequate laboratory facilities.

References

1. Barry M, Russi M, Armstrong L, Geller D, Tesh R, Dembry L, Gonzalez JP, Khan AS, Peters CJ. Treatment of a laboratory-acquired Sabia virus infection. New Eng J Med 1995; 333: 294-296.

2. Bausch DG, Rollin PE, Demby AH, Coulibaly M, Kanu J, Conteh AS, Wagoner KD, McMullan LK, Bowen MD, Peters CJ, Ksiazek TG. Clinical Virology of Lassa Fever: Evaluation of the Enzyme-Linked Immunosorbent Assay, Indirect Fluorescent-Antibody Test, and Virus Isolation on suspected Cases from West Africa, J Clin Micro. 2000 In press

3. Bray M. Martinez M. Smee DF. Kefauver D. Thompson E. Huggins JW. Cidofovir protects mice against lethal aerosol or intranasal cowpox virus challenge. Journal of Infectious Diseases. 181(1): 10-9, 2000

4. Briegel J, Forst H, Haller M, Schelling G, Kilger E, Kuprat G, Hemmer B, Hummel T, Lenhart A, Heyduck M, Stoll C, Peter K. Stress doses of hydrocortisone reverse hyperdynamic septic shock: a prospective, randomized, double-blind, single-center study. Crit Care Med. 1999; 27: 723-732.

5. Busico KM, McCormick JB, Parker L, Lloyd ES, Webb PA, Gary HE, Hill HA, Scribner CL, Craven RB, King IJ, Fisher-Hoch SP, Trippel S, Elliot LH, Demby A, Williams B, Khan AS, Johnson KM. Efficacy of ribavirin dose on outcome in adult Lassa fever aptients, Sierra Leone, 1980-1990. Presented 46th Annual Meeting of the American Society of Tropical Medicine and Hygiene, Lake Buena Vista, FL, 7-11 Dec, 1997

6. CDC. Health Information for International Travel, 1999-2000. US Govt Printing Office, Washington, DC, 1999 or www.cdc.gov/travel

7. CDC. Vaccinia (Smallpox) Vaccine Recommendations of the Immunization Practices Advisory Committee (ACIP) MMWR. 1991; 40(RR14): 1-10. available through www.cdc.gov/epo/mmwr/preview/mmwrhtml/00042032.htm

8. CDC. Fatal yellow fever in a traveler returning from Venezuela, 1999; 49: 303-305.

9. Chapman LE, Mertz GJ, Peters CJ, Jolson HM, Khan AS, Ksiazek TG, Koster FT, Baum KF, Rollin PE, Pavia AT, Holman RC, Christenson JC, Rubin PJ, Behrman RE, Wilson Bell LJ, Simpson GL, Sadek RF, and the Ribavirin Study Group. Intravenous Ribavirin for Hantavirus Pulmonary Syndrome: Safety and Tolerance During One Year of Open Label Experience. Antiviral Therapy 1999; 4: 211-219.

10. Chua KB, Bellini WJ, Rota PA, Harcourt BH, Temin A, Lam SK, Ksiazek TG, Rollin P, Zaki SR, Shieh W-J, Goldsmith CS, Roehrig JT, Eaton B, Gould R, Olson J, Field H, Daniel P, Ling AE, Peters CJ, Anderson LJ, Mahy BWJ. Nipah Virus: A Recently Emergent Deadly Paramyxovirus. Science 2000; 288(5470): 1432-1435.

11. Crowley MR. Katz RW. Kessler R. Simpson SQ. Levy H. Hallin GW. Cappon J. Krahling JB. Wernly J.

Successful treatment of adults with severe hantavirus pulmonary syndrome with extracorporeal membrane oxygenation Critical Care Medicine 1998; 26(2): 409-14.

12. Crumpacker, C, G Bubley, D Lucey, S Hussey, J Connor. Ribavirin enters cerebrospinal fluid. Lancet. 1986; ii: 45-46.

13. Eddy GA, Wagner FS, Scott SK, Mahlandt BJ. Protection of monkeys against Machupo virus by the passive administration of Bolivian haemorrhagic fever immunoglobulin (human origin). Bull World Health Organ 1975; 52: 723-727.

14. Enria DA, Briggiler AM, Fernandez NJ, et al. Importance of dose of neutralizing antibodies in treatement of Argentine haemorrhagic fever with immune plasma. Lancet 1984; 2: 255.

15. Enria DA, Briggiler AM, Levis S, et al. Preliminary report: Tolerance and antiviral effect of ribavirin in patients with Argentine hemorrhagic fever. Antiviral Res 1987; 7: 353-360.

16. Enria DA, Damilano AJ de, Briggiler AM, Ambrosio AM, Fernández NJ, Feuillade MR, Maiztegui JI. Sindrome neurologico tardio en enfermos de fiebre hemorrágica Argentina tratados con plasma immune. *Medicina (Buenos Aires)* 1985; 45: 615-620.

17. Enria DA, Maiztegui JI. Antiviral treatment of Argentine hemorrhagic fever. Antivir Res 1994; 23: 23-31.

18. Enria D, Bowen M, Mills JN, Shieh W-J, Bausch D, Peters CJ. Arenaviruses, Chapter 111, in Tropical Infectious Diseases: Principles, Pathogens & Practice. Eds: Richard L. Guerrant, David H. Walker, Peter F. Weller. W.B. Saunders, New York 1999; 1189-1212.

19. Feldmann H, Bugany H, Mahner F, Klenk H-D, Drenckhahn D, Schnittler HJ. Filovirus-induced endothelial leakage triggered by infected monocytes/ macrophages. Journal of Virology 1996; 70: 2208-2214.

20. Fenner F. Poxviruses, in Richman DD, Whitley RJ, Haydon FG, eds. Clinical Virology. Churchill Livingston, New York 1997; 27: 357-373.

21. Fisher-Hoch SP, Gborie S, Parker L, Huggins J. Unexpected adverse reactions clinical trial in rural west Africa. Antiviral Research 1992; 19: 139-47.

22. Fisher-Hoch SP, Khan JA, Rehman S, Mirza S, Khurshid M, McCormick JB. Crimean Congo Haemorrhagic Fever treated with oral ribavirin. Lancet 1995; 346: 472-475.

23. Gear JSS, Cassel GA, Gear AJ, Trappler B, Clansen L, Meyers AM, Kew MC, Bothwell TH, Sher R, Miller GB, Schneider J, Koornhoff HJ, Gomperts ED, Isaacson M, and Gear JHS (1975). Outbreak of Marburg virus disease in Johannesburg. British Medical Journal 4:489-493.

24. Goh KJ, Tan CT, Chew NK, Tan PS, Kamarulzaman A, Sarji SA, Wong KT, Abdullah BJ, Chua KB, Lam SK. Clinical features of Nipah virus encephalitis among pig farmers in Malaysia New England Journal of Medicine 2000; 42(17): 1229-35.

25. Halstead SB. Dengue and dengue hemorrhagic fever in Feigin and Cherry JD ed Textbook of Pediatric Infectious Disease. WB Saunders: Philadelphia 1987; 1510-1521.

26. Hedenstrom Mv, Heberle U, Theobald K. Vaccination against tick-borne encephalitis (TBE): influence of simultaneous application of TBE immunoglobulin on seroconversion and rate of adverse events. Vaccine. 1995; 13: 759-762.

27. Henderson DA, Inglesby TV, Bartlett JG, Ascher MS, Eitzen E, Jahrling PB, Hauer J, Layton M, McDade J, Osterholm MT, O'Toole T, Parker G, Perl T, Russell PK, Tonat K, for the Working Group on Civilian Biodefense. Smallpox as a Biological Weapon. JAMA. 1999; '281: 2127-2137.

28. Hubalek Z, Halouzka J. West Nile fever--a reemerging mosquito-borne viral disease in Europe. Emerging Infectious Diseases 1999; 5: 643-50.

29. Huggins JW, Hsiang CM, Cosgriff TM, Guang MY, Smith JI, Wu ZO, et al. Prospective, Double-Blind,

Concurrent, Placebo-Controlled Clinical Trial of Intravenous Ribavirin Therapy of Hemorrhagic Fever with Renal Syndrome. The Journal of Infectious Diseases 1991; 164: 1119-27.

30. Huggins JW, Kim GR, Brand OM, McKee KT. Ribavirin therapy for Hantaan virus infection in suckling mice. Journal of Infectious Diseases 1986; 153: 489-97

31. Huggins JW, Zhang Z, Bray M. Antiviral drug therapy of filovirus infections: S-adenosylhomocysteine hydrolase inhibitors inhibit Ebola virus *in vitro* and in a lethal mouse model. In Peters CJ, Leduc JW (eds): Ebola: the virus and the Disease, J Infect Dis 1999; 179 suppl 1: S240-247.

32. Jahrling PB, Geisbert J, Sweariengen JR, Jaax GP, Lewis T, Huggins JW, Schmidt JJ, LeDuc JW, Peters CJ. Passive immunization of Ebola virus-infected cynomolgus monkeys with immunoglobulin from hyperimmune horses. Arch Virol 1996; [Suppl]11: 135-140.

33. Jahrling PB, Hesse RA, Eddy GA, Johnson KM, Callis RT, Stephen EL. Lassa fever infection in rhesus monkeys. Pathogenesis and treatment with ribavirin. J Infect Dis 1980; 141: 580-589.

34. Jahrling PB, Geisbert TW, Geisbert JB, Swearengen JR, Bray M, Jaax NK, Huggins JW, LeDuc JW, Peters CJ. Evaluation of Immune Globulin and Recombinant Interferon alpha-2b for Treatment of Experimental Ebola Virus Infections. J Infect Dis 1999; 179 (Supp l): S224-234.

35. Jezek Z, Fenner F. Human Monkeypox. Monographs in Virology1st ed. Karger New York 1988; 17: 140.

36. Johnson KM, McCormick JB, Webb PA, Smith ES, Elliott LH, King IJ. Clinical virology of Lassa fever in hospitalized patients. J Infect Dis 1987; 155: 456-464.

37. Johnston RE, Peters CJ. Alphaviruses In Fields BN, Knipe DM, Howley PM, eds. Fields Virology, third edition. Philadelphia: Lippincott-Raven Publishers 1996; 28: 843-898.

38. Kenyon RH, Canonico PG, Green DE, Peters CJ. Effect of ribavirin and tributylribavirin on Argentine hemorrhagic fever (Junin virus) in guinea pigs. Antimicrob. Agents Chemother 1986; 29: 521-523.

39. Kesson AM, Ferguson JK, Rawlinson WD, Cunningham AL. Progressive vaccinia treated with ribavirin and vaccinia immune globulin. Clin Infect Dis 1997; 25: 911-14.

40. Kilgore PE, Ksiazek TG, Rollin PE, Mills JN, Villagra MR, Montenegro MJ, Costales MA, Paredes LC, Peters CJ. Treatment of Bolivian hemorrhagic fever with intravenous ribavirin. J Infect Dis 1997; 24: 718-722.

41. Koplan JP, Monsur KA, Foster SO, Huq F, Rahaman MM, Huq S, Buchanan RA, Ward NA. Treatment of variola major with adenine arabinoside. J Infect Dis 1975; 131: 34-39.

42. Lim TH, Chang KH, Han MC, Chang YB, Lim SM, Yu YS, Chun YH, Lee JS. Pituitary atrophy in Korean (epidemic) hemorrhagic fever: CT correlation with pituitary function and visual field. American Journal of Neuroradiology 1986; 7(4): 633-7.

43. Linthicum KJ, Anyamba A, Tucker CJ, Kelley PW, Myers MF, Peters CJ. Climate and satellite indicators to forecast Rift Valley fever epidemics in Kenya. Science 1999; 285: 397-400.

44. Maiztegui JI, McKee KT, Barrera Oro JG, Harrison LH, Gibbs PH, Feuillade MR, Enria DA, Briggiler AM, Levis SC, Ambrosio AM, Halsey NA, Peters CJ and the AHF Study Group. Protective efficacy of a live attenuated vaccine against Argentine hemorrhagic fever, J Infect Dis 1998; 177: 277-283.

45. Marta RF, Montero VS, Molinas FC. Systemic disorders in Argentine haemorrhagic fever. Bull Inst Pasteur 1998, 96: 115-24

46. Maruyama T, Rodriguez LL, Jahrling PB, Sanchez A, Khan AS, Nichol ST, Peters CJ, Parren PW, Burton DR. Ebola virus can be effectively neutralized by antibody produced in natural human infection. J Virol 1999; 73(7): 6024-30.

47. McCormick JB, King IJ, Webb PA, Scribner CL, Craven RB, Johnson KM, Elliott LH, Belmont-Williams R. Lassa fever. Effective therapy with ribavirin. *New Engl J Med* 1986: 314: 20-26.

48. McJunkin JE, Khan RR, Tsai TF. California-La Crosse encephalitis. in ed Hughes JM and Conte JE. Infect Dis Clinics North Amer. 1998; 12: 83.

49. Monath TP, Tsai TP, Flaviviruses TF. in Richman DD, Whitley RJ, Haydon FG, eds. Clinical Virology. Churchill Livingston, New York 1997; 49: 1133-1185.

50. Moolenaar RL, Dalton C, Lipman HB, et al. Clinical features that differentiate hantavirus pulmonary syndrome from three other acute respiratory illnesses. Clin Infect Dis 1995; 643-649.

51. Morrill JC, Mebus CA, Peters CJ. Safety of a mutagen-attenuated Rift Valley fever virus vaccine in fetal and neonatal bovids. AJVR 1997; 58: 1110-1114.

52. Morrill JC, Czarniecki CW, Peters CJ. Recombinant human inteferon-gamma modulates Rift Valley fever virus infection in the rhesus monkey. J Inteferon Res 1991; 11: 297-304.

53. Morrill JC, Jennings GB, Johnson AJ, Cosgriff TM, Gibbs PH, Peters CJ. Pathogenesis of Rift Valley fever in rhesus monkeys: Role of interferon response. Arch. Virol 1990; 110: 195-212.

54. Mupapa K, Masamba M, Kibadi K, Kuvula K, Bwaka A, Kipasa M, Colebunders R, Muyembe T on behalf of the International Scientific and Technical Committee, Centers for Disease Control (United States) Institute of Tropical Medicine and Médecins Sans Frontières (Belgium), and Pasteur Institute (France). Treatment of Ebola Hemorrhagic Fever with Blood Transfusions from Convalescent Patients. J Infect Dis 1999; Supp 1

55. Murray K, Eaton B, Hooper P, Wang L, Williamson M, Young P. Flying foxes, horses, and humans: a zoonosis caused by a new member of the Paramyxoviridae. in Emerging Infections I, ed WM Scheld, D Armstrong, JM Hughes, Washington DC ASM Press, 1998; 4: 43-58.

56. Nimmannitya, Suchitra. Dengue hemorrhagic fever: diagnosis and management. In Dengue and dengue hemorrhagic fever, ed DJ Gubler and G Kuno, CAB International 1997; 133-145.

57. Patterson JL, Fernandez-Larsson R. Molecular mechanisms of action of ribavirin. Rev Inf Dis 1990; 12: 1139-1146.

58. Peters CJ, GL Simpson, H Levy. Spectrum of Hantavirus Infection: Hemorrhagic fever with renal syndrome and hantavirus pulmonary syndrome. Annu Rev Med 1999; 50: 531-545.

59. Peters CJ, Jahrling PB, Khan AS. Management of patients infected with high-hazard viruses: scientific basis for infection control. Arch Virol 1996; Suppl 11: 1-28.

60. Peters CJ, Reynolds JA, Slone TW, Jones DE, Stephen EL. Prophylaxis of Rift Valley fever with antiviral drugs, immune serum, an interferon inducer, and a macrophage activator. Antiviral Res 1986; 6: 285-297.

61. Peters CJ, Huggins JW, Jahrling PB. Antiviral therapy for yellow fever. Annals of the International Symposium on Yellow Fever and Dengue, 15-19 May 1988, Rio de Janeiro, Brazil 1991; 134-152.

62. Peters CJ, Zaki SR. Viral Hemorrhagic Fever: An Overview Tropical Infectious Diseases: Principles, Pathogens & Practice. Eds: Richard L Guerrant, David H. Walker, Peter F Weller, WB Saunders, New York 1999; 10: 1180-1188.

63. Peters CJ. Pathogenesis of Viral Hemorrhagic Fevers. In Nathanson N, Ahmed R, Gonzalez-Scarano F, Griffin D, Holmes KV, Murphy FA, Robinson HL, eds. Viral Pathogenesis. Philadelphia: Lippincott-Raven Publishers, 1997; 32: 779-799.

64. Peters CJ, Zaki SR, Rollin PE. Viral Hemorrhagic Fevers, in Atlas of Infectious Diseases, External Manifestations of Systemic Infections. vol ed Robert Fekety, book ed GL Mandell Current Medicine, Philadelphia 1997; 8: 10.1-10.26

65. Peters CJ. Are the viral hemorrhagic fevers practical agents for biological terrorism? Emerging Infections, ASM Press ed Hughes, et al in press 2000; 4

66. Pittman PR, Liu CT, Cannon TL, Makuch RS, Mangiafico JA, Gibbs PH, Peters CJ Immunogenicity of

an inactivated Rift Valley fever vaccine in humans: a 12-year Vaccine. 1999; 18(1-2): 181-9,

67. Price ME, Fisher-Hoch SP, Craven RB, McCormick JB. A prospective study of maternal and fetal outcome in acute Lassa fever infection during pregnancy. Brit Med J 1988; 297: 584-587

68. Qian DY, Ding YS, Chen GF, Ding JJ, Chen YX, Lu TF, Wang ZX, Smego RA Jr. A placebo-controlled clinical trial of prednisone in the treatment of early hemorrhagic fever [letter]. J Infect Dis 1990; 162(5): 1213-4

69. Rosenberg RB, Waagner DC, Romano MJ, Kanase HN, Young RB. Hantavirus pulmonary syndrome treated with inhaled nitric oxide. Pediatr Infect Dis J 1998; 17: 749-52.

70. Sadek, RS, AS Khan, G Stevens, CJ Peters, TG Ksiazek. Ebola Hemorrhagic Fever, Democratic Republic of Congo, 1995: Determinants of Survival. J Infect Dis 1999; 179 (Supp l): S24-27

71. Sanchez A, Peters CJ, Zaki SR, Rollin PE. Filoviruses, in Tropical Infectious Diseases: Principles, Pathogens & Practice. Eds: Richard L. Guerrant, David H. Walker, Peter F, Weller WB Saunders, New York 1999; 115: 1240-1252.

72. Sayer WJ, Entwisle GM, Uyeno BT, Bignall RC. Cortisone therapy of early epidemic hemorrhagic fever: a preliminary report. Ann Int Med 1955; 42: 839

73. Sidley P. Fears over Ebola spread as nurse dies. Brit Med J 1996; 313: 1351.

74. Stephen EL, Jones DE, Peters CJ, Eddy GA, Loizeaux PS, Jahrling PB. Ribavirin treatment of toga-, arena-, and bunyavirus infections in subhuman primates and other laboratory animal species. In Ribavirin: A Broad Spectrum Antiviral Agent, Academic Press, New York, ed Smith RA and Kirkpatrick W. 1980; 169-183.

75. Swanepoel R, Gill DE, Shepherd AJ, Leman PA, Mynhardt JH, Harvey S. The Clinical Pathology of Crimean Congo Hemorrhagic Fever. Rev Infect Dis 1989: 11 (Supp 4): S794-S800.

76. Tignor GH, Hanman CA. Ribavirin efficacy in an *in vivo* model of Crimean-Congo hemorrhagic fever virus infection. Antiviral Res 1993; 22: 309-25.

77. Toro J, Vega JD, Khan AS, Mills JN, Padula P, Terry W, Yadon Z, Valderrama R, Ellis BA, Pavletic C, Cerda R, Zaki S, Wun-Ju S, Meyer R, Tapia M, Mansilla C, Baro M, Vergara JA, Concha M, Calderón G, Enria D, Peters CJ, Ksiazek TG. An outbreak of hantavirus pulmonary syndrome, Chile, 1997. Emerging Infectious Diseases in press, 1999.

78. Villinger F, Rollin PE, Brar SS, Chikkala NF, Winter J, Sundstrom JB, Zaki SR, Swanepoel R, Ansari AA, Peters CJ. Markedly Elevated Levels of Interferon (IFN)-gamma, IFN-alpha, Interleukin (IL)-2, IL-10, and Tumor Necrosis Factor-alpha Associated with Fatal Ebola Virus Infection. J Infect Dis 1999; 179 (Supp l): S188-191.

79. Wali JP, Biswas A, Chandra S, Malhotra A, Aggarwal P, Handa R, Wig N, Bahl VK. Cardiac involvement in Dengue Haemorrhagic Fever. Int J of Cardiology 64: 31-6, 1998

80. Watts DM, Ussery MA, Nash D, Peters CJ. 1989. Inhibition of Crimean-Congo hemorrhagic fever viral infectivity yields *in vitro* by ribavirin. Am J Trop Med Hyg 41: 581-585.

81. Wells RM, Sosa Estani S, Yadon ZE, Enria D, Padula P, Pini N, Mills JN, Peters CJ, Segura EL, the Hantavirus Pulmonary Syndrome Study Group for Patagonia. An unusual hantavirus outbreak in southern Argentina: Person-to-person transmission? Emerg Infect Dis 1997; 3: 171-174

82. Wells RM, Young J, Williams RJ, Armstrong LR, Busico K, Khan AS, Ksiazek TG, Rollin PE, Zaki SR, Nichol ST, Peters CJ. Hantavirus transmission in the United States. Emerging Infectious Diseases 1997; 3: 361-365.

83. Zaki SR, Goldsmith CS. Pathologic features of filovirus infections in humans in Klenk, Hans-Dieter, ed. Marburg and Ebola Viruses. Current Topics in Microbiology and Immunology. New York: Springer. 1999.

CHAPTER 13

IMMUNE PROPHYLAXIS AND VACCINATIONS

MARK A. FLETCHER and STANLEY A. PLOTKIN

Table of Contents

Practical Guidelines in Antiviral Therapy Ed. by Charles A.B. Boucher and George J. Galasso. 303 — 342
© 2002 *Elsevier Science. Printed in the Netherlands.*

Introduction

Vaccines have been without question the best antivirals. One virus disease, smallpox, has been eradicated by vaccination, and a second, polio, may be heading that way owing to the widespread application of live and killed vaccines. Cirrhosis and cancer due to hepatitis B virus infection could in principle be completely prevented by universal infant vaccination, and measles, rubella, and mumps virus vaccines have been shown to be capable of eliminating transmission in large geographical areas. Hepatitis A virus vaccine also may be capable of stopping virus circulation.

In addition, when the incubation period of a disease is sufficiently long (rabies being the classic case), vaccination on exposure can be quite successful, as likewise has been shown for hepatitis B and varicella-zoster.

Finally, therapeutic vaccination, a fringe concept until now, may turn out to be useful in suppressing persistent and chronic infections.

Vaccinology started as an empiric specialty, and immunology has played little role in vaccine development until recently. Indeed, it is still clearly the case that most vaccines work through induction of antiviral antibodies on mucosal surfaces and in the serum. Nevertheless, clinicians have appreciated for some time the importance of cellular immunity in such infections as measles and varicella-zoster, and future progress will undoubtedly depend on our ability to induce specific cellular immune responses. Some of these protective immune responses are presented in Table 1.

Table 1.   Target of the viral infection and some protective immune responses evoked

Target of the viral infection	Some protective immune responses evoked
Mucosa or skin	sIgA, intraepithelial lymphocytes (CD8+)
Bloodstream	Innate, IgG/IgM/IgE, T helper cells (CD4+ Th2)
Immunologically privileged sites*	Cytotoxic T lymphocytes (CD8+ Tc1), T helper cells (CD4+ Th1)

* "Immunological privilege" includes viruses that may remain latent or find refuge from the immune system
in sanctuary sites (i.e., brain, epididymis, and kidney; neurons, gametes, and red blood cells)

In this chapter, we will discuss the major viral vaccines, stressing points of practical importance in the prophylaxis of the corresponding infections. One area of particular relevance to public health officials, for example, is the "Target populations & other potential risk groups" that will be served by the vaccine. For this purpose, viral vaccines licensed for human use may be broken down into two broad categories. The first group is vaccines used throughout the world, without limitation to particular target populations or potential risk groups. Examples include vaccines for hepatitis B, influenza, measles, mumps, polio, and rubella. The second group is restricted to selected geographic areas or to special risk groups. For instance, there are the vaccines against hepatitis A, Japanese encephalitis, rabies, tick-borne encephalitis, varicella-zoster, and yellow fever.

Although the convenience of the reader dictates that the viral vaccines discussed in this chapter will be presented in alphabetic order, vaccinologists often find it convenient to class vaccines by other means, such as by the "Region of the body infected" (Table 2) or by the "Type of vaccine" (Table 3).

Table 2. Transmission of viral pathogens

Region of the body infected	Route of transmission	Examples
Mucosa or skin	Direct contact	Touching, biting, kissing, sexual intercourse, droplet spread
	Airborne	Aerosols, droplet nuclei, dust
	Vehicle-borne	Food, water, formites
Bloodstream	Arthropod vectors	*Culex tritaeniorhynchus, Aedes aegypti, Ixodes ricinus*
	Blood or biological products	Serum, plasma, tissues, organs

Table 3. Viral vaccines, classified by region of the body infected and by type of vaccine

Type of vaccine

Live-attenuated	Killed	Subunit/protein	Virus	Region of the body infected
×			Measles virus	Mucosa or skin
×			Mumps virus	Mucosa or skin
×			Rubella virus	Mucosa or skin
×			Varicella-zoster virus	Mucosa or skin
×			Yellow fever virus	Bloodstream
×	×		Japanese encephalitis virus	Bloodstream
×	×		Poliovirus	Mucosa or skin
	×		Hepatitis A virus	Mucosa or skin
	×		Rabies virus	Mucosa or skin
	×		Tick-borne encephalitis virus	Bloodstream
	×	×	Influenza virus	Mucosa or skin
		×	Hepatitis B virus	Mucosa or skin/Bloodstream

Hepatitis A Virus Vaccine

Target Populations & Other Potential Risk Groups

The hepatitis A virus vaccine is indicated for high-risk groups, including sexually active homosexuals, intravenous drug abusers, people with chronic liver diseases, hemophiliac patients (or other recipients of clotting-factor concentrates), and selected food handlers [1]. International voyagers to hepatitis A-endemic countries (which excludes the USA, Canada, Australia, New Zealand, Japan, Western Europe, and Scandinavia) should be vaccinated. People who are occupationally exposed to hepatitis A virus (such as animal care workers or certain laboratory personnel) should receive vaccine. Health care workers might be indicated if there is a risk of exposure to the feces of infected patients and proper precautions are not respected [2]. In regions marked by a high carriage rate for hepatitis B virus or for hepatitis C virus, clinical studies suggest that it may be advisable to vaccinate chronic carriers of either virus with the hepatitis A virus vaccine.

Administration of The Vaccine

Vaccine Composition
The hepatitis A virus vaccine is an inactivated, whole-virus vaccine (which is prepared from strain HM175, strain CR326F, strain GBM, or strain RG-SB of the hepatitis A virus) that has been grown on one of the human diploid cell strains, then formalin inactivated and adsorbed on aluminum hydroxide or onto a liposome adjuvant.

Contraindications & Recommendations
Vaccine should not be given if there has been a history of an immediate anaphylactic reaction to a previous dose of any hepatitis A virus vaccine or be given to a person who has had hypersensitivity reactions either to the adjuvant (alum) or to the preservative (phenoxyethanol) [3]. Hepatitis A virus vaccine may be administered to immunocompromised people. Furthermore, immunization with this inactivated viral vaccine in not contra-indicated during pregnancy.

Dose, Route & Schedule
The vaccine is injected intramuscularly into the deltoid. Two injections are required, with the second dose being administered 6 to 18 months after the first dose. For each of the hepatitis A virus vaccines, the pediatric dose is one half of the adult dose [4].

Post-Exposure Prophylaxis & Outbreak Control

Human immune globulin (HIG) prophylaxis should be administered within 2 weeks of close contact with a person infected with the hepatitis A virus. For rapid protection after possible hepatitis A virus exposure, hepatitis A virus vaccine in the first dose also can be given along with (HIG). To interrupt an outbreak of hepatitis A, administration of the vaccine to particular target groups may be more effective than relying on post-exposure.

Immune Response To The Vaccine

Protective Immune Responses & Duration of Immunity
Seroprotection upon hepatitis A virus vaccination is defined as an antibody concentration measured by enzyme - linked immunosorbant assay (ELISA) that is at least 10 mIU per ml, relative to a World Health Organization (WHO) human immune globulin preparation standard. The initial dose of hepatitis A virus vaccine induces seroconversion in 90 percent of vaccinees within four weeks, and there is nearly complete seroconversion after the second dose [5]. Calculations show that protective antibody concentrations will persist at least 20 years [6].

Causes of Primary Vaccine Failure
Vaccine is less immunogenic after the first dose in persons older then 40 years and in the obese.

Vaccine Reactogenicity & Reported Adverse Events
The minor side effects in adults are local soreness and headache. There have been rare reports of an adverse event following inoculation.

Some Public Health Issues & Further Trends

A field trial in Thailand with over 39,000 children who received two injections either of hepatitis A virus vaccine or of hepatitis B virus vaccine (as the control) demonstrated a protective efficacy of 97 percent [7].

Sanitation has been improving in some of the formerly hepatitis A endemic regions of the world, leading to an "epidemiological shift," in which a larger fraction of children enter adolescence without having been exposed to the hepatitis A virus. Recent examples include Israel and certain countries of Southeast Asia such as Hong Kong and Australia. In locales where there now is a sizable population of seronegative adolescents, public health officials are being called upon for advice about the most appropriate hepatitis A virus vaccination strategy. Recommendations range from continued targeting of certain risk groups to universal vaccination of children. In the USA, for example, many states have added hepatitis A virus vaccination to the childhood immunization schedule [8], a policy that is under consideration by other countries.

Hepatitis B Virus Vaccine

Target Populations & Other Potential Risk Groups

Among adults, there are many high-risk categories that are indicated for pre-exposure hepatitis B virus vaccination. These include certain health care workers, institutionalized persons, hemodialysis patients, hemophiliacs, persons in contact with carriers of the hepatitis B virus (e.g., household or via institutions for developmentally disabled persons), intravenous drug users, persons engaging in homosexual behaviors, persons with multiple heterosexual partners, and prison inmates. The hepatitis B endemic areas are Southeast Asia, Africa, the Middle East, the islands of the South and Western Pacific, and the Amazon basin of Latin America. International voyagers to these regions should be vaccinated.

The Expanded Programme on Immunization (EPI) of the WHO recommends universal hepatitis B virus immunization of infants beginning at birth to 2 months of age. Many national vaccination programs also target previously unvaccinated adolescents (11 to 12 years of age) [9].

Although not included in any official recommendations, there are studies to suggest that hepatitis B virus vaccination be encouraged among patients with chronic hepatitis C, among sewer workers, and among chronic liver disease patients awaiting transplantation.

Administration of The Vaccine

Vaccine Composition

All hepatitis B virus vaccines use the surface protein as antigen. Some of these vaccines are derived from the plasma of infected humans [10]; however, the major vaccine manufacturers produce recombinant protein vaccines, in which the hepatitis B virus surface antigen (HBsAg) has been produced by recombinant DNA expression systems [11]. Each recombinant HBsAg (rHBsAg) vaccine differs by the particular surface and presurface components contained within the expressed surface protein. Lately, regional vaccine manufacturers have begun exploiting this recombinant DNA technology to produce rHBsAg vaccines. The recombinant protein hepatitis B virus vaccines contain from 5 to 40 μg rHBsAg per ml adsorbed onto aluminum hydroxide. The antibacterial agent thiomersal is no longer used in rHBsAg vaccines available in the USA.

Contraindications & Recommendations

If a person has had an immediate anaphylactic reaction to a dose of any hepatitis B virus vaccine, a following dose is contraindicated. Likewise, anyone with a known history of an anaphylactic reaction to "Bakers yeast" should not receive a rHBsAg vaccine prepared on *Saccharomyces cerevisiae* [12]. Vaccination ought to be deferred in case of mild to moderate illness, with or without fever. On the other hand, pregnant or lactating women may be vaccinated, and there is no specific contraindication to vaccination of someone who already may be infected with the hepatitis B virus.

Dose, Route & Schedule

In general, the pediatric dose of hepatitis B virus vaccine contains half of the adult dose. Persons who undergo kidney dialysis, and other immunocompromised persons, are given twice the standard dose. Vaccine is injected via the intramuscular route.

Previously unvaccinated adolescents and adults may be immunized using a 0-, 1-, and 6-month schedule [13]. The schedule of an infant's immunization depends upon the HBsAg status of the mother. Infants born to HBsAg-negative mothers can receive their first immunization at birth or at 2 months of age; the second injection should be at least 1 month after the first; and the third injection should be no sooner than 2 months after the second dose, but not before the child is 6 months old. (In practice, infants are vaccinated at birth, 1, and 6 months, or at 2, 4, and 12 months of age) On the other hand, infants that are born to HBsAg-positive mothers must be vaccinated within 12 hours of birth and should receive hepatitis B immune globulin (HBIG), which may be given simultaneously but at a different anatomic site. The second dose of vaccine should be administered at 1 to 2 months of age, and the third dose should be given at 6 months of age.

Given the broad indications for hepatitis B virus vaccination, and the importance of immunizing populations living in endemic regions, much clinical research has been devoted to alternative, possibly more convenient schedules. Examples include a two-dose schedule instead of the currently recommended three-dose schedule, single dose priming followed by a booster years later, or vaccine administered in yearly intervals.

Route of Administration
Vaccine is given intramuscularly into the anterolateral thigh muscle of neonates and children and into the deltoid for persons of any age. Some clinical investigators study intradermal vaccination with smaller doses as an equally immunogenic (but less costly) route of administration.

Post-Exposure Prophylaxis & Outbreak Control

HBIG should be given in association with hepatitis B virus vaccine to any infant within 12 hours of delivery who is born to a mother who is HBsAg positive (i.e., a hepatitis B virus carrier); however, such immune globulin prophylaxis strategies are rarely possible in under-industrialized countries.

Other indications for post-exposure prophylaxis with HBIG for a seronegative person include intimate exposure (e.g., household or sexual) with a person who is a HBsAg carrier or any other percutaneous or permucosal exposure to the hepatitis B virus. Some investigators have described prophylaxis strategies to be used in cases of reactivation of endogenous hepatitis B virus infection in the course of transplantation surgery.

Attempts are being made at "vaccine therapy" to cure patients with chronic hepatitis B virus infection.

Immune Response To The Vaccine

Protective Immune Responses & Duration of Immunity
The protective serum titer to hepatitis B virus vaccination has been established at 10 mIU per ml; nonetheless, recent studies suggest that a vigorous cellular immune response is equally necessary, such that the post-vaccination serum titers > 10 mIU per ml may best be considered as differentiating vaccine responders from vaccine non-responders [14]. Plasma-derived hepatitis B virus vaccines induce immune responses that are equivalent to those obtained from the recombinant protein vaccines, and the intradermal route of immunization appears to be as immunogenic as the intramuscular route.

Children infected by the hepatitis B virus during perinatal exposure have a poorer prognosis then those that have been infected later in life. Consequently, much clinical work has been devoted to demonstrating that the hepatitis B virus vaccines are appropriately safe and immunogenic when administered to neonates, either preterm or full term.

Studies of antibody decay among vaccinees indicate decades-long persistence. Immune memory is also maintained: long-term follow up of vaccinees in a hepatitis B endemic region uncovered cases of occult infection that were only revealed by increases in the serum anti-HBsAg antibody titers. It appears that booster vaccinations are unnecessary to maintain lifelong protective immunity [15].

Causes of Primary Vaccine Failure
Studies show that some of the causes of primary vaccine failure are a history of being a smoker, increased age, and extreme obesity. By contrast, hepatitis B virus vaccine remains safe and immunogenic when given to malnourished children. People with HIV/AIDS have a sub-optimal response to hepatitis B virus vaccination that can be overcome by increasing the number of vaccine doses. Other immunocompromised persons are likely to be hyporesponsive, including those with chronic hepatitis C, those requiring hemodialysis, those with leukemia, and those with diabetes mellitus. In other instances, a poor response to hepatitis B virus immunization might have an immunogenetic explanation.

The humoral immune response to hepatitis B virus is directed at the "a" determinant of the surface antigen; the prevalence of viral mutants may increase under the selective pressure of a systematic program of vaccination [16]. A scientific debate is now underway about the emergence of vaccine-resistant hepatitis B virus. The argument is that large-scale vaccination efforts may favor the rise of HBsAg mutants, both within the "a" determinant [17] and outside of the "a" determinant region of the HBsAg. Infection by an "a" determinant HBsAg mutant, for example, is claimed to have been the cause of certain failures of perinatal post-exposure prophylaxis. Nevertheless, hepatitis B virus vaccination programs continue to be highly effective in the prevention of hepatitis B and of hepatocellular carcinoma, and it is reassuring that in a chimpanzee model the rHBsAg vaccine protected against infection by an "a" determinant hepatitis B virus variant.

Vaccine Reactogenicity & Reported Adverse Events
There have been rare occurrences of anaphylaxis following hepatitis B virus immunization [18]. Case reports of adverse events alleged to be linked to injection with the rHBsAg vaccine fall into two general categories: dermatological disorders, such as eczema, mastocytoma, lichen planus, or granuloma annulare; or particular immunologic diseases, such as demyelinating polyneuropathy vasculitis, rheumatic disorder, thrombocytopenic purpura, or nephrotic syndrome. In France, in the wake of a national campaign of hepatitis B virus vaccination directed at adolescents, media pressure fueled allegations of a temporal link between vaccination and first episodes of multiple sclerosis. The large-scale pharmaco-epidemiologic studies published so far do not support such a supposition [19]. Correspondingly, the WHO is continuing its ambitious program of global hepatitis B virus vaccination, which already has led to a remarkable fall in the incidence of hepatocellular carcinoma in Taiwan [20].

Some Public Health Issues & Further Trends

As a wide-ranging public health policy, neonatal immunization has been incorporated into the EPI and has been adopted by many countries, with noteworthy reductions in the incidence and prevalence of chronic hepatitis B virus infections and of hepatocellular carcinomas [21]. (Taiwan is perhaps the best documented example to date.) Upon completing an initial vaccination program aimed at high-risk adults, the USA turned to immunization of all infants with hepatitis B virus vaccine, complemented by an adolescent "catch up" program [22]. For other countries with a low prevalence of hepatitis B virus infection, public health officials may favor selective vaccination programs, centered--not on infants--but on particular at-risk adult groups or on adolescents.

The effectiveness of HBIG prophylaxis to prevent perinatal hepatitis B virus infection proves that hepatitis B virus antibodies are needed to protect such children at the time of birth. In regions where hepatitis B immune globulin is unavailable, hepatitis B virus immunization during pregnancy has been used, especially in countries having a high prevalence of chronic hepatitis B virus infection. Universal vaccination of all neonates, regardless of the hepatitis B virus status of the mother, is an alternate "maternal - infant" approach that has been used in under-industrialized countries that lack the resources to engage in systematic screening of mothers (for the presence of serum markers of chronic hepatitis B virus infection) and that do not have access to hepatitis B immune globulin. This approach has been highly successful in The Gambia, for instance.

Influenza Virus Vaccine

Target Populations & Other Potential Risk Groups

Influenza virus vaccination is a yearly indication in selected groups living at increased risk for morbidity and mortality. These include persons who are older than 65 years [23], who have a chronic cardiopulmonary disease, who are immunocompromised (for example, by cancer, for transplantation, or by diabetes), who are on long-term aspirin therapy [24], or who are entering the second or third trimester of pregnancy during the influenza season. Health care workers may be important vectors of infection; hence, they should receive yearly influenza vaccinations. Influenza vaccination is highly recommended as well for those adults in good health wishing to limit morbidity (e.g., community workers, people subject to high exposure, and frequent travelers) [25]. While there are no universal recommendations for children, those falling within one of the many risk groups mentioned above ought to be vaccinated each year [26].

Administration of The Vaccine

Vaccine Composition
The influenza virus vaccine is a killed virus. Each vaccine contains representative antigens from the two influenza A subtypes and from the single influenza B type

(e.g., A-H1N1, A-H3N2, and B), with the particular virus strains chosen each year by WHO-designated influenza monitoring laboratories. To prepare the vaccine, virus is grown on embryonated chicken eggs and then inactivated chemically. The vaccine virus may be presented in its inactivated whole virus form, or it may be presented as an inactivated split virus (also referred to as a subvirion or purified surface antigen vaccine). Chemical splitting agents currently in use include Triton X-100, Triton N-101, ether, or tri-n-butyl-phosphate.

Contraindications & Recommendations
Influenza vaccine should not be readministered in instances of an immediate anaphylactic reaction to a preceding dose, and should be not be given to someone having a history of anaphylactic hypersensitivity to eggs or egg proteins [27]. (Cautious immunization is acceptable in instances of food allergy to eggs.) Other limitations to influenza virus vaccination include moderate to severe illness (with or without a fever), young age (less than 6 months old), and the occurrence of neurological signs and symptoms following previous immunization. Asthma sufferers may be vaccinated against influenza.

Dose, Route & Schedule
A single, intramuscular injection is given to adults, customarily before the influenza season starts. For immunologically naive children less than nine years of age, the preferred schedule is two doses of vaccine given one-month apart. Only the split virus vaccine should be used for children younger than 13 years [28].

Post-Exposure Prophylaxis & Outbreak Control

Chemoprophylaxis, while not an alternative to influenza virus vaccination, may be indicated during community outbreaks of influenza A, particularly among unvaccinated health care workers or among immunocompromised persons who may not have had an adequate immune response to vaccination.

Immune Response To The Vaccine

Protective Immune Responses & Duration of Immunity
The humoral immune response to vaccination, particularly the presence of antibodies to the viral hemagglutinin as measured by the haemagglutination inhibition test, represents immunoconversion to vaccination and predicts immunoprotection. Influenza virus vaccination also produces a mucosal and a cellular immune response that may be equally important in the protective immune response [29].

The influenza virus undergoes continual mutation leading to yearly "drifts", with numerous "shifts" in the course of a century. Yearly vaccination is obligatory as this may prime the immune memory to respond more effectively to these "drifts" and "shifts". On the other hand, the concept of "original antigenic sin" has been elaborated to account for variations that have been noted in the humoral immune response to yearly vaccination [30]. For example, an influenza virus vaccination may provoke cross-reactive anamnestic antibody responses that date either from immunization with preceding influenza virus vaccines or from exposure to strains that had been in circulation years before [31]. For certain investigators, this misdirection of the humoral immune response explains, in part, the variable effectiveness of influenza virus vaccination from year to year [32].

Causes of Primary Vaccine Failure
The elderly population is particularly vulnerable to influenza virus infection; they also tend to respond poorly to influenza virus vaccination. Active cigarette smokers, to a lesser extent, fall within the same conundrum, particularly among older cigarette smokers. Children and adults suffering from HIV/AIDS, being immunocompromised, often mount an inadequate response to influenza virus vaccination. Although appropriate immune responses may be restored by highly active retroviral therapy, influenza virus vaccination may promote HIV replication, leaving this an area under intensive clinical investigation.

Vaccine Reactogenicity & Reported Adverse events
There are rare examples of anaphylactic reaction because of egg-sensitivity [27]. Whole-virion vaccines produce more local and systemic reactogenicity then do the split-virion vaccines. An elevation in the incidence of cases of the Guillain-Barré syndrome occurred within eight weeks of immunization during the swine influenza virus vaccination campaign of 1976 (i.e., between 4.9 and 5.9 reported cases per million doses of vaccine), but this phenomenon was not duplicated following other seasons' influenza vaccination campaigns. Vasculitis as a complication of influenza virus vaccination has been documented, and there are case reports in the literature of neurological signs and symptoms coinciding temporally with influenza virus vaccination.

Some Public Health Issues & Further Trends

Some of the over-riding themes of influenza virus vaccination include: (i) enlarging the vaccine coverage for the elderly and the institutionalized (as well as those that care for them), (ii) continuing to demonstrate the positive economic impact of immunizing working adults, (iii) documenting the impact of influenza virus infections on the under-industrialized world, and (iv) preparing for newer influenza virus vaccines (such as the intra-nasal and the live attenuated approaches).

The elderly and the institutionalized as a group bear the largest burden of influenza, in terms of morbidity, hospitalization, and mortality [33, 34]. Vaccination programs directed at the elderly are effective, and efforts are underway to improve the vaccination coverage among these populations, as well as to encourage vaccination of the health care workers who serve these populations [35]. Numerous clinical trials have demonstrated the economic benefits of vaccination of healthy adults to lower workplace absenteeism rates and to improve workplace efficiency [36]. The recommendations by industrialized countries for influenza virus vaccine are becoming broader [37], while the global impact of influenza on morbidity and mortality in under-industrialized countries also is becoming better appreciated. One future for influenza virus vaccination will be to encourage wider application of the current vaccine, while new approaches to influenza virus vaccination include other routes of administration, new adjuvants, and the clinical development of live attenuated influenza virus vaccines.

Japanese Encephalitis Virus Vaccine

Target Populations & Other Potential Risk Groups

In broad areas of Asia, Japanese encephalitis virus vaccination is included in the national pediatric immunization schedules, so children expatriating to endemic areas also should be considered for immunization. Furthermore, this vaccine is presently indicated for adult travelers to endemic areas, for the U.S. military, and for particular research laboratory workers.

Aministration of The Vaccine

Vaccine Composition
Killed virus vaccines are made in many countries of Asia from the Nakayama-Beijing-1 (P1) strain of Japanese encephalitis virus, which is grown on mouse brain and then formalin inactivated [38]. In China, two Japanese encephalitis vaccines are available, one that is an inactivated virus vaccine (P3 strain grown on primary hamster kidney cells and then formalin inactivated) and the other that is a live attenuated virus vaccine (SA14-14-2 strain) grown on primary hamster kidney cells [39].

Contraindications & Recommendations
Japanese encephalitis virus vaccination should not be continued in persons who may have experienced a hypersensitivity reaction to a preceding dose.

Dose, Route & Schedule
For children in Asia, the schedules of vaccination vary by country, but in general two doses are given 1 to 4 weeks apart (half dose in children less than 3 years of age), then an initial booster one year later, with additional boosters at 1- to 3-year intervals. All doses are given subcutaneously. For the live attenuated virus vaccine, a half dose is administered subcutaneously to children at 1 and 2 years of age (with a possible booster at 6 years of age), although other schedules are being tested that are more compatible with the established pediatric vaccination schedules. For travelers originating from areas without endemic transmission, three doses of vaccine (half dose for children 1 to 3 years old) are given subcutaneously on days 0, 7, and 30. A booster dose is recommended two years later [40].

Post-Exposure Prophylaxis & Outbreak Control

There is no post-exposure immunoprophylaxis against Japanese encephalitis. In certain provinces of China, vaccine is administered to children each spring in order to eliminate the yearly seasonal outbreaks of Japanese encephalitis.

Immune Response To The Vaccine

Protective Immune Responses & Duration of Immunity

A serum titer of neutralizing antibodies greater than 1:10 is sign of seroconversion and is taken to be indicative of protection. The Japanese encephalitis virus vaccines are more immunogenic in Asian subjects than in subjects from non-endemic areas, probably because of previous exposures to the other Flaviviruses that are prevalent in Asia. Therefore, after an initial immunization series with the killed virus vaccine, there are positive neutralizing antibody responses in 94 to 100% of Asian subject (2-dose primary series) and in greater than 90% of non-Asians (3-dose primary series). Available field data suggests that the inactivated virus vaccine (2-dose primary series) provides protective immunity that persists for 1 to 3 years, so Asian children usually receive booster immunizations about every 2 years. For the 3-dose series used for persons originating outside of Asia, studies of the persistence of vaccine-derived immunity suggest that a first booster may be needed 2 to 3 years after the primary series.

Causes of Primary Vaccine Failure

Neither the possible effects of concurrent anti-malaria medication nor of the presence of maternal antibodies have been tested.

Vaccine Reactogenicity & Reported Adverse Events

There are important side effects associated with vaccination with mouse brain-derived killed Japanese encephalitis virus vaccine, which include allergic adverse events, the Guillain-Barré syndrome, and acute disseminated encephalomyelitis [38]. The allergic adverse events are generalized urticaria/angioedema (Quincke's edema), erythema multiforme, erythema nodosum, joint swelling, and wheezing–particularly with the possibility of a delayed onset following the second or third dose [41].

Some Public Health Issues & Further Trends

Post-licensure field trials in different Asian countries produce an estimate of vaccine effectiveness in the order of 74 to 95% for the inactivated vaccines, and from 96 to 100% for the live attenuated vaccine [39].

Japanese encephalitis is a severe problem in endemic areas of Asia. Efforts are being made to incorporate Japanese encephalitis virus vaccination into the EPI of more countries in Asia and to widen the use of the live attenuated vaccine produced in China.

Measles Virus Vaccine

Target Populations & Other Potential Risk Groups

Measles vaccine is intended for all children, as well as for adults (in particular, health care workers) who do not have a history of measles infection or do not have evidence of measles immunity [42].

Administration of The Vaccine

Vaccine Composition
The measles vaccine is a live attenuated virus vaccine, which was derived from the original wild virus isolated by Enders and Peebles in 1954, called Edmonston. By further serial passages of the Edmonston strain through cell lines (e.g., human kidney, human amnion, sheep kidney, and chick embryo) the vaccine strains, AIK-C, Edmonston A, and Edmonston B, were developed [43]. (Other measles vaccine virus strains also are available.) To prepare vaccine batches, the vaccine virus is grown on chick embryo fibroblast cell culture [44]. In industrialized countries, measles virus vaccine is usually combined with mumps and rubella virus vaccine [45] or with rubella virus vaccine alone [46].

Contraindications & Recommendations
Measles virus vaccine should not be administered to anyone who had an immediate anaphylactic reaction to a previous dose of measles (or measles - rubella, or measles - mumps - rubella) virus vaccine, who is allergic to a component of the vaccine, or who has a history of anaphylactic reactions to gelatin or gelatin-containing products [47]. Other vaccine contraindications include moderate or severe illness (with or without a fever) [48], an episode of thrombocytopenia within 6 weeks of a previous dose of vaccine, or having recently received immune globulin. A history of hypersensitivity to eggs or egg products is not always a contraindication to measles virus vaccination, although care should be exercised during the inoculation [49]. HIV-infected persons who are not severely immunocompromised may be vaccinated.

Dose, Route & Schedule
Measles virus vaccine is intended for all children, ranging in age from 9 months (i.e., as part of the EPI, where a monovalent measles virus vaccine is used) to 12 months (for most national immunization schedules, where measles vaccine is contained in a combined measles - rubella or in a combined measles - mumps - rubella vaccine). Many of these national immunization schedules require that a second vaccination be given during childhood: either at 4 to 6 years of age or at the beginning of adolescence. Measles virus vaccine is most often injected by the subcutaneous route, although clinical studies and field trials have shown that the vaccine also may be administered successfully as an aerosol.

Post-Exposure Prophylaxis & Outbreak Control

For countries having a well-established national program of two-dose measles virus immunization, isolated foyers of under-vaccination or of non-vaccination remain challenges. Measles virus is easily transmitted; a few isolated cases may rapidly explode into an outbreak in a susceptible community. Furthermore, imported measles virus infections continue to appear in Canada, Europe, and the USA. HIG may be administered prophylactically, within 6 days of exposure to infants less than 6 months of age born of measles non-immune mothers, to children too young to have received their first dose of vaccine (i.e., 6 to 12 months of age), to pregnant women, or to severely immunocompromised persons. Exposed children older than 6 months of age should receive measles virus vaccine, as well as HIG. In emergency situations (e.g., refugee and displaced-persons camps), mass measles virus vaccination has been counseled, since certain studies show that targeted measles virus vaccination has proven to be useful in controlling measles outbreaks.

Immune Response To The Vaccine

Protective Immune Responses & Duration of Immunity

Measles virus vaccine induces both a humoral and a cellular immune response. Many methods are used to establish measles antibody titers, but measles virus vaccine immunogenicity and vaccination effectiveness appears to be best established by determination of neutralizing antibodies. After a first measles virus vaccine immunization, detectable antibody titers persist for many years, and upon boosting (either with vaccine or by infection) there is an increase in serum antibody titers. IgM antibody appears initially for those persons who did not mount an immune response to the primary immunization; on the other hand, muted humoral immune response to vaccine or infection has been noted in individuals retaining an elevated level of circulating serum IgG measles antibodies.

Causes of Primary Vaccine Failure

After a single immunization under even the most opportune conditions, 2 to 5% of children remain unprotected, emphasizing the need for a booster [42]. Residual maternal antibodies may substantially reduce the humoral immune response of the infant to vaccination; hence, children are vaccinated after they reach 9 to 12 months of age. Even in the absence of confounding maternal antibodies, however, infants younger than 6 months of age respond poorly to measles vaccination. In addition, there are intrinsic differences in the immunogenicity of the different measles vaccine virus strains that are used for infant vaccinations.

Vaccine Reactogenicity & Reported Adverse Events

The most frequent side effects of measles virus immunization are fever (temperature greater than 39.4°C, occurring 7 to 12 days after vaccination), transient rashes, and transient thrombocytopenia. Rarely, in less than one instance per million vaccine doses, vaccine-associated CNS conditions have occurred. Other infrequent side effects of vaccination are allergic reactions to eggs or gelatin [50] and hypersensitivity to the neomycin used in the manufacture of the vaccine. The measles virus vaccination program in the United Kingdom was temporarily disrupted by allegations that measles vaccination enhanced susceptibility to inflammatory bowel disease and to autism. These claims have been largely disproven [51].

Clinical trials to evaluate vaccination of young infants with high-titer measles virus vaccines were performed over the past decade. Unfortunately, after Edmonston-Zagreb high-titer or Schwarz high-titer virus vaccine was administered to 5 month olds in Senegal, a significantly elevated risk of death from respiratory or diarrheal disease was noted during the 24- to 39-month follow-up. High dose Edmonston-Zagreb measles virus vaccine (100-fold greater than standard titer) also was given to 6 month olds in Haiti. There was greater mortality in girls than boys. These results led to the subsequent discontinuation of use of high titer measles virus vaccine in infants. Succeeding studies suggested that augmented immunosuppression occurred, although others explain that there had been a "non-specific beneficial effect of the standard measles vaccine rather than a harmful effect of the high-titre vaccines" [52].

Some Public Health Issues & Further Trends

The current EPI provides for only one dose of the Schwarz strain measles virus vaccine, given at 9 months of age, but this been enough to prevent millions of measles deaths per year.

Measles virus vaccine effectiveness for a two-dose schedule has been calculated to be greater than 90%. Correspondingly, as has been demonstrated in numerous national vaccination programs (e.g., Canada, Finland [53], Spain, Taiwan, and the USA), a second dose of measles virus vaccine is required to control the burden of disease fully. Due to rigorous adherence to the two-dose immunization approach, endogenous measles has been eliminated from the Scandinavian countries and from Latin America [54]. An issue for each country that adopts the use of a second measles virus vaccine dose will be to fix the appropriate age group for receipt of this second immunization [55]. For example, it has been argued that revaccination may be of greater value at 11 to 12 years of age than at 4 to 6 years of age [56].

Waning of maternal-derived immunity leaves non-immunized infants particularly vulnerable to measles virus infection during their first year of life, which has been demonstrated by field studies in Ghana and in Nigeria. On the other hand, the presence of maternal antibodies may block the induction of a protective response to immunization among the group most at risk from infection, infants below 9 months of age. The challenges for measles virus vaccine include (i) vaccination of infants younger than 6 months of age, (ii) the eventual eradication of measles, and (iii) measles surveillance within established immunization programs. Infants less than 6 months of age who receive maternal antibodies supplied by measles immunized mothers may be less protected against infection than infants receiving antibodies from naturally infected (i.e., convalescent) mothers. Correspondingly, measles vaccination at an early age may become more accessible. After the eradication of smallpox, and a recent redoubling of efforts to control and then eradicate polio, the next global target is measles [57]. Furthermore, seroprevalence surveys will be a keystone to the construction of such programs because subclinical measles occurs regularly within vaccinated populations.

Mumps Virus Vaccine

Target Population & Other Potential Risk Groups

Mumps is a childhood vaccine, which is administered on the same schedule as measles virus and rubella virus vaccines. Mumps virus immunization also is important for remaining susceptible children who are approaching puberty and for any susceptible international travelers. Healthcare workers and others having close contact with children might receive special consideration for mumps virus vaccination.

Administration of The Vaccine

Vaccine Composition
The live attenuated mumps vaccine, based upon one of different mumps virus vaccine strains (e.g., Jeryl Lynn, Urabe, Rubini, etc.), is grown on either chick embryo fibroblast, human embryo fibroblast, or quail embryo fibroblast cell culture [58].

Contraindications & Recommendations
Care should be taken with potential vaccine recipients who have an anaphylactic sensitivity to gelatin, gelatin-containing products, or neomycin [47]. Immunization may be deferred in case of an acute febrile illness. Vaccination of pregnant women should be avoided, and women should refrain from becoming pregnant for 3 months after immunization. Mumps vaccine should not be given to persons with suppressed immunity, with the exception of children with HIV/AIDS.

Dose, route & Schedule
In industrialized countries, the mumps virus vaccine, like the measles and the rubella virus vaccines, is often administered in two doses, the first given on or after the first birthday, and the second given at 4 to 6 years of age or at 11 to 12 years of age. Mumps virus vaccination is not included in the EPI.

Post-Exposure Prophylaxis & Outbreak Control

HIG is not a useful post-exposure prophylaxis. On the other hand, selective mumps virus vaccination may stem the course of an outbreak.

Immune Response To The Vaccine

Protective Immune Responses & Duration of Immunity
Mumps virus vaccination induces neutralizing antibodies within a few weeks of immunization, that appear to persist until the age of booster vaccination.

Causes of Primary Vaccine Failure
Most of the mumps virus vaccines are highly effective in protecting against mumps disease with the exception of the Rubini strain mumps virus vaccine that appears to have been less effective in the field [59].

Vaccine Reactogenicity & Reported Adverse Events
Very rare cases of allergic reactions have been noted for all measles - mumps - rubella virus vaccines [47]. The Urabe strain mumps virus vaccine is highly immunogenic but there have been reports of vaccine associated meningoencephalitis and orchitis.

Some Public Health Issues & Further Trends

A single dose of live attenuated mumps virus vaccine (Jeryl Lynn strain) was at least 95% effective in preventing mumps disease during a clinical trial. Post-licensure studies of outbreaks have allowed the vaccine effectiveness to be calculated at between 75 and 91% for the two most widely used mumps virus vaccine strains (Jeryl Lynn and Urabe).

Among well-vaccinated populations, the incidence of mumps disease continues to decline. With the effort now being invested in the global eradication of measles, and the transitional introduction into many countries of the measles - rubella vaccine, later being followed by measles - mumps - rubella vaccine, the eradication of mumps may become possible one day [58].

Poliovirus Vaccine

Target Populations & Other Potential Risk Groups

All children should be vaccinated against poliomyelitis, beginning at infancy. Poliovirus vaccine is also indicated for adult healthcare workers who may be in contact with patients excreting poliovirus, as well as for travelers to a polio-endemic region.

Administration of The Vaccine

Vaccine Composition
The oral poliovirus vaccine (OPV) uses attenuated forms of the three strains of poliovirus. Type 1 (SO + 2) comes from the Mahoney strain; type 2 (SO + 2) is derived from the P 712 strain; and type 3 (SOR + 1) is of Leon strain origin. Each is grown on cell culture, as exemplified by the monkey kidney cell culture system. The WHO standards, in TCID50, for each of the three strains of attenuated poliovirus in the trivalent OPV vaccine are 105.9 ± 0.5 for type 1, 105.0 ± 0.5 for type 2, and 105.7 ± 0.5 for type 3.

To prepare the killed poliovirus vaccine, the most widely used being the enhanced potency inactivated poliovirus vaccine (eIPV), three strains of poliovirus, Type 1 (Mahoney), Type 2 (MEF-I), and Type 3 (Saukett), are grown on continuously propagating, Vero strain, monkey kidney cells or are raised on human diploid cell strain culture [60].

Contraindications & Recommendations
OPV must not be given to persons with a known immunodeficiency or with an altered immune status (e.g., leukemias or solid tumors, congenital immunodeficiencies, long-term immunosuppressive therapy, or HIV infection), or to persons living in a household with an HIV/AIDS patient or living with someone who might not be immune to poliovirus. IPV contains trace amounts of antibiotics (i.e., streptomycin, polymyxin B, and neomycin), so care must be taken to avoid vaccination of persons having an allergy to any of these components. For either poliovirus vaccine, vaccine should not

be readministered to anyone who might have experienced an immediate anaphylactic reaction to a previous dose, and vaccination should be deferred in persons having a mild to severe acute illness (with or without fever). Pregnant women may be vaccinated against poliovirus: eIPV is preferred, but OPV may be given if rapid immunity is necessary [61].

Dose, Route & Schedule

OPV is a mainstay of the EPI, where it is administered using a birth, 6-, 10-, and 14-week schedule. It is given by month in the form of drops.

Enhanced IPV is the primary poliovirus vaccine in much of Europe and in North America [62]. Although each country has its own recommended pediatric vaccination schedule, in general, eIPV has been incorporated into the four-dose diphtheria and tetanus toxoid - pertussis vaccine series. (A three-dose primary series, at 2, 4, and 12-months, for example, may be sufficient, however.) A supplementary, booster injection of eIPV is given between 4 and 6 years of age. Furthermore, some European countries require regular eIPV boosters throughout adulthood.

The subcutaneous route of eIPV administration is used (while the intradermal route has been recently tested clinically).

Post-Exposure Prophylaxis & Outbreak Control

Focused poliovirus vaccination may be able to block transmission of wild-type virus and to shorten the duration of an outbreak.

Immune Response To The Vaccine

Protective Immune Responses & Duration of Immunity

The protective immune response to eIPV immunization is measured by the titer of neutralizing serum antibodies that are produced. (A cut-off of 1:8 is commonly accepted as indicating seroconversion.) After three doses, almost all vaccine recipients become seropositive [60]. A serum neutralizing antibody response will be mounted to OPV because of exposure to live virus; on the other hand, there is little induction of mucosal immunity after primary eIPV immunization [63]. OPV induces neutralizing serum antibodies, like eIPV, but a broader immune response follows, which is characterized by secretary IgA from the gastrointestinal tract [64]. Immunity from OPV is believed to persist throughout the life of the vaccinee.

Causes of Primary Vaccine Failure

Immune responses to OPV have been sub-optimal following mass vaccination campaigns in many developing countries. Explanations for these failures of vaccination include interference from concurrent infections of the gastrointestinal tract, suppression due to secretory IgA in colostrum for breast-fed infants, interference from maternal antibodies, and breakdowns in the cold chain [65].

Vaccine Reactogenicity & Reported Adverse Events

As it replicates in the intestinal tract, the strains of poliovirus vaccine contained in OPV may revert to virulence. The risk of vaccine associated paralytic poliomyelitis (VAPP) because of OPV reversion was estimated for the USA at one case of paralytic disease (i.e., in the OPV recipient or a vaccine-associated contact) for every 2.5 million doses distributed, with the greatest risk after the first dose (by a factor of 9.7) compared with the subsequent doses. VAPP has been reported after mass vaccination campaigns, so in under-industrialized countries where pediatric HIV/AIDS may be widespread, there are correspondingl risks associated with OPV administration.

Based upon indications that some of the OPV produced in the 1960s had been contaminated with a mouse virus (SV40), and subsequent hypotheses that this virus might be neoplastic in man, extensive biomedical and epidemiological studies were conducted, with no evidence that the presence of this adventitious virus in early batches the OPV had detrimental effects to human health.

For eIPV, there are no major side effects, with the exception of rare hypersensitivity reactions to the antibiotics used during the production of this vaccine.

Some Public Health Issues & Further Trends

Many studies have shown the effectiveness of the EPI schedule of OPV administration in the under-industrialized world, with a calculated protective efficacy ranging from 81 to 93 percent [66-68].

In May 1988, the World Health Assembly of the WHO adopted a resolution "to eradicate poliomyelitis globally by the year 2000." The EPI recommends the use of OPV as the center of a poliomyelitis eradication program that includes national immunization days, "mopping-up" activities, and surveillance for acute flaccid paralysis.

In 1994, the independent International Commission for the Certification of Poliomyelitis Eradication in the Americas declared the Western Hemisphere free of wild-type poliomyelitis [69].

In France, eIPV was recommended by the French Ministry of Health in 1983. With 95 percent vaccine coverage (four doses by 24 months of age), there have been no reported cases of paralytic poliomyelitis since 1990 [70]. The Netherlands uses a three dose eIPV series. During 1992/93, a focal outbreak of 67 poliomyelitis cases devastated a religious community in Holland that refuses vaccination, but the poliovirus did not spread to the unvaccinated in the general Dutch population.

It has been argued that combined use of eIPV with OPV may be most efficacious in the global eradication of poliomyelitis because fewer doses of vaccine (eIPV and OPV) will ultimately be needed to achieve consistent induction of serum neutralizing antibodies, and there would be a boosting of secretory antibody responses in the nasopharynx and in the gastrointestinal tract. A combined poliovirus immunization program, eIPV/OPV, has been used in Israel (i.e., the West Bank and the Gaza Strip) since 1978, and there have been no subsequently reported cases of poliomyelitis.

How will we know when poliomyelitis has been eradicated and we may prudently stop administering vaccine [71]? In industrialized countries free of poliomyelitis, continued serosurveys are needed to establish the level of immunity in the population, perhaps indicating groups that might require targeted eIPV booster immunizations. If an outbreak occurs, the responsible virus has to be characterized, in one part to establish its source and in another part to determine if there has been a vaccine failure. Furthermore, although the reservoir of the poliovirus is man, the vaccine viruses also may be found widely in nature. It is still an open question how long OPV will persist in the environment after the mass vaccination campaigns in under-industrialized countries have ceased [72]. Once poliovirus has been declared eradicated, there will most likely be a protracted period of continued vaccination with eIPV [73].

Rubella Virus Vaccine

Target Populations & Other Potential Risk Groups

Rubella virus vaccine is intended to provide sufficient immunity during pregnancy in order to protect the fetus from infection and to prevent the congenital rubella syndrome. In order to achieve this goal, public health policies have used both childhood vaccination (usually in a vaccine combination that includes the measles virus vaccine) and targeted adult vaccination. In the latter approach, all non-immune, prepubertal males and females should be vaccinated [74]. In some instances, college students and military recruits have been targeted for immunization. Furthermore, any opportunity to determine immune status and to immunize seronegative women against rubella, such as at the time of marriage, immediately after delivery, or following an induced abortion, should be pursued.

Administration of The Vaccine

Vaccine Composition
The rubella virus vaccine is a live attenuated rubella virus (the most widely used vaccine strain is RA27/3) that is grown on a human diploid cell strain culture.

Contraindications & Recommendations
A second dose is not advisable if the vaccinee had an immediate anaphylactic reaction to the previous rubella virus immunization. Women customarily have been counseled to avoid pregnancy for 3 months after receiving a rubella virus vaccine.

Dose, Route & Schedule
Pediatric rubella virus vaccination follows the same schedule as measles and mumps virus vaccination: two doses, the first given on or after the first birthday, and the second given at 4 to 6 years of age or at 11 to 12 years of age. Subcutaneous injection is the recommended route.

Post-Exposure Prophylaxis & Outbreak Control

Rapid vaccination of susceptibles can stem a rubella outbreak [75].

Immune Response To The Vaccine

Protective Immune Responses & Duration of Immunity
The seroprotective level is 10 IU per ml, and protective antibody responses persist for decades following immunization.

Causes of Primary Vaccine Failure
Although there are few episodes of primary vaccine failure and protective immunity remains dependable for decades, the specter of the congenital rubella syndrome has driven the acceptance of a two-dose rubella virus vaccination schedule in many industrialized countries [76].

Vaccine Reactogenicity & Reported Adverse Events
The most often observed side effect of rubella virus vaccination is rash, fever, and adenopathy occurring 5 to 12 days after vaccination. Joint pain and swelling, particularly in the smaller, peripheral joints, has been described in seronegative women [77]. Transient peripheral neuritic complaints occur rarely.

Some Public Health Issues & Further Trends

Focused programs of rubella virus vaccination targeting women of childbearing age substantially lower the incidence of the congenital rubella syndrome, as has been demonstrated in Australia, Japan, and the United Kingdom. Universal programs of childhood vaccination would seem to be more convenient to apply, and they may reach the same goal. But great care must be observed to avoid the creation of a vulnerable non-immune cohort of children and adolescents that has been neither infected naturally nor immunized with vaccine. This requires sustained vaccination of each new birth cohort, high levels of vaccine coverage, and vigilant follow-up immunization of older children born before initiation of the program. With the intensive efforts that are being directed at measles eradication, and the increasing availability of measles virus vaccines that also contain a rubella virus vaccine component (e.g., measles - rubella, or measles - mumps - rubella), it could be the moment to begin considering the eradication of rubella [78].

Rabies Virus Vaccine

Target Populations & Other Potential Risk Groups

Prophylactic rabies virus immunization is essential for all professions that involve danger of animal bite [79]. Groups at risk include veterinarians, animal handlers (hunters and dogcatchers), spelunkers, and certain lab workers. Areas endemic for dog rabies are most of Africa, the countries of Latin America, the Indian subcontinent, and Southeast Asia (with the exception of Japan and Taiwan). So prophylactic rabies virus vaccination is also recommended for children living in areas with endemic rabies or for persons moving to these areas.

Administration of The Vaccine

Vaccine Composition

All available rabies virus vaccines are prepared from the killed, whole virus [80]. Many cell culture rabies vaccines are available, differing by rabies vaccine virus strain and by cell substrate. For the human diploid cell vaccine (HDCV), the Pitman-Moore L503 3M rabies virus strain is grown on the human embryo fibroblast cell culture (type MRC-5). The virus is then β-propiolactone inactivated. Newer versions of this vaccine are the purified Vero-cell rabies vaccine (PVRV) and the chromatographically purified Vero-cell rabies vaccine (CPRV) [81, 82]. The purified chick embryo cell vaccine (PCEC) uses the Flury strain, the RVA vaccine uses the Kissling strain that has been raised on fetal rhesus lung cells, the purified duck embryo vaccine (PDEV) uses the Pittman-Moore strain, the primary Syrian hamster kidney cell culture vaccine (PHKCV) uses the Beijing strain, and the purified chick embryo cell culture vaccine (PCECV) uses the Flury LEP-C25 strain. In contrast to these cell culture derived vaccines, most of the non-industrialized world depends upon the traditional nerve tissue vaccines, such as the Fuenzalida-Palacios rabies virus vaccine raised on suckling mouse brain (which is used in Latin America and the former Soviet Union) or the Semple rabies virus vaccine derived from sheep, goat, or rabbit brains (which is used in Africa and in Asia).

Contraindications & Recommendations

Concurrent administration of serum or antimalarial medication (e.g., chloroquine, mefloquine, or other structurally related antimalarial agents) may interfere with the rabies virus vaccine immune response. Rabies vaccine can be administered during pregnancy and to persons with HIV/AIDS.

Dose, Route & Schedule

For pre-exposure vaccination, three doses are given on day 0, 7, and 21 or 28 by the intramuscular route (anterolateral aspect of the mid-thigh, for children younger than 24 months, and deltoid, for children older than 24 months and for adults). An intradermal route of administration is available with HDCV rabies virus vaccine, which uses one-tenth of the intramuscular dose. For either route of administration, a first booster dose should be given a year later.

Post-Exposure Prophylaxis & Outbreak Control

Following a potentially rabid animal bite, the treatment protocol to be followed depends upon the vaccination status of the bite victim.

If the victim has received previous pre-exposure immunization with a cell culture rabies vaccine, has had previous post-exposure prophylaxis with a cell culture rabies vaccine, or has a history of previous vaccination with any other type of rabies vaccine and a documented history of antibody response to this prior vaccination, then intramuscular vaccination with two doses of a cell culture rabies vaccine at day 0 and 3, without rabies immune globulin (RIG), is adequate.

If the bite victim has not been previously vaccinated, five doses of the vaccine are given on day 0, 3, 7, 14, and 28. Both the WHO and U.S. recommendations are for intramuscular inoculation. Many developing countries have chosen an intradermal route of administration, which uses other schedules, to lower treatment costs and to ensure better compliance. Two examples are the Thai schedule (i.e., day 0, 3, 7 (two doses), 28, and 90, used with PVRV, PCECV, or PDEV) and an alternative developing country schedule (i.e., day 0 (eight doses), 7 (four doses), 28, and 90, used with cell culture vaccines). Post-exposure vaccination should be given in conjunction with RIG on day 0 (in all cases according to American recommendations, but only in the more serious categories of rabies exposure according to the World Health Organization). Following possible exposure to rabies virus, vaccine must be promptly administered, combined with vigorous washing of the wound with soap or iodine solution. As much as possible of the RIG should be infiltrated into and around the wound. The remainder should be injected intramuscularly, at an anatomical site distant from the wound. In the industrialized world, RIG of human origin (human rabies immune globulin, HRIG) is generally used, while purified and pepsin-treated equine rabies immune globulin (ERIG) is the alternative for much of the rest of the world.

In countries where RIG is unavailable for post-exposure prophylaxis, a vaccine-only injection schedule is used that relies on four doses on day 0 (two doses), 7, and 21.

Immune Response To The Vaccine

Protective Immune Responses & Duration of Immunity
After pre-exposure rabies virus vaccination, antibodies directed against the G protein of the viral envelope appear 10 to 14 days after the first injection. Three doses of vaccine have been found to provide 100 percent seroconversion; furthermore, the dose at day 21 or later is essential for persistent high antibody titers. The minimum acceptable antibody level is complete virus neutralization at a 1: 5 serum dilution as determined by rapid fluorescent focus inhibition test (RFFIT). This dilution is approximately equal to the minimum titer of 0.5 IU per ml, established by the WHO serum neutralization test.

Persons at continuously high risk of exposure, such as specialized laboratory workers, must have their serum titers for rabies antibodies checked every 6 months. Other high-risk groups (e.g., veterinarians and animal handlers) should have antibody levels tested every 2 years. In all circumstances, the rabies serum antibody titer must surpass 0.5 IU per ml [83].

Causes of Primary Vaccine Failure

If the person presenting for pre-exposure immunization is also taking an antimalarial agent that is structurally related to chloroquine, the HDCV rabies virus vaccine must not be given by the intradermal route; the intramuscular route of vaccination should be used. Post-exposure rabies virus vaccine failures are uncommon for the cell culture vaccines. They are usually the result of inadequately applied treatment, such as neglecting to apply RIG to the wound. By contrast, there appears to be a greater risk of vaccine failure for the nerve tissue vaccines, which is compounded by the fact that RIG infrequently is administered conjointly.

Vaccine Reactogenicity & Reported Adverse Events

HDCV has been linked to allergic reactions (i.e., Type III hypersensitivity reactions), particularly 2 to 21 days after a subsequent injection. These reactions are due to contaminating proteins in the vaccine [84]. The Semple rabies virus vaccine contains adult nerve tissue antigen (i.e., myelin basic protein), leading to a non-negligible risk of post-vaccination allergic "encephalomyelitis". The Fuenzalida-Palacios rabies virus vaccine is made from suckling mouse brains, and the allergic "encephalomyelitis" risk, while still present, is much less than for the Semple rabies virus vaccine.

Some Public Health Issues & Further Trends

A few of the major issues confronting rabies vaccination are (i) bat rabies, (ii) the global paucity of RIG, and (iii) the possibility of including rabies virus vaccine in the calendar of childhood vaccination for certain countries.

While human rabies is most immediately associated with dog bites, many other mammals may carry rabies, including cats, skunks, raccoons, foxes, woodchucks, and bats. Bat rabies is an increasingly recognized but difficult to handle problem, as the potential exposure is not always evident [85]. Medical practitioners ought to reasonably consider that a contact occurred if a sleeping person awakens to find a bat in the room, or if an adult witnesses a bat in the room with a previously unattended child, with a mentally disturbed person, or with an intoxicated person. Unless the bat can be caught and tests negative for the rabies virus, post-exposure prophylaxis is warranted. The cell culture rabies virus vaccines provide protection against the rabies virus strains found in bats [86].

The cost of HRIG is prohibitive, and the global supplies of the less expensive, but equally effective, ERIG are limited, meaning that potential rabies patients in the under-industrialized world may not be receiving the complete post-exposure prophylaxis series (i.e., rabies vaccine plus rabies immune globulin).

Cell culture rabies virus vaccines may be safely and effectively administered in association with the EPI vaccines. The risk of rabies infection is particularly elevated for small children living in an area endemic for dog rabies, so childhood rabies virus vaccination is being considered for inclusion in the pediatric schedule of some countries.

Smallpox Virus Vaccine

Target Populations & Other Potential Risk Groups

With the global eradication of smallpox (variola), the only remaining indications for smallpox vaccination (vaccinia) are for workers in laboratories researching the orthopoxviruses. Until March 1990, the Pentagon mandated routine vaccination of US military recruits. Some military forces continue to vaccinate their personnel [87].

Administration of The Vaccine

Vaccine Composition
The remaining stocks of smallpox virus vaccine (vaccinia) that are available were raised on the skin of calves, harvested, purified, and then freeze-dried. (The two most commonly used strains were the Lister strain and the New York City Board of Health strain.)

Contraindications & Recommendations
Vaccinia virus should not be administered to a person suffering from an immune disorder (e.g., agammaglobulinemia or hypogammaglobulinemia, leukemia, and lymphoma) or an exfoliative skin condition (e.g., eczema, atopic dermatitis, impetigo, or chickenpox). Patients under immunosuppressive drug treatment and pregnant women should not be vaccinated.

Dose, Route & Schedule
Vaccinia is administered by scarification (i.e., intradermal inoculation with a bifurcated needle by multiple rapid strokes across the lateral surface of the upper arm). Booster doses of 15 punctures are given every 10 years.

Post-Exposure Prophylaxis & Outbreak Control

Primary smallpox vaccination, applied after exposure, was occasionally found to modify or even stop an attack of smallpox.

Immune Response To The Vaccine

Protective Immune Responses & Duration of Immunity
The vaccinia virus is introduced directly into the basal cell layer of the skin, where the virus multiplies. The immune response in marked by both serum antibodies (particularly neutralizing antibodies, but also complement fixation and haemagglutination inhibition antibodies) and by a delayed-type hypersensitivity reaction. Immune protection seems to persist for at least 10 to 20 years.

Causes of Primary Vaccine Failure
In order to inhibit the reactogenicity associated with vaccinia vaccination, attenuated smallpox virus vaccine strains were developed, but these appeared to have been less immunogenic.

Vaccine Reactogenicity & Reported Adverse Events
A number of important side effects were associated with the massive smallpox eradication program: eczema vaccinatum, progressive vaccinia, generalized vaccinia, and post-vaccination encephalopathy or encephalitis.

Some Public Health Issues & Further Trends

Smallpox was certified by the WHO Global Commission on 9 December 1979 to have been eradicated from the Earth.

Tick-borne Encephalitis Virus Vaccine

Target Populations & Other Potential Risk Groups

Tick-borne encephalitis virus vaccine is indicated for inhabitants of an area endemic for any of the tick vectors (i.e., *Ixodes ricinus, Dermacentor* spp., and *Haemaphysalis* spp.). Particularly affected countries are Austria, the Czech Republic, Finland, Germany, Hungary, Italy, Sweden, Switzerland, and the Russian Republic, as well as the Baltic republics and the countries of the former Yugoslavia. People having outdoor occupations or hobbies are at high risk of tick bites and hence infection.

Administration of The Vaccine

Vaccine Composition
The tick-borne encephalitis vaccine is a formaldehyde-killed virus that had been grown on primary chicken embryo cells. It is adsorbed on aluminum hydroxide.

Contraindications & Recommendations
The vaccine is not indicated for persons who may have had an immediate anaphylactic reaction to a previous dose of vaccine or for those with a history of anaphylactic hypersensitivity to one of the vaccine components (e.g., human albumin, thimerosal, or gelatin).

Dose, Route & Schedule
The primary series is composed of three doses, at 0, 1 to 3 months, and then 10 to 15 months, with booster doses recommended once every 3 years, following the primary series. An accelerated three-dose schedule of immunizations on day 0, 7, and 28 has been shown to be also safe and immunogenic.

Post-Exposure Prophylaxis & Outbreak Control

Tick-borne encephalitis immune globulin, containing specific immunoglobulins against the virus, can be given intramuscularly up to 4 days after the tick bite. Conversely, the immune globulin must not be given 4 or more days after the suspected tick bite because the treatment may enhance infection by the tick-borne encephalitis virus. For the same reason, neither should there be a repeat administration of immune globulin for 28 days following the initial treatment.

Immune Response To The Vaccine

Protective Immune Responses & Duration of Immunity
After the third injection, almost all vaccine recipients demonstrate seroconversion, as indicated by ELISA antibody titers. High antibody titers persist for at least 3 to 5 years, which is the recommended moment for a booster vaccination.

Causes of Primary Vaccine Failure
Although no controlled clinical trials of vaccine efficacy have been carried out, the protective effectiveness of this vaccine after the three-dose primary series has been estimated at over 97% from post-marketing data.

Vaccine Reactogenicity & Reported Adverse Events
Tick-borne encephalitis virus vaccine induces local immune responses characteristic of a killed virus vaccine that is absorbed, and it produces some systemic effects (e.g., fatigue, fever, and headache).

Some Public Health Issues & Further Trends

Unresolved public health aspects of the tick-borne encephalitis virus vaccine include (i) the geographic distribution of the disease, (ii) its inclusion in pediatric vaccination schedules, and (iii) suspicions of immune enhancement between Flavivirus infections. Tick-borne encephalitis cases have been diagnosed from continental Europe, across Eastern Europe and the Russian interior, and in China. But the true extent of this illness has yet to be appreciated, particularly in the Russian Federation and in China. In some countries such as Austria, tick-borne encephalitis vaccination has been incorporated into the pediatric immunization schedule, whereas in most others it is only indicated for at-risk occupations (i.e., foresters, woodcutters, farmers, or military personnel) and for those practicing outdoor hobbies. Finally, clinical studies continue to explore the possibility that a vaccine against one Flavivirus, the tick-borne encephalitis virus, might induce a state of immune enhancement with respect to other Flaviviruses such as dengue fever virus or yellow fever virus.

Varicella-zoster Virus Vaccine

Target Populations & Other Potential Risk Groups

Following the early lead of Japan, the USA has established an aggressive schedule for varicella-zoster virus (VZV) immunization [88] that targets younger children (between 12 and 18 months of age), older children (between 19 months and 12 years of age) without a reliable history of having had chickenpox, susceptible household contacts of immunocompromised individuals, and all healthcare workers. Furthermore, it is strongly recommended that adults at elevated risk of infection or transmission (e.g., people working with children, college students, members of the penal system, and military personnel) should be vaccinated. Finally, women of childbearing age who are not pregnant should consider being vaccinated.

In immunocompromised children, the effects of VZV infection may be particularly grave. Although children suffering from a state of immunodeficiency–such as leukemic children–risk the development of a varicella-zoster-like illness following administration of this live attenuated virus, clinical studies reveal that their immunization has been both safe and effective. Consequently, some countries, notably in Europe, have reserved VZV vaccination to immunocompromised children.

Administration of The Vaccine

Vaccine Composition
VZV vaccine contains the Oka strain of attenuated varicella-zoster virus, which has been passaged in human embryo lung cells, guinea pig embryo cells, and human diploid cells. After production, the vaccine virus is lyophilized, and the vaccine is stored at -20 to 5°C until it is reconstituted for use.

Contraindications & Recommendations
The clinical issues surrounding VZV vaccination fall into five categories: hypersensitivity, concurrent illnesses, pregnancy, immunodeficiencies, and association with the measles - mumps - rubella virus vaccine [89].

VZV vaccination is contraindicated in persons having had an immediate anaphylactic reaction to a previous dose of VZV vaccine, or in those that have a history of anaphylactic reaction to neomycin or gelatin. Vaccination should be deferred in cases of moderate or severe illness (with or without fever), and no salicylates should be taken for 6 weeks after vaccination (to lessen the risk of Reye syndrome). VZV vaccine is contraindicated if the subject had had varicella zoster or herpes zoster within the previous 21 days, and in persons with untreated active tuberculosis. Women should be counseled to avoid pregnancy for 1 month after vaccination. As a general rule, VZV vaccine is not administered to immunocompromised individuals, which includes patients with leukemia, lymphoma, or other malignancies, patients receiving radiotherapy or chemotherapy, patients with HIV/AIDS, or someone receiving a course of high-dose corticosteroids. If the potential vaccinee has a family history of a primary immunodeficiency, he or she should be evaluated for immune competence before inoculation.

Newly vaccinated persons are advised to avoid close contact with high-risk susceptible individuals for 6 weeks after vaccination. Although unlikely, there is a theoretical risk that the vaccine virus may be transmitted from healthy vaccinees to varicella-zoster-susceptible persons, for example, the immunocompromised, pregnant women [90], fetuses (i.e., congenital varicella syndrome), or new-born infants (i.e., neonatal chickenpox). The immune responses to each vaccine will be affected if measles - mumps - rubella virus vaccine and VZV vaccines are given within 1 to 30 days of each other.

Dose, Route & Schedule

Children should receive the VZV vaccine between 12 and 18 months of age. It is given by subcutaneous injection. Unvaccinated children who have an uncertain history of chickenpox should be immunized at the 11- to 12-year-old visit. Adolescents and adults without a history of varicella-zoster should be vaccinated twice because they have been found to be in general less responsive to immunization than children.

Post-Exposure Prophylaxis & Outbreak Control

VZV vaccine may stem an outbreak if administered soon after exposure.

Immune Response To The Vaccine

Protective Immune Responses & Duration of Immunity

Immunization with the VZV vaccine induces both a humoral immune response (serum IgG antibodies) and a cellular immune response (exemplified by assays of cell mediated immunity). Infants show seroconversion rates surpassing 90% after receipt of a single inoculation of the VZV vaccine. Adults, on the other hand, manifest a poorer vaccine response; therefore, two injections are necessary to induce approximately the same level of post-vaccination immunity. Both humoral and cellular immune responses appear to persist for at least a decade, even in the absence of exposure to exogenous VZV.

Causes of Primary Vaccine Failure

Among vaccinated children, breakthrough varicella-zoster usually is observed at a rate of 0 to 4% per year. Nevertheless, the clinical signs of infection are less severe in the vaccine recipients. In adults who have been vaccinated, there has been no increase over years of follow up in the incidence or severity of VZV infection.

Vaccine Reactogenicity & Reported Adverse Events

Other then the anticipated local reactogenicity, VZV vaccination has been associated with a mild varicella-zoster-like rash. There has been a single case report of a vaccinated child spreading the varicella-zoster vaccine virus to his pregnant mother; otherwise, there have been no other reported clinical instances of transmission of the virus to a non-vaccinated susceptible. Post-marketing studies strongly suggest that induction of herpes zoster because of VZV vaccination is rare.

Some Public Health Issues & Further Trends

When healthy children who had received the Oka/Merck varicella-zoster vaccine were followed for seven years, 95 percent of the vaccine recipients remained free of varicella-zoster [91]. In this study, the varicella-zoster that did occur in less than 5 percent of the vaccine recipients was considerably milder than natural chicken pox. In a second American study that compared clinical cases of natural varicella-zoster with breakthrough varicella-zoster, live attenuated Oka/Merck virus vaccination provided significant lessening of the number of lesions, of the incidence of fever, and of the duration of illness in the breakthrough cases [92]. A third study, which followed vaccinated children (ages 12 months to 17 years) for five to ten years, established an 18.6 percent rate of breakthrough disease (nevertheless, with shorter duration, lower fever temperatures, and less skin lesions observed), which is greater than previously reported [93].

Varicella-zoster virus immunization may ultimately reduce the incidence of herpes zoster in adulthood. For instance, VZV vaccinated leukemic children have a subsequently lower incidence of herpes zoster, perhaps because the vaccine virus leaves less latency than the wild virus [94]. In addition, vaccination may boost the cellular immune responses to VZV in the elderly, potentially providing protection from the reactivation of herpes zoster.

The remarkable examples of Japan and the USA have compelled public health authorities in other countries to debate the introduction of chickenpox vaccination in their own countries, for example, in New Zealand and in Mexico. Economic models of cost benefit and cost effectiveness often overshadow the arguments, however.

To be an effective public health intervention, both parents and practitioners need to be appropriately educated to the likely benefits and the possible risks of VZV vaccination. A combination vaccine with measles - mump - rubella vaccine will augment the utility of VZV vaccination [95].

Yellow Fever Virus Vaccine

Target Populations & Other Potential Risk Groups

Yellow fever virus vaccine is included in the EPI for the most heavily affected countries of West Africa. Immunization is recommended for travelers to areas where yellow fever is endemic or enzootic, particularly in Africa (e.g., Nigeria, Cameroon, Angola, and Niger) and South America (e.g., Peru, Bolivia, Brazil, and Columbia). It is the only disease for which an International Certificate of Vaccination may be required, as per WHO guidelines, both for travelers into yellow fever endemic areas and for inhabitants of yellow fever endemic areas leaving their countries for non-endemic areas.

Administration of The Vaccine

Vaccine Composition
Yellow fever vaccine is a live attenuated virus, most often produced from the 17D strain

of yellow fever virus, which has been raised on fertilized hens' eggs.

Contraindications & Recommendations

The vaccine should not be given to people who are allergic to eggs. It also is contraindicated in pregnant women (because of a small risk of vaccine-related congenital infection), in immunocompromised persons, and in children younger than 4 months of age [96]. Of particular relevance to the EPI, yellow fever virus vaccine may be administered in association with measles virus vaccine without interfering with the appropriate immune responses.

Dose, Route & Schedule

The single dose of vaccine can be given by the subcutaneous route or by scarification. International travel regulations require a booster immunization every ten years.

Post-Exposure Prophylaxis & Outbreak Control

There is no immune globulin available to treat exposure to the yellow fever virus. Few nations in West African nations apply yellow fever virus vaccination systematically and regularly, so it is fortunate that mass vaccination has been such an effective response to yellow fever epidemics.

Immune Response To The Vaccine

Protective Immune Responses & Duration of Immunity

A single injection of the yellow fever virus vaccine induces neutralizing serum antibodies in over 90% of vaccine recipients, which are complete within 10 days of inoculation. Mild viremia of brief duration has been noted in about half of vaccinees. Although International Health Regulations insist on revaccination every 10 years, field evidence suggests that yellow fever virus vaccine immunity is lifelong.

Causes of Primary Vaccine Failure

Although a few yellow fever virus vaccine failures have been traced to irregularities in the storage of the vaccine or of the cold chain, field studies suggest that host factors such as malnutrition, pregnancy, and HIV/AIDS are responsible for most episodes of vaccine failure.

Vaccine Reactogenicity & Reported Adverse Events

As a vaccine produced on eggs, the risk of anaphylaxis among egg-sensitive individuals is always present. There have been rare reports after yellow fever virus vaccination of vaccine-associated encephalitis, some with neurological complications.

Some Public Health Issues & Further Trends

The recent history of yellow fever virus immunization is marked by particular trends: reemergence in West Africa, expansion into East Africa, prevalence growing in Latin America, and urbanization of the disease. The WHO recommends that the administration of yellow fever virus vaccine to 9 month olds be incorporated into the national immunization schedules of the most affected African nations. A cost-effectiveness analysis in Nigeria, for example, suggests that routine EPI vaccination is preferable to the present situation, which relies on emergency control of epidemics [97].

Combination Viral Vaccines

Some of the viral vaccines that have been presented in this chapter are combinations. For instance, both the poliovirus vaccine and the influenza virus vaccine are prepared by combining strains of the same viral species. Other viral vaccine combinations that are detailed in Table 4 present different viral species in the same vaccine.

Table 4. Some combination viral vaccines

Type of combination	Vaccines licensed for human use	References
Strains of the same virus species		
	Poliovirus	[98, 99]
	Influenza virus	[100]
Different viral species		
	Hepatitis B virus - hepatitis A virus	[101]
	Measles virus - rubella virus	[102]
	Measles virus - mumps virus	[103]
	Measles virus - mumps virus - rubella virus	[45]
	Measles virus - mumps virus - rubella virus - varicella zoster virus	[95]

REFERENCES

1. [No authors listed]. Prevention of hepatitis A through active or passive immunization: Recommendations of the Advisory Committee on Immunization Practices (ACIP). MMWR.Morb.Mortal. Wkly.Rep. 1996; 45(RR-15): 1-30.

2. Lerman Y, Chodik G, Aloni H, Ribak J, Ashkenazi S. Occupations at increased risk of hepatitis A: a 2-year nationwide historical prospective study. Am.J.Epidemiol. 1999; 150(3): 312-20.

3. Clemens R, Safary A, Hepburn A, Roche C, Stanbury WJ, Andre FE. Clinical experience with an inactivated hepatitis A vaccine. J.Infect.Dis. 1995; 171 Suppl 1: S44-S49

4. Halsey NA, Chesney PJ, Gerber MA, Gromisch DS, Kohl S, Marcy SM, Marks MI, Murray DL, Overall JC, Pickering LK, et al. Prevention of hepatitis A infections: Guidelines for use of hepatitis A

vaccine and immune globulin. Committee on Infectious Diseases. Pediatrics. 1996; 98(6): 1207-15.

5. Dagan R, Greenberg D, Goldenbertg-Gehtman P, Vidor E, Briantais P, Pinsk V, Athias O, Dumas R. Safety and immunogenicity of a new formulation of an inactivated hepatitis A vaccine. Vaccine 1999; 17(15-16): 1919-25.

6. Van Herck K, Beutels P, Van Damme P, Beutels M, Van den Dries J, Briantais P, Vidor E. Mathematical models for assessment of long-term persistence of antibodies after vaccination with two inactivated hepatitis A vaccines. J.Med.Virol. 2000; 60(1): 1-7.

7. Innis BL, Snitbhan R, Kunasol P, Laorakpongse T, Poopatanakool W, Kozik CA, Suntayakorn S, Suknuntapong T, Safary A, Tang DB. Protection against hepatitis A by an inactivated vaccine. J.Am.Med.Assoc. 1994; 271(17): 1328-34.

8. Bell BP, Shapiro CN, Alter MJ, Moyer LA, Judson FN, Mottram K, Fleenor M, Ryder PL, Margolis HS. The diverse patterns of hepatitis A epidemiology in the United States - implications for vaccination strategies. J.Infect.Dis. 1998; 178(6): 1579-84.

9. [No authors listed]. Update: recommendations to prevent hepatitis B virus transmission — United States. MMWR.Morb.Mortal.Wkly.Rep. 1999; 48(RR-2): 33-4.

10. Liao SS, Li RC, Li H, Yang JY, Zeng XJ, Gong J, Wang SS, Li YP, Zhang KL. Long-term efficacy of plasma-derived hepatitis B vaccine: a 15-year follow-up study among Chinese children. Vaccine 1999; 17(20-21): 2661-6.

11. Adkins JC, Wagstaff AJ. Recombinant hepatitis B vaccine: A review of its immunogenicity and protective efficacy against hepatitis B. BioDrugs 1998; 10(2): 137-58.

12. Grotto I, Mandel Y, Ephros M, Ashkenazi I, Shemer J. Major adverse reactions to yeast-derived hepatitis B vaccines - A review. Vaccine 1998; 16(4): 329-34.

13. Kane M. Implementing universal vaccination programmes: USA. Vaccine 1995; 13 Suppl 1: S75-S76

14. Jack AD, Hall AJ, Maine N, Mendy M, Whittle HC. What level of hepatitis B antibody is protective? J.Infect.Dis. 1999; 179(2): 489-92.

15. Kane M, Banatvala J, Da Villa G, Esteban R, Franco E, Goudeau A, Grob P, Jilg W, Rizzetto M, Van Damme P, et al. Are booster immunisations needed for lifelong hepatitis B immunity? Lancet 2000; 355(9203): 561-5.

16. Hsu HM, Lu CF, Lee SC, Lin SR, Chen DS. Seroepidemiologic survey for hepatitis B virus infection in Taiwan: The effect of hepatitis B mass immunization. J.Infect.Dis. 1999; 179(2): 367-70.

17. Hsu HY, Chang MH, Liaw SH, Ni YH, Chen HL. Changes of hepatitis B surface antigen variants in carrier children before and after universal vaccination in Taiwan. Hepatology 1999; 30(5): 1312-7.

18. Stratton KR, Howe CJ, Johnston RB, Jr. Adverse events associated with childhood vaccines other than pertussis and rubella. Summary of a report from the Institute of Medicine. J.Am.Med.Assoc. 1994; 271(20): 1602-5.

19. Levy-Bruhl D, Rebière I, Desenclos JC, Drucker J. Comparaison entre les risques de premières atteintes démyélisantes centrales aiguës et les bénéfices de la vaccination contre l'hépatite B. Bull.Epidémiol.Hebd. 1999; (9): 33-5.

20. Hall A, Kane M, Roure C, Meheus A. Multiple sclerosis and hepatitis B vaccine? Vaccine 1999; 17(20-21): 2473-5.

21. Kane MA. Status of hepatitis B immunization programmes in 1998. Vaccine 1998; 16 Suppl: S104-S108

22. Cassidy W. School-based adolescent hepatitis B immunization programs in the United States: strategies and successes. Pediatr.Infect.Dis.J. 1998; 17 Suppl 7: S43-S46

23. Nichol KL, Margolis KL, Wuorenma J, von Sternberg T. The efficacy and cost effectiveness of

vaccination against influenza among elderly persons living in the community. N.Engl.J.Med. 1994; 331(12): 778-84.

24. [No authors listed]. Recommendations for prevention and control of influenza. Recommendations of the Immunization Practices Advisory Committee. Centers For Disease Control, Department of Health and Human Services. Ann.Intern.Med. 1986; 105(3): 399-404.

25. [No authors listed]. Prevention and control of influenza: recommendations of the Advisory Committee on Immunization Practices (ACIP). MMWR.Morb.Mortal.Wkly.Rep. 1999; 48(RR-4): 1-28.

26. Izurieta HS, Thompson WW, Kramarz P, Shay DK, Davis RL, DeStefano F, Black S, Shinefield H, Fukuda K. Influenza and the rates of hospitalization for respiratory disease among infants and young children. N.Engl.J.Med. 2000; 342(4): 232-9.

27. James JM, Zeiger RS, Lester MR, Fasano MB, Gern JE, Mansfield LE, Schwartz HJ, Sampson HA, Windom HH, Machtinger SB, et al. Safe administration of influenza vaccine to patients with egg allergy. J.Pediatr. 1998; 133(5): 624-8.

28. Groothuis JR, Levin MJ, Rabalais GP, Meiklejohn G, Lauer BA. Immunization of high-risk infants younger than 18 months of age with split-product influenza vaccine. Pediatrics 1991; 87(6): 823-8.

29. el-Madhun AS, Cox RJ, Soreide A, Olofsson J, Haaheim LR. Systemic and mucosal immune responses in young children and adults after parenteral influenza vaccination. J.Infect.Dis. 1998; 178(4): 933-9.

30. de Bruijn IA, Remarque EJ, Jol-van der Zijde CM, van Tol MJ, Westendorp RG, Knook DL. Quality and quantity of the humoral immune response in healthy elderly and young subjects after annually repeated influenza vaccination. J.Infect.Dis. 1999; 179(1): 31-6.

31. Gross PA, Sperber SJ, Donabedian A, Dran S, Morchel G, Cataruozolo P, Munk G. Paradoxical response to a novel influenza virus vaccine strain: the effect of prior immunization. Vaccine 1999; 17(18): 2284-9.

32. Beyer WEP, de Bruijn IA, Palache AM, Westendorp RGJ, Osterhaus ADME. Protection against influenza after annually repeated vaccination - A meta-analysis of serologic and field studies. Arch.Intern.Med. 1999; 159(2): 182-8.

33. Bradley SF. Prevention of influenza in long-term-care facilities. Infect.Control Hosp.Epidemiol. 1999; 20(9): 629-37.

34. Barker WH, Borisute H, Cox C. A study of the impact of influenza on the functional status of frail older people. Arch.Intern.Med. 1998; 158(6): 645-50.

35. Carman WF, Elder AG, Wallace LA, McAulay K, Walker A, Murray GD, Stott DJ. Effects of influenza vaccination of health-care workers on mortality of elderly people in long-term care: a randomised controlled trial. Lancet 2000; 355(9198): 93-7.

36. Saxen H, Virtanen M. Randomized, placebo-controlled double blind study on the efficacy of influenza immunization on absenteeism of health care workers. Pediatr.Infect.Dis.J. 1999; 18(9): 779-83.

37. Ambrosch F, Fedson DS. Influenza vaccination in 29 countries: An update to 1997. Pharmacoeconomics 1999; 16 Suppl 1: 47-54.

38. [No authors listed]. Inactivated Japanese encephalitis virus vaccine. Recommendations of the Advisory Committee on immunization Practices (ACIP). MMWR.Morb.Mortal.Wkly.Rep. 1993; 42(RR-1): 1-15.

39. Hennessy S, Liu Z, Tsai TF, Strom BL, Wan CM, Liu HL, Wu TX, Yu HJ, Liu QM, Karabatsos N, et al. Effectiveness of live-attenuated Japanese encephalitis vaccine (SA14-14-2): a case-control study. Lancet 1996; 347(9015): 1583-6.

40. DeFraites RF, Gambel JM, Hoke CH, Jr., Sanchez JL, Withers BG, Karabatsos N, Shope RE, Tirrell S, Yoshida I, Takagi M, et al. Japanese encephalitis vaccine (Inactivated, BIKEN) in US soldiers: Immunogenicity and safety of vaccine administered in two dosing regimens. Am.J.Trop.Med.Hyg.

1999; 61(2): 288-93.

41. Berg SW, Mitchell BS, Hanson RK, Olafson RP, Williams RP, Tueller JE, Burton RJ, Novak DM, Tsai TF, Wignall FS. Systemic reactions in U.S. Marine Corps personnel who received Japanese encephalitis vaccine. Clin.Infect.Dis. 1997; 24(2): 265-6.

42. Orenstein WA, Markowitz LE, Atkinson WL, Hinman AR. Worldwide measles prevention. Isr.J.Med.Sci. 1994; 30(5-6): 469-81.

43. Lepow ML, Nankervis GA. Eight-year serologic evaluation of Edmonston live measles vaccine. J.Pediatr. 1969; 75(3): 407-11.

44. Gellin BG, Katz SL. Measles: state of the art and future directions. J.Infect.Dis. 1994; 170 Suppl 1: S3-S14

45. Broliden K, Leven B, Arneborn M, Bottiger M. Immunity to measles before and after MMR booster or primary vaccination at 12 years of age in the first generation offered the 2-dose immunization programme. Scand.J.Infect.Dis. 1998; 30(1): 23-7.

46. Skinner R, Christie P, Cowden JM. The measles/rubella immunisation campaign in Scotland. Health Bull. 1996; 54(1): 88-98.

47. Miyazawa H, Saitoh S, Kumagai T, Yamanaka T, Yasuda S, Tsunetsugu-Yokota Y, Inouye S, Sakaguchi M. Specific IgG to gelatin in children with systemic immediate- and nonimmediate-type reactions to measles, mumps and rubella vaccines. Vaccine 1999; 17(17): 2176-80.

48. Scott S, Cutts FT, Nyandu B. Mild illness at or after measles vaccination does not reduce seroresponse in young children. Vaccine 1999; 17(7-8): 837-43.

49. Khakoo GA, Lack G. Guidelines for measles vaccination in egg-allergic children. Clin.Exp.Allergy 2000; 30(2): 288-93.

50. Kelso JM, Jones RT, Yunginger JW. Anaphylaxis to measles, mumps, and rubella vaccine mediated by IgE to gelatin. J.Allergy Clin.Immunol. 1993; 91(4): 867-72.

51. Afzal MA, Minor PD, Schild GC. Clinical safety issues of measles, mumps and rubella vaccines. Bull.World Health Organ. 2000; 78(2): 199-204.

52. Aaby P, Samb B, Simondon F, Knudsen K, Seck AMC, Bennett J, Markowitz L, Whittle H. Five year follow-up of morbidity and mortality among recipients of high-titre measles vaccines in Senegal. Vaccine 1996; 14(3): 226-9.

53. Paunio M, Peltola H, Valle M, Davidkin I, Virtanen M, Heinonen OP. Twice vaccinated recipients are better protected against epidemic measles than are single dose recipients of measles containing vaccine. J.Epidemiol.Community Health 1999; 3(3): 173-8.

54. de Quadros CA, Hersh BS, Nogueira AC, Carrasco PA, da Silveira CM. Measles eradication: experience in the Americas. Bull.World Health Organ. 1998; 76 Suppl 2: 47-52.

55. Thomas A, Xu D, Wooten K, Morrow B, Redd S. Timing and effectiveness of requirements for a second dose of measles vaccine. Pediatr.Infect.Dis.J. 1999; 18(3): 266-70.

56. Wittler RR, Veit BC, Mcintyre S, Schydlower M. Measles revaccination response in a school-age population. Pediatrics 1991; 88(5): 1024-30.

57. Cutts FT, Henao-Restrepo AM, Olivé JM. Measles elimination: Progress and challenges. Vaccine 1999; 17 Suppl 3: S47-S52

58. Galazka AM, Robertson SE, Kraigher A. Mumps and mumps vaccine: A global review. Bull.World Health Organ. 1999; 77(1): 3-14.

59. Goh KT. Resurgence of mumps in Singapore caused by the Rubini mumps virus vaccine strain. Lancet 1999; 354(9187): 1355-6.

60. Murdin AD, Barreto L, Plotkin S. Inactivated poliovirus vaccine: past and present experience. Vaccine

1996; 14(8): 735-46.

61. Englund J, Glezen WP, Piedra PA. Maternal immunization against viral disease. Vaccine 1998; 16(14-15): 1456-63.

62. Halsey NA, Abramson JS, Chesney PJ, Fisher MC, Gerber MA, Marcy SM, Murray DL, et al. Poliomyelitis prevention: Revised recommendations for use of inactivated and live oral poliovirus vaccines. Pediatrics 1999; 103(1): 171-2.

63. Herremans TM, Reimerink JHJ, Buisman AM, Kimman TG, Koopmans MPG. Induction of mucosal immunity by inactivated poliovirus vaccine is dependent on previous mucosal contact with live virus. J.Immunol. 1999; 162(8): 5011-8.

64. Kaul D, Ogra PL. Mucosal responses to parenteral and mucosal vaccines. Dev.Biol.Stand. 1998; 95: 141-6.

65. Cirne MD, Duarte MNDR, Nobrega DD, Desouza EMD, Monteiro D, Oliveira MJC, Dantas MCD, et al. Factors affecting the immunogenicity of oral poliovirus vaccine: A prospective evaluation in Brazil and the Gambia. J.Infect.Dis. 1995; 171(5): 1097-106.

66. Deivanayagam N, Nedunchelian K, Ahamed SS, Rathnam SR. Clinical efficacy of trivalent oral poliomyelitis vaccine: a case-control study. Bull.World Health Organ. 1993; 71(3-4): 307-9.

67. Deming MS, Jaiteh KO, Otten MWJ, Flagg EW, Jallow M, Cham M, Brogan D, N'Jie H. Epidemic poliomyelitis in The Gambia following the control of poliomyelitis as an endemic disease. II. Clinical efficacy of trivalent oral polio vaccine. Am.J.Epidemiol. 1992; 135(4): 393-408.

68. Singh J, Kumar K, Bora D, Chawla U, Bilochi NC, Sharma RS, Kapur ML, Kumar S, Aggarwal BK, Dhaon JK. Epidemiological evaluation of oral polio vaccine efficacy in Delhi. Indian J.Pediatr. 1992; 59(3): 321-3.

69. [No authors listed]. Certification of the eradication of poliomyelitis. Bull.World Health Organ. 1996; 74(1): 109-10.

70. Malvy DJ, Drucker J. Elimination of poliomyelitis in France: epidemiology and vaccine status. Public Health Rev 1993; 21(1-2): 41-9.

71. Hull HF, Aylward RB. Invited commentary: The scientific basis for stopping polio immunization. Am.J.Epidemiol. 1999; 150(10): 1022-5.

72. Fine PEM, Carneiro IAM. Transmissibility and persistence of oral polio vaccine viruses: Implications for the global poliomyelitis eradication initiative. Am.J.Epidemiol. 1999; 150(10): 1001-21.

73. Sutter RW, Prevots DR, Cochi SL. Poliovirus vaccines - Progress toward global poliomyelitis eradication and changing routine immunization recommendations in the United States. Pediatr.Clin.North Am. 2000; 47(2): 287-308.

74. Ukkonen P. Rubella immunity and morbidity: impact of different vaccination programs in Finland 1979-1992. Scand.J.Infect.Dis. 1996; 28(1): 31-5.

75. Greaves WL, Orenstein WA, Stetler HC, Preblud SR, Hinman AR, Bart KJ. Prevention of rubella transmission in medical facilities. J.Am.Med.Assoc. 1982; 248(7): 861-4.

76. Fogel A, Barnea BS, Aboudy Y, Mendelson E. Rubella in pregnancy in Israel: 15 years of follow-up and remaining problems. Isr.J.Med.Sci. 1996; 32(5): 300-5.

77. Mitchell LA, Tingle AJ, Grace M, Middleton P, Chalmers AC. Rubella virus vaccine associated arthropathy in postpartum immunized women: Influence of preimmunization serologic status on development of joint manifestations. J.Rheumatol. 2000; 27(2): 418-23.

78. Plotkin SA, Katz M, Cordero JF. The eradication of rubella. J.Am.Med.Assoc. 1999; 281(6): 561-2.

79. [No authors listed]. Human rabies prevention — United States, 1999. Recommendations of the Advisory Committee on Immunization Practices (ACIP). MMWR.Morb.Mortal.Wkly.Rep. 1999; 48(RR-1): 1-21.

80. Plotkin SA. Rabies. Clin.Infect.Dis. 2000; 30(1): 4-12.

81. Sabchareon A, Lang J, Attanath P, Sirivichayakul C, Pengsaa K, Le Mener V, Chantavanich P, Prarinyanuphab V, Pojjaroen-Anant C, Nimnual S, et al. A new Vero cell rabies vaccine: results of a comparative trial with human diploid cell rabies vaccine in children. Clin.Infect.Dis. 1999; 29(1): 141-9.

82. Lang J, Cetre JC, Picot N, Lanta M, Briantais P, Vital S, Le Mener V, Lutsch C, Rotivel Y. Immunogenicity and safety in adults of a new chromatographically purified Vero-cell rabies vaccine (CPRV): a randomized, double-blind trial with purified Vero-cell rabies vaccine (PVRV). Biologicals 1998; 26(4): 299-308.

83. Strady A, Lang J, Lienard M, Blondeau C, Jaussaud R, Plotkin SA. Antibody persistence following preexposure regimens of cell-culture rabies vaccines: 10-year follow-up and proposal for a new booster policy. J.Infect.Dis. 1998; 177(5): 1290-5.

84. Fishbein DB, Dreesen DW, Holmes DF, Pacer RE, Ley AB, Yager PA, Sumner JW, Reid-Sanden FL, Sanderlin DW, Tong TC. Human diploid cell rabies vaccine purified by zonal centrifugation: a controlled study of antibody response and side effects following primary and booster pre-exposure immunizations. Vaccine 1989; 7(5): 437-42.

85. Gardner SD. Bat rabies in Europe. J.Infect. 1999; 38(3): 205-8.

86. Dietzschold B, Hooper DC. Human diploid cell culture rabies vaccine (HDCV) and purified chick embryo cell culture rabies vaccine (PCECV) both confer protective immunity against infection with the silver-haired bat rabies virus strain (SHBRV). Vaccine 1998; 16(17): 1656-9.

87. Henderson DA, Inglesby TV, Bartlett JG, Ascher MS, Eitzen E, Jahrling PB, Hauer J, Layton M, McDade J, Osterholm MT, et al. Smallpox as a biological weapon: Medical and public health management. J.Am.Med.Assoc. 1999; 281(22): 2127-37.

88. American Academy of Pediatrics (AAP). Varicella vaccine update. Pediatrics 2000; 105(1): 136-41.

89. Chartrand SA. Varicella vaccine. Pediatr.Clin.North Am. 2000; 47(2): 373-94.

90. Huang W, Hussey M, Michel F. Transmission of varicella to a gravida via close contacts immunized with varicella-zoster vaccine - A case report. J.Reprod.Med. 1999; 44(10): 905-7.

91. Kuter BJ, Weibel RE, Guess HA, Matthews H, Morton DH, Neff BJ, Provost PJ, Watson BA, Starr SE, Plotkin SA. Oka/Merck varicella vaccine in healthy children: final report of a 2-year efficacy study and 7-year follow-up studies. Vaccine 1991; 9(9): 643-7.

92. Bernstein H, Rothstein E, Watson BM, Reisinger K, Blatter M, Wellman CO, Chartrand S, Cho I, Ngai A, White CJ. Clinical survey of natural varicella compared with breakthrough varicella after immunization with live attenuated Oka/Merck varicella vaccine. Pediatrics 1993; 92(6): 833-7.

93. Clements DA, Armstrong CB, Ursano AM, Moggio MM, Walter EB, Wilfert CM. Over five-year follow-up of Oka/Merck varicella vaccine recipients in 465 infants and adolescents. Pediatr.Infect.Dis.J. 1995; 14(10): 874-9.

94. Hardy I, Gershon AA, Steinberg SP, LaRussa P. The incidence of zoster after immunization with live attenuated varicella vaccine. A study in children with leukemia. Varicella Vaccine Collaborative Study Group. N.Engl.J.Med. 1991; 325(22): 1545-50.

95. Berger R, Just M. Interference between strains in live virus vaccines. II: Combined vaccination with varicella and measles-mumps-rubella vaccine. J.Biol.Stand. 1988; 16(4): 275-9.

96. Robert E, Vial T, Schaefer C, Arnon J, Reuvers M. Exposure to yellow fever vaccine in early pregnancy. Vaccine 1999; 17(3): 283-5.

97. Monath TP, Nasidi A. Should yellow fever vaccine be included in the expanded program of immunization in Africa? A cost-effectiveness analysis for Nigeria. Am.J.Trop.Med.Hyg. 1993; 48(2): 274-99.

98. Sabin AB. Properties of attenuated polioviruses and their behavior in human beings. Special Publ.N.Y.Acad.Sci. 1957; 5: 128-33.

99. Vidor E, Meschievitz C, Plotkin SA. Fifteen years of experience with Vero-produced enhanced potency inactivated poliovirus vaccine. Pediatr.Infect.Dis.J. 1997; 16(3): 312-22.

100. Cox NJ, Subbarao K. Influenza. Lancet 1999; 354(9186): 1277-82.

101. Thoelen S, Van Damme P, Leentvaar-Kuypers A, Leroux-Roels G, Bruguera M, Frei PC, Bakasenas V, Safary A. The first combined vaccine against hepatitis A and B: an overview. Vaccine 1999; 17(13-14): 1657-62.

102. Ramos-Alvarez M, Miller BH, Jackson JE. Immunization of children with attenuated measles rubella bivalent vaccine. Am.J.Dis.Child. 1975; 129(4): 474-7.

103. Popow-Kraupp T, Kundi M, Ambrosch F, Vanura H, Kunz C. A controlled trial for evaluating two live attenuated mumps-measles vaccines (Urabe Am 9-Schwarz and Jeryl Lynn-Moraten) in young children. J.Med.Virol. 1986; 18(1): 69-79.

CONTRIBUTOR ADDRESSES

Practical Guidelines in Antiviral Therapy
Edited by Charles A.B. Boucher and George J. Galasso
Contributing Editors: David A. Katzenstein and David A. Cooper

CHARLES A.B. BOUCHER, Eykman-Winkler Institute, Department of Virology
Heidelberglaan 100 (G04.515), 3584 CX Utrecht, The Netherlands

RICHARD J. WHITLEY, M.D., Dept. Pediatrics, Div. Clinical Virology,
616 Children's Hospital, 1600 7th Ave. So., Birmingham, AL 35233-0011

ANN ARVIN, Stanford Univ. Sch. Med., Dept. Pediatrics G312,
300 Pasteur Drive, Stanford, CA 94305

MENNO D. DE JONG, Dept. of Medical Microbiology Academic Medical Center,
University of Amsterdam, Meibergdreef 9, 1105 AZ Amsterdam, The Netherlands

DAVID J. BACK, Dept. Pharmacology & Therapeutics, University of Liverpool,
Ashton Street, Liverpool, L69 3GE, United Kingdom

JOHN TREANOR, Infectious Disease Unit, University of Rochester,
School of Medicine, 601 Elmwood Ave. Box 689, Rochester, NY 14642

SAYE KHOO, Dept. Pharmacology & Therapeutics, University of Liverpool, Ashton
Street, Liverpool, L69 3GE, United Kingdom

MARK HOLODNIY, VA Palo Alto Health Care System, 3801 Miranda Ave.
(132), Palo Alto, CA 94304

MARK A. FLETCHER, Aventis Pasteur SA, 2 avenue Pont Pasteur,
69367 Lyon, France

MICHAEL LEDERMAN, Div. of Infectious Diseases, University Hospitals of Cleveland, 10900 Euclid Ave., Cleveland, OH 44106-4984

PAUL GRIFFITHS, Royal Free and Univ. College Med. Sch., Dept. Virology, Pond Street, London, NW3 2PF, United Kingdom

C.J. PETERS, Professor of Pathology and Microbiology/Immunology, 3.146 Keiller Building, 301 University Boulevard, Galveston, TX 77555-0609

RICHARD REICHMAN, Infectious Diseases Unit, University of Rochester, School of Medicine, 601 Elmwood Ave. Box 689, Rochester, NY 14642

ROB SCHUURMAN, Utrecht University Hospital, Eykman Winkler Institute, Dept. of Virology, Heidelberglaan 100, 3584 CX Utrecht, The Netherlands

STANLEY PLOTKIN, 4650 Wismer Rd., Douglastown, PA 18901

TERESA WRIGHT, GI Section 111B, VAMC, 4150 Clement Street, San Francisco, CA 94121

DOUGLAS M. FLEMING, OBE, PhD, FRCGP, Director, Birmingham Research Unit, The Royal College of General Practitioners, Lordswood House, Birmingham, G17 9DB, United Kingdom

DAVID A. COOPER, MD, Natl. Cntr. in HIV Epidemiol. & Clin. Res., 2nd Floor, 376 Victoria Str., Sydney, NSW, Austalia 2010
e-mail dcooper@nchecr.unsw.edu.au

DAVID A. KATZENSTEIN, MD, Stanford Univ. Med. Cntr., Division of Infectious Dis., 300 Pasteur Drive, S-156, Stanford, CA 94305
e-mail davidkk@leland.stanford.edu

GEORGE J. GALASSO, Ph.D., Health Sciences Consultant, 636 Crocus Drive, Rockville, MD 20850-2045, Tel. +(301) 762-7864, Fax +(301) 762-1574
e-mail galassog@att.net

Printed and bound by CPI Group (UK) Ltd, Croydon, CR0 4YY

03/10/2024

01040330-0002